Imaging of the Hip

Editor

MIRIAM A. BREDELLA

MAGNETIC RESONANCE IMAGING CLINICS OF NORTH AMERICA

www.mri.theclinics.com

Consulting Editors
SURESH K. MUKHERJI
LYNNE STEINBACH

February 2013 • Volume 21 • Number 1

ELSEVIER

1600 John F. Kennedy Boulevard • Suite 1800 • Philadelphia, Pennsylvania 19103-2899

http://www.theclinics.com

MRI CLINICS OF NORTH AMERICA Volume 21, Number 1
February 2013 ISSN 1064-9689, ISBN 13: 978-1-4557-7114-1

Editor: Pamela Hetherington

Magnetic Resonance Imaging Clinics of North America (ISSN 1064-9689) is published quarterly by Elsevier Inc., 360 Park Avenue South, New York, NY 10010-1710. Months of issue are February, May, August, and November. Business and Editorial Offices: 1600 John F. Kennedy Blvd., Ste. 1800, Philadelphia, PA 19103-2899. Customer Service Office: 3251 Riverport Lane, Maryland Heights, MO 63043. Periodicals postage paid at New York, NY and additional mailing offices. Subscription prices are $337.00 per year (domestic individuals), $541.00 per year (domestic institutions), $172.00 per year (domestic students/residents), $376.00 per year (Canadian individuals), $678.00 per year (Canadian institutions), $488.00 per year (international individuals), $678.00 per year (international institutions), and $249.00 per year (international and Canadian students/residents). International air speed delivery is included in all *Clinics* subscription prices. All prices are subject to change without notice. **POSTMASTER:** Send address changes to *Magnetic Resonance Imaging Clinics*, Elsevier Health Sciences Division, Subscription Customer Service, 3251 Riverport Lane, Maryland Heights, MO 63043. Customer Service (orders, claims, online, change of address): Elsevier Health Sciences Division, Subscription Customer Service, 3251 Riverport Lane, Maryland Heights, MO 63043. Tel:1-800-654-2452 (U.S. and Canada); 314-447-8871 (outside U.S. and Canada). Fax: 314-447-8029. E-mail: journalscustomerservice-usa@elsevier.com (for print support); journalsonlinesupport-usa@elsevier.com (for online support).

Reprints. For copies of 100 or more of articles in this publication, please contact the Commercial Reprints Department, Elsevier Inc., 360 Park Avenue South, New York, NY 10010-1710. Tel.: 212-633-3812; Fax: 212-462-1935; E-mail: reprints@elsevier.com.

Magnetic Resonance Imaging Clinics of North America is covered in the *RSNA Index of Imaging Literature, MEDLINE/PubMed (Index Medicus),* and *EMBASE/Excerpta Medica.*

Printed and bound by CPI Group (UK) Ltd, Croydon, CR0 4YY

Transferred to digital print 2012

Contributors

CONSULTING EDITOR

SURESH K. MUKHERJI, MD, FACR
Department of Radiology, University of
Michigan Health System, Ann Arbor, Michigan

GUEST EDITOR

MIRIAM A. BREDELLA, MD
Associate Professor of Radiology, Harvard
Medical School, Division of Musculoskeletal
Radiology and Interventions, Department of
Radiology, Massachusetts General Hospital,
Boston, Massachusetts

AUTHORS

SUZANNE E. ANDERSON, MD
School of Medicine Sydney, The University of
Notre Dame Australia, Sydney, New South
Wales, Australia

LAURA W. BANCROFT, MD
Adjunct Professor, Florida Hospital, University
of Central Florida School of Medicine; Clinical
Professor, Florida State University School of
Medicine, Orlando, Florida

JENNY T. BENCARDINO, MD
Department of Radiology, NYU Langone
Medical Center, Hospital for Joint Diseases,
New York, New York

DONNA G. BLANKENBAKER, MD
Professor, Department of Radiology, University
of Wisconsin School of Medicine and Public
Health, Madison, Wisconsin

ITAMAR BOTSER, MD
Sports Medicine Fellow, Orthopaedic Surgery,
Stanford University, Redwood City, California

MIRIAM A. BREDELLA, MD
Associate Professor of Radiology, Division of
Musculoskeletal Radiology and Interventions,
Department of Radiology, Massachusetts
General Hospital, Harvard Medical School,
Boston, Massachusetts

CARSON B. CAMPE, MD
Resident Physician, Division of
Musculoskeletal Imaging, Department of
Radiology, Massachusetts General Hospital,
Boston, Massachusetts

CONNIE Y. CHANG, MD
Division of Musculoskeletal Imaging and
Intervention, Department of Radiology;
Assistant Radiologist, Massachusetts General
Hospital; Instructor of Radiology, Harvard
Medical School, Boston, Massachusetts

TALIA FRIEDMAN, MD
Fellow, Department of Radiology and Imaging,
Hospital for Special Surgery, New York,
New York

YULIYA GOMBAR III, MS
Philadelphia College of Osteopathic Medicine,
Philadelphia, Pennsylvania

AMBROSE J. HUANG, MD
Division of Musculoskeletal Imaging and
Intervention, Department of Radiology;
Assistant Radiologist, Director of
Musculoskeletal Intervention, Massachusetts
General Hospital; Instructor of Radiology,
Harvard Medical School, Boston,
Massachusetts

WASEEM KHAN, MD
Clinical Fellow in Musculoskeletal Radiology, Thomas Jefferson University Hospital, Philadelphia, Pennsylvania

YOUNG-JO KIM, MD, PhD
Associate Professor, Harvard Medical School, Massachusetts; Director, Child and Adult Hip Program, Boston Children's Hospital, Boston, Massachusetts

KHALDOUN KOUJOK, MD
Department of Diagnostic Imaging, Pediatric Radiologist, Children's Hospital of Eastern Ontario; Assistant Professor of Radiology, University of Ottawa, Ottawa, Ontario, Canada

LUKE MAJ, MD, MHA
Fellow, Division of Musculoskeletal Imaging and Intervention, Thomas Jefferson University Hospital, Philadelphia, Pennsylvania

WILLIAM C. MEYERS, MD, MBA
President, Vincera Core Physicians; Professor of Surgery, Drexel University College of Medicine; Adjunct Professor of Surgery, Thomas Jefferson University Hospital, Philadelphia, Pennsylvania

THEODORE T. MILLER, MD
Professor of Radiology, Weill Medical College of Cornell University, New York, New York

WILLIAM B. MORRISON, MD
Professor of Radiology, Director, Division of Musculoskeletal Imaging and Intervention, Thomas Jefferson University Hospital, Philadelphia, Pennsylvania

WILLIAM E. PALMER, MD
Director, Division of Musculoskeletal Imaging, Department of Radiology, Massachusetts General Hospital, Boston, Massachusetts

CATHERINE N. PETCHPRAPA, MD
Department of Radiology, NYU Langone Medical Center, Hospital for Joint Diseases, New York, New York

CHRISTOPHER PETTIS, MD
Assistant Professor, Florida Hospital, University of Central Florida School of Medicine; Clinical Assistant Professor, Florida State University School of Medicine, Orlando, Florida

MARC R. SAFRAN, MD
Professor, Orthopaedic Surgery, Stanford University, Redwood City, California

MARCOS LORETO SAMPAIO, MD
Musculoskeletal Radiologist, The Ottawa Hospital; Assistant Professor of Radiology, University of Ottawa, Ottawa, Ontario, Canada

MARK E. SCHWEITZER, MD
Musculoskeletal Radiologist, The Ottawa Hospital; Professor and Chair of Radiology, University of Ottawa, Ottawa, Ontario, Canada

ADNAN SHEIKH, MD
Musculoskeletal Radiologist, The Ottawa Hospital, Associate Professor of Radiology, University of Ottawa, Ottawa, Ontario, Canada

DAVID W. STOLLER, MD
Director, National Orthopaedics Imaging Associates and MRI at California Pacific Medical Center, San Francisco, California; Adjunct Professor of Radiology, Johns Hopkins University School of Medicine, Baltimore, Maryland

ATUL K. TANEJA, MD
Musculoskeletal Imaging and Intervention, Massachusetts General Hospital, Harvard Medical School, Boston, Massachusetts

MARTIN TORRIANI, MD, MSc
Musculoskeletal Imaging and Intervention, Massachusetts General Hospital, Harvard Medical School, Boston, Massachusetts

MICHAEL J. TUITE, MD
Professor, Department of Radiology, University of Wisconsin School of Medicine and Public Health, Madison, Wisconsin

ERIKA J. ULBRICH, MD
Department of Diagnostic and Interventional Radiology, University Hospital Zurich, Zurich, Switzerland

CHRISTOPHER WASYLIW, MD
Assistant Professor, Florida Hospital, University of Central Florida School of Medicine; Clinical Assistant Professor, Florida State University School of Medicine, Orlando, Florida

ADAM C. ZOGA, MD
Associate Professor of Radiology, Director, Musculoskeletal MRI and Ambulatory Imaging Centers, Thomas Jefferson University Hospital, Philadelphia, Pennsylvania

Contents

Understanding normal anatomy of the hip is important for diagnosing its pathology. MR arthrography is more sensitive for the detection of intra-articular pathology than noncontrast MR imaging. Important elements of the osseous structures on MR imaging include the alignment and the marrow. Acetabular ossicles may be present. Normal variations involving the cartilage include the supra-acetabular fossa and the stellate lesion. Important muscles of the hip are the sartorius, rectus femoris, iliopsoas, gluteus minimus and medius, adductors, and hamstrings. The iliofemoral, ischiofemoral, and pubofemoral ligaments represent thickenings of the joint capsule that reinforce and stabilize the hip joint. Normal variations in the labrum include labral sulcus and absent labrum. The largest nerves in the hip and thigh are the sciatic nerve, the femoral nerve, and the obturator nerve.

Acetabular labral tears are a mechanical cause of hip pain. Hip MR imaging should be performed on 1.5-T or 3-T magnets using small field-of-view and high-resolution imaging. The following should be used in the assessment for labral tear abnormalities on MR arthrography: labral morphology and contrast extension into the labral substance or between the labral base and acetabulum. Description of the labral tear and extent of tear is useful for hip arthroscopists. Understanding the pitfalls around the acetabular labral complex helps avoids misinterpretation of labral tears.

Hip deformity such as acetabular dysplasia and cam and pincer deformities are thought to be a major cause of hip osteoarthritis. Currently, clinically effective surgical procedures such as pelvic osteotomies and femoral and acetabular osteoplasties are available to correct the underlying deformity. These procedures are most effective in the presence of minimal chondral damage in the joint. Currently, and more so in the future, high-resolution morphologic imaging and biochemical imaging techniques such as Delayed gadolinium-enhanced MR imaging of cartilage, T2, and T1rho will have a clinically important role in diagnosing and staging chondral damage in the hip.

and imaging findings of important congenital and acquired osseous disorders of the pediatric and adult hip.

Luke Maj, Yuliya Gombar III, and William B. Morrison

Inflammation of the hip may be due to infectious and noninfectious causes. Furthermore, involvement is categorized based on the origin and spread to adjacent structures involving the soft tissues, the joint, and underlying bone to refine the differential diagnosis. Magnetic resonance (MR) imaging is highly effective in establishing the presence and underlying cause of inflammatory and degenerative arthropathies. This article discusses the use of MR imaging for evaluation of various inflammatory conditions of the hip, both infectious and noninfectious. The number of hip prostheses is increasing, and inflammatory conditions involving the postoperative hip is also detailed separately.

Laura W. Bancroft, Christopher Pettis, and Christopher Wasyliw

After initial evaluation with radiography, magnetic resonance (MR) imaging is the most common modality used to establish the diagnosis and characterize osseous and soft tissue tumors of the hip. Tumors involving the proximal femur are often benign, and MR imaging can be specific in diagnosing solitary bone cyst, osteochondroma, and chondroblastoma. Benign and malignant soft tissue tumors about the hip are often nonspecific in their MR imaging appearances, but knowledge of the patient's age may direct a more limited differential diagnosis. In the setting of malignancy, MR imaging is commonly used to stage tumors and follow patients postoperatively.

Carson B. Campe and William E. Palmer

Metal-on-metal (MoM) hip arthroplasty was expected to provide benefits over metal-on-polyethylene systems. After widespread placement of MoM implants, outcomes have been disappointing. MoM implants are associated with higher serum levels of metal ions, adverse periarticular soft tissue reactions, and increased long-term failure rates. In light of these findings, it is crucial that patients with MoM implants be closely monitored for adverse effects. MR imaging is ideally suited for assessment of these patients and complements standard clinical evaluation and laboratory testing. This article reviews the background of MoM implants, emerging data on complications, strategies for using MR imaging, and MR imaging findings in patients with reaction to metal.

Itamar Botser and Marc R. Safran

MR imaging of the hip is frequently used in symptomatic patients before hip preservation surgery; it is used as a decision-making tool and as a planning tool. The MRI can confirm the preliminary working diagnosis, identify other possible sources of pain, and highlight anatomic areas that are not routinely viewed during surgery. In addition, MR imaging is capable of illustrating normal and abnormal bony morphology of the femur and pelvis; and in the case that arthrography is used, diagnostic injection can be administrated concurrently. This article highlights a surgeon's perspective on the use of MR imaging in the patient with nonarthritic hip pain.

Magnetic resonance (MR) imaging has become the workhorse in the imaging evaluation of the painful or clinically abnormal hip. It provides an excellent anatomic overview and demonstration of the bony structures, articular surfaces, and surrounding soft tissues. Conversely, sonography can also demonstrate superficial intraarticular structures and the periarticular soft tissues, is quickly performed, allows dynamic evaluation of tendons and muscles, and can guide percutaneous procedures. These two modalities are complementary, and this article concentrates on the MR imaging–sonographic correlations of several entities about the hip.

MAGNETIC RESONANCE IMAGING CLINICS OF NORTH AMERICA

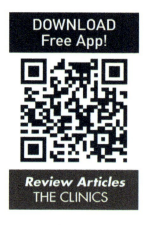

PROGRAM OBJECTIVE:

The goal of Magnetic Resonance Imaging Clinics of North America is to keep practicing physicians up to date with current clinical practice by providing timely articles reviewing the state of the art in patient care.

TARGET AUDIENCE

All practicing physicians and healthcare professionals who provide patient care utilizing findings from Magnetic Resonance Imaging.

ACCREDITATION

The Elsevier Office of Continuing Medical Education (EOCME) is accredited by the Accreditation Council for Continuing Medical Education (ACCME) to provide continuing medical education for physicians.

The EOCME designates this journal-based CME activity for a maximum of 13 *AMA PRA Category 1 Credit*(s)™. Physicians should claim only the credit commensurate with the extent of their participation in the activity.

All other health care professionals completing continuing education credit for this activity will be issued a certificate of participation.

DISCLOSURE OF CONFLICTS OF INTEREST

The EOCME assesses conflict of interest with its instructors, faculty, planners, and other individuals who are in a position to control the content of CME activities. All relevant conflicts of interest that are identified are thoroughly vetted by EOCME for fair balance, scientific objectivity, and patient care recommendations. EOCME is committed to providing its learners with CME activities that promote improvements or quality in healthcare and not a specific proprietary business or a commercial interest.

The planning committee, staff, authors and editors listed below have identified no financial relationships or relationships to products or devices they or their spouse/life partner have with commercial interest related to the content of this CME activity:

Suzanne E. Anderson, MD; Laura W. Bancroft, MD; Jenny T. Bencardino, MD; Donna G. Blankenbaker, MD; Itamar Botser, MD; Miriam A. Bredella, MD; Carson B. Campe, MD; Connie Y. Chang, MD; Nicole Congleton, Talia Friedman, MD; Yuliya Gombar III, MS; Ambrose J. Huang, MD; Waseem Khan, MD; Khaldoun Koujok, MD; Luke Maj, MD, MHA; Jill McNair; William C. Meyers, MD, MBA; Theodore T. Miller, MD; William B. Morrison, MD; William E. Palmer, MD; Catherine N. Petchprapa, MD; Christopher Pettis, MD; Marcos Loreto Sampaio, MD; Mark E. Schweitzer, MD; Adnan Sheikh, MD; Katelynn Steck; David W. Stoller, MD; Atul K. Taneja, MD; Martin Torriani, MD, Msc; Michael J. Tuite, MD; Erika J. Ulbrich, MD; Shankar Veerubhotla; Christopher Wasyliw, MD; and Adam C. Zoga, MD.

The planning committee, staff, authors and editors listed below have identified financial relationships or relationships to products or devices they or their spouse/life partner have with commercial interest related to the content of this CME activity:

Young-Jo Kim, MD, PhD has received a research grant and is a consultant or advisor for Siemens Health Care.
Suresh K. Mukherji, MD, FACR is a consultant or adivsor for Philips.
Marc R. Safran, MD has received fellowship support from Smith and Nephew, and ConMed Linvatec; is a consultant/advisor for Biomimedica, Cool Systems Inc, and Arthrocare; and received a research grant from Ferring Pharmaceuticals.

UNAPPROVED/OFF-LABEL USE DISCLOSURE

The EOCME requires CME faculty to disclose to the participants:

1. When products or procedures being discussed are off-label, unlabelled, experimental, and/or investigational (not US Food and Drug Administration (FDA) approved; and
2. Any limitations on the information presented, such as data that are preliminary or that represent ongoing research, interim analyses, and/or unsupported opinions. Faculty may discuss information about pharmaceutical agents that is outside of DA-approved labelling. This information is intended soley for CME and is not intended to promote off-label use of these medications. If you have any questions, contact the medical affairs department of the manufacturer for the most recent prescribing information.

TO ENROLL

To enroll in the *Magnetic Resonance Imaging Clinics of North* Continuing Medical Education program, call customer service at 1-800-654-2452 or sign up online at http://www.theclinics.com/home/cme. The CME program is available to subscribers for an additional annual fee of $223.00.

METHOD OF PARTICIPATION

In order to claim credit, participants must complete the following:

1. Complete enrolment as indicated above.
2. Read the activity.
3. Complete the CME Test and Evaluation. Participants must achieve a score of 70% on the test. All CME Tests and Evaluations must be completed online.

CME INQUIRIES/SPECIAL NEEDS

For all CME inquiries or special needs, please contact elsevierCME@elsevier.com.

Foreword

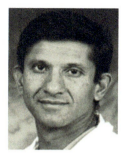

Suresh K. Mukherji, MD, FACR
Consulting Editor

It is with great delight that I welcome Dr Miriam A. Bredella, MD as the guest editor of this issue of *Magnetic Resonance Imaging Clinics of North America*. She has chosen the very important topic of hip imaging and has done an outstanding job of creating a very comprehensive issue that covers anatomy, various pathologic abnormalities, and postoperative imaging. She also includes a surgeon's perspective on using MRI for patients with nonarthritic hip pain, which I can certainly appreciate, being a rapidly aging middle-age man and an occasional sports "weekend warrior."

She has assembled an *outstanding* group of contributing authors who are a virtual "who's who" of musculoskeletal imaging with special expertise in the hip. All of us at *Magnetic Resonance Imaging Clinics of North America* congratulate and

thank all of the authors for their contributions and thank Dr Bredella for creating such an outstanding issue. Residents, fellows, and staff will find this issue very helpful regardless of to whether they come from a background of imaging or surgery. I am sure this edition will become an "instant classic" and an issue that will be referred to for many years to come.

Suresh K. Mukherji, MD, FACR
Department of Radiology
University of Michigan Health System
1500 East Medical Center
Ann Arbor, MI 48109-0030, USA

E-mail address:
mukherji@med.umich.edu

1064-9689/13/$ – see front matter © 2013 Published by Elsevier Inc

Preface

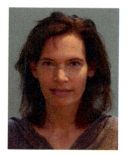

Miriam A. Bredella, MD
Guest Editor

The hip is a complex joint and challenging to image. Due to its high spatial resolution, multiplanar capability, and excellent tissue contrast, MRI has become the modality of choice for evaluating intra-articular and extra-articular pathology of the hip. Heightened interest in hip impingement syndromes and developments in biochemical cartilage imaging as well as metal artifact reduction sequences have further established MRI as an essential tool in the workup of hip pain. In this issue of *Magnetic Resonance Imaging Clinics of North America*, world-renowned authors discuss topics ranging from tendon, labral, neoplastic, and osseous pathology to femoroacetabular and ischiofemoral impingement, sports hernia, biochemical cartilage imaging, and imaging of metal-on-metal hip arthroplasty.

Drs Chang and Huang begin by beautifully illustrating normal intra-articular and extra-articular anatomy of the hip and anatomic variants, followed by Drs Blankenbaker and Tuite's comprehensive review of acetabular labral pathology and the role of MR arthrography. A surgeon's perspective on the assessment of hip cartilage is given by Dr Kim, who also discusses cutting-edge biochemical cartilage imaging techniques. Drs Ulbrich, Stoller, Anderson, and I further explore cartilage and labral pathology in a thorough review of state-of-the-art imaging and novel concepts in femoroacetabular impingement.

Ischiofemoral impingement, a recently described entity associated with hip pain, is reviewed by Drs Taneja, Torriani, and I with detailed imaging findings and an up-to-date discussion. A systematic review of tendon injuries with a focus on an anatomy-based search process is provided by Drs Petchprapa and Bencardino, which can be of immense practical value for most radiologists. Athletic pubalgia and sports hernia are challenging diagnoses requiring a thorough knowledge of the anatomy and are discussed in detail by Drs Khan, Zoga, and Meyers.

Drs Sheikh, Koujok, Sampaio, and Schweitzer report on pathology and MRI findings of relevant congenital and acquired osseous disorders of the pediatric and adult hip. Drs Maj, Gombar, and Morrison discuss important infectious and noninfectious inflammatory conditions of the hip. Drs Bancroft, Pettis, and Wasyliw illustrate MRI findings of neoplasms around the hip and provide clinical and imaging guidelines to arrive at the correct diagnosis.

Metal-on-metal hip arthroplasties have recently been found to cause adverse soft tissue reactions and high long-term failure rates, prompting recalls and specific follow-up recommendations. Drs Campe and Palmer discuss the role of MRI in the

Magn Reson Imaging Clin N Am 21 (2013) xiii–xiv
http://dx.doi.org/10.1016/j.mric.2012.09.007
1064-9689/13/$ – see front matter © 2013 Elsevier Inc. All rights reserved.

evaluation of patients with a reaction to metal and the use of metal artifact reduction sequences. Last, Drs Botser and Safran highlight the surgeon's perspective on using MRI for patients with nonarthritic hip pain, and Drs Friedman and Miller review the role of ultrasound in hip pain with MRI correlation.

I would like to thank all the authors for their outstanding contributions to this issue. I would also like to thank Pamela Hetherington and Sarah Barth of Elsevier for their support.

Miriam A. Bredella, MD
Department of Radiology
Musculoskeletal Imaging and Interventions
Massachusetts General Hospital and
Harvard Medical School
55 Fruit Street, Yawkey 6E
Boston, MA 02114, USA

E-mail address:
mbredella@partners.org

Dedication

To my father, Lothar Bredella, with love.

Magn Reson Imaging Clin N Am 21 (2013) xv
http://dx.doi.org/10.1016/j.mric.2012.09.010
1064-9689/13/$ – see front matter © 2013 Elsevier Inc. All rights reserved.

MR Imaging of Normal Hip Anatomy

Connie Y. Chang, MD*, Ambrose J. Huang, MD

KEYWORDS

- Hip • Normal • Anatomy • Labrum • Anatomic variant

KEY POINTS

- Understanding normal anatomy is important for diagnosing pathology of the hip.
- MR arthrography is more sensitive for the detection of intra-articular pathology than noncontrast MR imaging.
- Important components of hip anatomy include the osseous structures, cartilage, muscles and tendons, capsular ligaments, labrum, nerves, and vessels.

IMAGING THE HIP

Hip pain is a common complaint, especially in athletes, and it has a broad differential diagnosis. MR imaging has improved the radiologist's ability to diagnose causes of hip pain, especially soft tissue pathology.[1]

The hip joint is difficult to image because it is not oriented in the standard axial, coronal, and sagittal planes of the body, and there is significant variation in hip joint orientation from person to person. Acetabular version, for example, can range from −10.8 to +22.1 degrees.[2,3]

At the authors' institution, MR imaging is performed on 1.5- and 3-T scanners using a phased-array surface coil. One fluid-sensitive sequence is obtained with a large field of view that includes the proximal femurs, the pelvis, and the sacrum. The remaining sequences use a small field of view focused on the symptomatic hip and are acquired in the standard axial, coronal, and sagittal imaging planes. They also use an oblique axial imaging plane (also known as the "sagittal oblique" imaging plane by some authors[4,5]), oriented parallel to the long axis of the femoral neck, to evaluate for labral tears and femoroacetabular impingement.[6,7] These images are prescribed using a coronal localizer image that includes the superior labrum and the transverse acetabular ligament; the oblique axial images are then acquired perpendicular to the line that connects these two structures (**Fig. 1**).[8] The imaging parameters used at the authors' institution on the 1.5- and 3-T MR imaging scanners are detailed in **Tables 1** and **2**.

The authors also inject intra-articular contrast to perform MR arthrography. The intra-articular contrast distends the joint, separates the soft tissue structures, and increases the contrast resolution, all of which help to increase the conspicuity of intra-articular pathology, such as labral tears, osteocartilaginous bodies, and osteochondral and cartilage defects.[8,9]

Using fluoroscopic guidance, a 22-gauge needle, and an anterior or anterolateral approach, the authors position the needle within the joint and inject 10 to 12 mL of a 1:250 mixture of dilute gadolinium (10 mL of a mixture consisting of 0.4 mL of gadopentetate dimeglumine [Magnevist; Bayer Healthcare Pharmaceuticals, Wayne, NJ] diluted

Funding Sources: None.
Conflict of Interest: None.
Division of Musculoskeletal Imaging and Intervention, Department of Radiology, Massachusetts General Hospital, Harvard Medical School, 55 Fruit Street, Yawkey 6E, Boston, MA 02114, USA
* Corresponding author.
E-mail address: cychang@partners.org

Magn Reson Imaging Clin N Am 21 (2013) 1–19
http://dx.doi.org/10.1016/j.mric.2012.08.006
1064-9689/13/$ - see front matter © 2013 Elsevier Inc. All rights reserved.

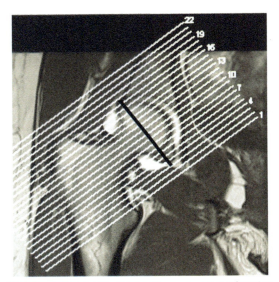

Fig. 1. Coronal MR image from a scout planning sequence shows the method for acquiring oblique axial images (*solid white lines*), which are prescribed perpendicular to a line connecting the superolateral labrum and the transverse acetabular ligament (*black line*).

in 50 mL of normal saline, 5 mL of iopamidol 41% [Isovue-M-200; Bracco Diagnostics, Princeton, NJ], and 5 mL of preservative-free lidocaine 1%). They target the superolateral aspect of the femoral head/neck junction to minimize the possibility of injecting into the femoral vessels or the iliopsoas tendon sheath. The imaging digital detector may be angled laterally by approximately 15 degrees to further avoid puncturing these structures and also to create a trajectory approximately perpendicular to the target injection location. Alternatively, if the digital detector cannot rotate, the toes can be taped inward, which places the hip

at approximately 15 degrees of internal rotation. Care is taken to remove all bubbles from the syringe, tubing, and needle, because air bubbles create MR imaging blooming artifact, which may mimic intra-articular osteocartilaginous bodies or otherwise obscure pathology. The capacity of the hip joint varies from 8 to 20 mL.[9,10] During the injection, they use fluoroscopy to look for a "rings of Saturn" pattern of contrast around the femoral neck to confirm that the injection is intra-articular (**Fig. 2**). When the injection is complete, the patient is brought directly to the MR imaging scanner; imaging should commence within 30 minutes of contrast injection to maximize joint distention and to minimize contrast resorption. All MR arthrography sequences use a small field of view focused on the injected hip. The imaging parameters used at the authors' institution for MR arthrography on the 1.5- and 3-T MR imaging scanners are detailed in **Tables 3** and **4**.

OSSEOUS STRUCTURES

The hip joint is a ball-and-socket joint composed of the femoral head articulating with the acetabulum. The acetabulum is the junction of the three bones of the pelvis: (1) the ilium, (2) the ischium, and (3) the pubis. It is important to evaluate all of these bones and the sacrum in routine hip MR imaging because fractures of any of these bones can present as "hip pain."[11,12] The acetabulum approximates the surface of two-thirds of a sphere, which is incomplete at the inferior aspect; the transverse acetabular ligament, a soft tissue structure, spans the inferior margin of the acetabulum and thus completes the "socket," which holds the femoral head ("ball") in place (**Fig. 3**).[10]

There is a spectrum of morphologies of the proximal femur and the acetabulum and the

Table 1 1.5-T hip MR imaging parameters								
Sequence	TR	TE	TI	NEX	Matrix	ST × Sk	FOV	Flip Angle
Coronal FMPIR	3800	45	150	1	320 × 192	5 × 6	360	90
Axial PD	1933	27		2	320 × 256	4 × 5	180	90
Coronal T1	483	10		1	384 × 224	4 × 5	200	90
Coronal T2 FS	4150	76		1.5	320 × 224	4 × 5	200	90
Sagittal PD	2267	44		1	320 × 224	4 × 5	200	90
Oblique axial PD FS	2583	35		1	512 × 256	4 × 5	180	90

Abbreviations: FMPIR, fast multiplanar inversion recovery; FOV, field of view (mm); FS, fat suppressed; NEX, number of excitations; PD, proton density; Sk, skip (mm); ST, slice thickness (mm); TE, echo time (milliseconds); TI, inversion time (milliseconds); TR, repetition time (milliseconds).

Table 2
3-T hip MR imaging parameters

Sequence	TR	TE	TI	NEX	Matrix	ST × Sk	FOV	Flip Angle
Coronal FMPIR	4250	48	200	1	320 × 192	4 × 4.4	360	120
Axial PD	2730	9		1	256 × 256	4 × 4.4	200	140
Coronal T1	931	15		2	384 × 307	4 × 4.6	199	140
Coronal T2 FS	3070	60		1	256 × 256	4 × 5	200	150
Sagittal PD	3500	43		2	384 × 307	4 × 4.4	199	170
Oblique axial PD FS	4000	69		2	256 × 154	3 × 3	200	150

Abbreviations: FMPIR, fast multiplanar inversion recovery; FOV, field of view (mm); FS, fat suppressed; NEX, number of excitations; PD, proton density; Sk, skip (mm); ST, slice thickness (mm); TE, echo time (milliseconds); TI, inversion time (milliseconds); TR, repetition time (milliseconds).

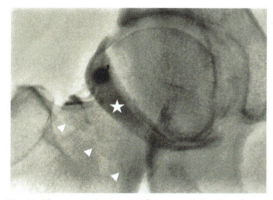

Fig. 2. Fluoroscopic image from an injection for an MR arthrogram of the right hip shows the typical appearance of intra-articular contrast, including a "rings of Saturn" pattern over the upper femoral neck (*asterisk*) and a collar of contrast that extends to the lower femoral neck (*arrowheads*). The needle was placed at the superolateral aspect of the femoral head/neck junction.

geometric relationships between the two. Developmental dysplasia of the hip (DDH) is a condition in which the morphologies or geometric relationships deviate substantially from the normal. Although DDH is typically diagnosed using radiography or ultrasound, some measurements derived from cross-sectional imaging can improve characterization or increase the specificity of the diagnosis of DDH. Acetabular version and femoral version are two measurements commonly used to diagnose DDH,[13] although abnormal measurements are often present in asymptomatic healthy people.[14] Abnormalities of the anterior and posterior acetabular sector angles are more specific for the diagnosis of DDH (**Fig. 4**). The normal anterior and posterior acetabular sector angles are greater than 50 degrees and greater than 90 degrees, respectively. In DDH, these angles are decreased.[14]

The medullary spaces of the normal proximal femoral epiphysis and apophysis contain yellow

Table 3
1.5-T hip MR arthrogram parameters

Sequence	TR	TE	NEX	Matrix	ST × Sk	FOV	Flip Angle
Axial T2 FS	2250	53	3	320 × 192	4 × 4	160	180
Coronal T1	660	14	2	320 × 192	4 × 4	160	180
Coronal T1 FS	563	12	2	320 × 224	4 × 4	160	180
Coronal T2 FS	2250	53	3	320 × 192	4 × 4	160	180
Sagittal T1 FS	550	11	2	320 × 192	3.5 × 3.5	160	180
Oblique axial T1 FS	600	15	2	320 × 192	3.5 × 3.5	160	180

Abbreviations: FMPIR, fast multiplanar inversion recovery; FOV, field of view (mm); FS, fat suppressed; NEX, number of excitations; PD, proton density; Sk, skip (mm); ST, slice thickness (mm); TE, echo time (milliseconds); TI, inversion time (milliseconds); TR, repetition time (milliseconds).

Table 4
3-T hip MR arthrogram parameters

Sequence	TR	TE	NEX	Matrix	ST × Sk	FOV	Flip Angle
Axial T2 FS	3500	82	2	384 × 307	4 × 4	159	150
Coronal T1	663	15	1	448 × 336	4 × 4	160	140
Coronal T1 FS	570	15	1	448 × 318	4 × 4	160	140
Coronal T2 FS	4320	82	3	384 × 311	4 × 4	159	150
Sagittal T1 FS	640	13	2	448 × 318	3.5 × 3.5	160	170
Oblique axial T1 FS	550	14	1	448 × 318	3.5 × 3.5	160	140

Abbreviations: FMPIR, fast multiplanar inversion recovery; FOV, field of view (mm); FS, fat suppressed; NEX, number of excitations; PD, proton density; Sk, skip (mm); ST, slice thickness (mm); TE, echo time (milliseconds); TI, inversion time (milliseconds); TR, repetition time (milliseconds).

marrow, which follows fat signal intensity on all pulse sequences. The medullary spaces of the femoral neck and intertrochanteric region typically contain red marrow, which on T1-weighted MR images is lower in signal intensity compared with normal fat and yellow marrow and higher in signal intensity compared with skeletal muscle.[15] The bony pelvis is a common reservoir for red marrow.[16]

Ossific fragments adjacent to the acetabular rim are known as os acetabuli or os acetabulare, and their clinical significance is unclear. They are present in approximately 2% to 3% of asymptomatic patients. They may represent ununited secondary acetabular ossification centers, incompletely healed acetabular fractures, fragmented osteophytes, or labral ossification caused by prior or repeated acetabular trauma.[17] In addition, there are accessory ossification centers, which may persist as unfused accessory ossicles surrounded by intact cartilage. Rarely, these may project into the acetabular fossa, where they could be misinterpreted as intra-articular osteocartilaginous bodies.[18]

Lien and colleagues[19] described blind-ending, tubular tracks of contrast material on hip MR arthrography and CT arthrography that originate from the acetabular fossa at or near its junction with the acetabular cartilage (**Fig. 5**). Tracks were on average 11 mm long and 1.2 mm wide. They were seen in 15% of symptomatic hips and 18% of asymptomatic hips, suggesting that tubular tracks of contrast are incidental findings rather than sources of hip pain. Their study was limited by the study population, however, because the number of asymptomatic hips in their study was much smaller than the number of symptomatic hips.

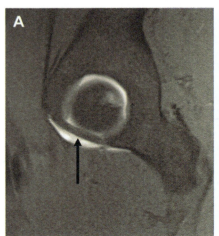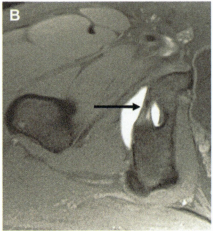

Fig. 3. (*A*) Sagittal and (*B*) oblique axial T1-weighted fat-suppressed MR images after the injection of intra-articular dilute gadopentetate dimeglumine show the transverse acetabular ligament (*arrows*) as a linear low signal intensity structure that extends from the anteroinferior to the posteroinferior corners of the acetabulum.

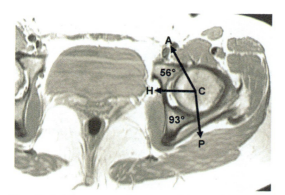

Fig. 4. Axial proton density weighted MR image showing measurements of the anterior and posterior acetabular sector angles. CA is a line between the center of the femoral head and the anterior acetabular rim. CP is a line between the center of the femoral head and the posterior acetabular rim. CH is a line through the center of the femoral head that parallels the horizontal lie of the pelvis. The anterior acetabular sector angle is the angle between CA and CH and is normally greater than 50 degrees. The posterior acetabular sector angle is the angle between CP and CH and is normally greater than 90 degrees. The acetabular sector angles are decreased in DDH.

CARTILAGE

A horseshoe-shaped articular cartilage called the "lunate" lines the acetabulum. A central depression within the acetabulum known as the acetabular fossa lacks this cartilage lining and is instead lined by synovium and filled with fibrofatty tissue.[9]

In the weight-bearing portion of the superior acetabulum, at approximately the 12-o'clock position, there can be a normal variant called the supra-acetabular fossa. This is an indentation in the acetabular roof that may be filled with cartilage or fibrous tissue, and it may fill with contrast during MR arthrography or CT arthrography. Importantly, the supra-acetabular fossa has smooth margins and no underlying or surrounding marrow edema (**Fig. 6**).[17,20]

Located slightly more medial than the supra-acetabular fossa, there can be a linear area of discontinuity, thinning, or absence of the acetabular cartilage. This normal variant is known as the stellate crease or stellate lesion. The stellate lesion is sometimes associated with a subchondral osseous fragment. One of the hip plicae (the "ligamental plica"), a low signal intensity structure, may attach to the medial aspect of the stellate lesion or the osseous fragment and extend toward the acetabular fossa (**Fig. 7**). The stellate lesion should be distinguished from the triradiate cartilage remnant or physeal scar, which is located in the acetabular fossa itself.[17,21]

Other than the fovea capitus, a central surface depression of the femoral head where the ligamentum teres femoris arises, cartilage covers the entire femoral head.[9,10,22] A femoral head chondral crease may be seen in DDH.[21,22]

Assessment of the articular cartilage of the hip has been found to be challenging on MR imaging.[23,24] The curved morphology of the femoral head and acetabulum, the close apposition of the articular surfaces, the use of body coils or phased array coils rather than dedicated small surface coils, and the relatively thin cartilage of the hip as compared with the knee present

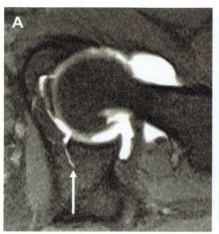
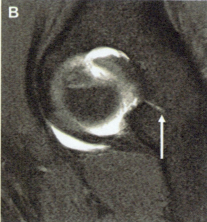

Fig. 5. (A) Oblique axial and (B) sagittal T1-weighted fat-suppressed MR images after the injection of intra-articular dilute gadopentetate dimeglumine show a tubular track of contrast (*arrows*), seen as a linear, blind-ending, contrast-filled structure that arises from the acetabular fossa near its junction with the acetabular cartilage and extends into the ischium.

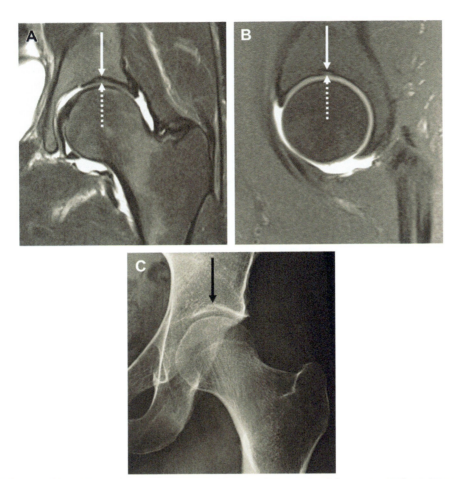

Fig. 6. (*A*) Coronal T2-weighted fat-suppressed and (*B*) sagittal T1-weighted fat-suppressed MR images after the injection of intra-articular dilute gadopentetate dimeglumine show a supra-acetabular fossa, seen as an indentation in the acetabular roof at the 12-o'clock position (*solid arrow*). The indentation is filled in with intermediate signal intensity cartilage (*dotted arrow*). (*C*) Radiograph in the same patient depicts the cortex of the supra-acetabular fossa (*arrow*).

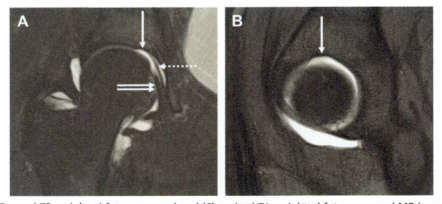

Fig. 7. (*A*) Coronal T2-weighted fat-suppressed and (*B*) sagittal T1-weighted fat-suppressed MR images after the injection of intra-articular dilute gadopentetate dimeglumine show a stellate lesion, seen as a bare cartilage area over the superomedial aspect of the acetabulum (*solid arrow*). Attached to the medial aspect of the stellate lesion is one of the hip plicae (the "ligamental plica") (*dotted arrow*), a linear low signal intensity structure that heads inferomedially toward the acetabular fossa. *Double arrows* depict the ligamentum teres femoris lateral to the plica.

difficulties for identifying cartilage defects of the hip. The sensitivity and specificity of MR arthrography for the detection of hip cartilage defects is 50% to 79% and 77% to 84%, respectively.[23] The sensitivity and specificity of CT arthrography are similar, at 67% to 89% and 67% to 82%, respectively.[25] Continuous leg traction to separate the acetabulum and femur may be helpful for evaluating the cartilage, but results are preliminary, and more research needs to be performed to determine the clinical usefulness of this technique.[25,26]

MUSCLES, TENDONS, AND BURSAE

There are many muscles and tendons that surround the hip and allow it to perform a wide range of motions, including flexion, extension, abduction, adduction, and internal and external rotation. The muscles of the hip and proximal thigh are generally well-delineated from one another by well-defined fascial and fatty planes (**Fig. 8**). Normal skeletal muscle is intermediate in signal intensity on all pulse sequences.[27] T1-weighted MR images are best for evaluating muscle bulk and signal intensity. On these images, muscles have a "marbled" appearance because of high signal intensity fat located between intermediate signal intensity muscles and interspersed between fibers of individual muscles. The appearance of fatty infiltration ranges from high T1 signal intensity marbling to complete high T1 signal intensity replacement. A decrease in muscle bulk reflects atrophy. Focal muscle atrophy suggests chronic full-thickness tendon tear but is also consistent with prior severe muscle trauma, chronic disuse,

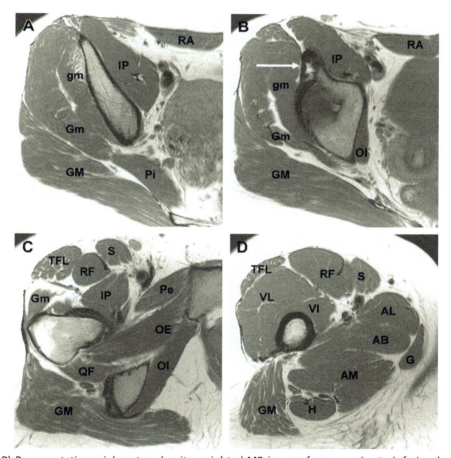

Fig. 8. (*A–D*) Representative axial proton density weighted MR images from superior to inferior depict normal muscle anatomy: AB, adductor brevis; AL, adductor longus; AM, adductor magnus; G, gracilis; gm, gluteus minimus; Gm, gluteus medius; GM, gluteus maximus; H, hamstrings; IP, iliopsoas; OE, obturator externus; OI, obturator internus; Pe, pectineus; Pi, piriformis; QF, quadratus femoris; RA, rectus abdominis; RF, rectus femoris; S, sartorius; TFL, tensor fascia lata; VI, vastus intermedius; VL, vastus lateralis. (*B*) Reflected head of the rectus femoris (*arrow*), which attaches to the superolateral aspect of the acetabulum.

muscle denervation, or chronic corticosteroid use.[27,28] Tendons, being tightly bound fascicles of collagen, appear as thin bands of low signal intensity on all pulse sequences.[27]

Important tendon attachments include the sartorius origin (anterior superior iliac spine), the rectus femoris origin (anterior inferior iliac spine and superior acetabular rim), the iliopsoas insertion (lesser trochanter of the femur), the gluteus minimus and medius insertions (greater trochanter of the femur), the adductor group origin (pubis), and the hamstring group origin (ischial tuberosity) because they are sites of common avulsion injuries.

The hamstrings are the most commonly injured muscles in the lower extremities.[29,30] Although all hamstring tendons have a common origin on the posterolateral ischial tuberosity, the semimembranosus attaches to the superolateral facet, and the long head of the biceps femoris and semitendinosus form a conjoint tendon that originates from the inferomedial facet. On rare occasions, the semitendinosus and biceps femoris arise separately.[10,31,32]

Quadriceps injuries are second to hamstring injuries among lower-extremity muscular injuries, and the rectus femoris is the most commonly injured muscle in the quadriceps group.[29] The rectus femoris has two origins: a direct or straight head as a round tendon from the anterior inferior iliac spine, and an indirect or reflected head as a broad, flat tendon from the superior acetabular ridge and the superior hip capsule more posteriorly and superiorly (see Fig. 8B). The two tendons join a few centimeters distal to their origins, where the direct head tendon merges with the anterior rectus femoris fascia and the indirect head tendon enters into the muscle belly and forms the deep myotendinous junction. The direct head initiates flexion, whereas the indirect head has a greater role during mid-flexion. The rectus femoris also extends the knee.[33,34]

The insertional anatomy of the gluteus minimus and medius is complex and has muscular and tendinous components. There are four bony facets on the greater trochanter: (1) anterior, (2) lateral, (3) superoposterior, and (4) posterior. The gluteus minimus has a tendon attachment at the anterior facet of the greater trochanter and a muscle and tendon attachment at the anterior and superior capsule of the hip joint. The gluteus medius has a tendon attachment at the superoposterior facet and a muscular attachment lateral to the anterior facet, superficial to the gluteus minimus tendon (Fig. 9). There is no tendon attachment at the posterior facet; the greater trochanteric bursa lies superficial to this facet.[35] The gluteus maximus has one insertion on the iliotibial band and

a second on the gluteal tuberosity of the proximal posterior aspect of the femur.[36]

An accessory iliacus tendon is a relatively common anatomic variant, not usually symptomatic, that occurs in 66% of hip MR arthrography.[17,37] The linear separation between the two tendons at their common insertion on the lesser trochanter should not be misconstrued as a longitudinal split tear of the iliopsoas tendon (Fig. 10). Other variant muscle slips of the iliopsoas can also be seen but are relatively rare. All of these may cause compression of the femoral nerve or its component nerve roots.[38]

There are three important bursae in the region of the pelvis and hip: (1) the greater trochanteric bursa, which is composed of three discrete components underlying each of the three gluteal tendons; (2) the iliopsoas bursa; and (3) the ischiogluteal bursa.[8] These bursae may become inflamed because of tendon friction syndromes. Fluid in the iliopsoas bursa, however, may be a normal finding, because it communicates directly with the hip joint in 10% to 15% of individuals.[9] The normal iliopsoas bursa is collapsed and appears as a thin low signal intensity structure. It is bordered by the iliopsoas muscle anterolaterally, the femoral vessels anteriorly or anteromedially, the pectineal eminence of the pubic bone medially, and the joint capsule and labrum posteriorly (Fig. 11A). A distended iliopsoas bursa is a rounded or tear-drop shaped structure in the same location. It can be multiloculated or multilobed and appear as a horseshoe-shaped collection surrounding each side of the iliopsoas tendon, and it may extend more proximally into the pelvis (see Fig. 11B).[9,10,17,39]

LIGAMENTS AND SYNOVIUM/CAPSULE

The iliofemoral, ischiofemoral, and pubofemoral ligaments represent thickenings of the joint capsule that reinforce and stabilize the hip joint. They are named for the bones that they connect. The Y-shaped iliofemoral ligament is one of the strongest ligaments in the body. It reinforces the anterior capsule by limiting anterior translation during extension and external rotation. It originates between the anterior inferior iliac spine and the superior acetabulum and spirals toward the femur, where it fans out and attaches along the intertrochanteric line (Fig. 12).[36,40]

The ischiofemoral ligament reinforces the posterior capsule by resisting internal rotation and posterior translation. It originates from the ischium posteroinferior to the acetabulum and also spirals toward the femur, where it attaches on the medial base of the greater trochanter,

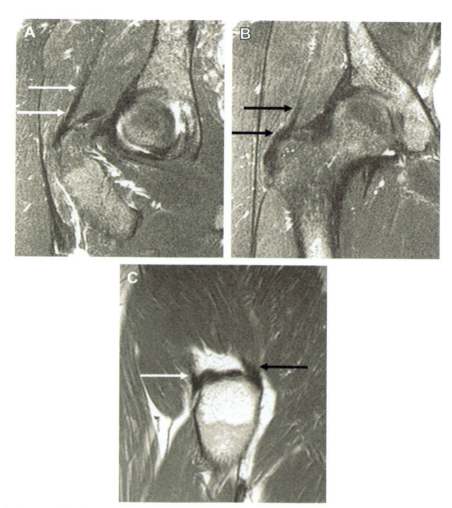

Fig. 9. (*A, B*) Coronal T2-weighted fat-suppressed and (*C*) sagittal proton density weighted MR images show the bony attachment sites of the gluteus minimus (*white arrows*) and gluteus medius (*black arrows*) tendons at the anterior and superoposterior facets of the greater trochanter of the femur, respectively.

along the superolateral aspect of the femoral neck (**Fig. 13**).[36,40]

The pubofemoral ligament is relatively weak, but it also helps to reinforce the anterior inferior and inferior capsule by resisting hyperextension and hyperabduction. It originates from the pectineal eminence and obturator crest of the pubic bone, the superior pubic ramus, and the obturator membrane, and it spirals toward the femoral head where it blends with the iliofemoral ligament. It attaches near the lesser trochanter, medial to the iliofemoral ligament attachment (**Fig. 14**). These capsular ligaments increase the stability of the joint not only because of the translational and rotational motions they restrict, but because the spiraling courses of the iliofemoral and pubofemoral ligaments serve to "screw"

the femoral head into the acetabulum during extension.[36,40]

A deeper layer of fibers called the zona orbicularis encircles the base of the femoral neck. It does not have a direct attachment to bone but instead merges with the fibers of the iliofemoral and ischiofemoral ligaments.[21,41] It acts as a collar for the joint capsule and femoral neck, helps to secure the femoral neck within the acetabulum, and resists inferior distraction (see **Figs. 12** and **13**).[9,18,40]

The ligamentum teres femoris arises from the fovea of the femoral head and courses inferiorly where it inserts onto the transverse acetabular ligament (**Fig. 15**). It can have multiple bundles, but they can be difficult to resolve on routine MR imaging. It may be absent in patients with

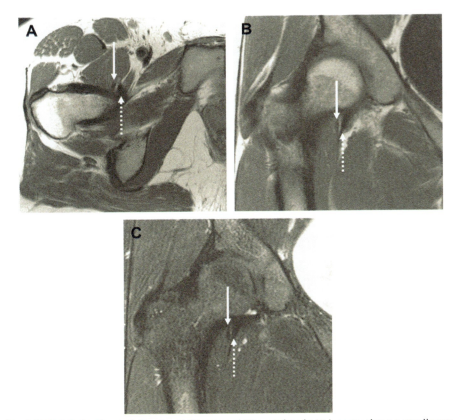

Fig. 10. (*A*) Axial proton density weighted and (*B*) coronal T1-weighted MR images show a small accessory iliacus tendon (*solid arrow*) immediately lateral to the iliopsoas tendon proper (*dotted arrow*). A linear focus of high signal intensity separating the two tendons mimics an iliopsoas tendon longitudinal split tear. This linear focus between the two tendons loses signal intensity on the coronal T2-weighted fat-suppressed MR image (*C*), indicating that it represents fat separating the two tendons and not a longitudinal split tear.

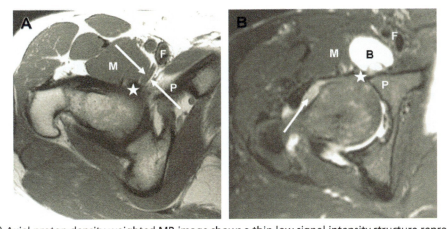

Fig. 11. (*A*) Axial proton density weighted MR image shows a thin low signal intensity structure representing the coapted walls of a nondistended iliopsoas bursa (between the two *arrows*). (*B*) Axial T2-weighted fat-suppressed MR image in a different patient with right hip osteoarthritis shows a small hip joint effusion, synovitis (*arrow*), and fluid distention of the iliopsoas bursa with minimal loculation (B). In (*A*) and (*B*), the iliopsoas bursa is bordered by the iliopsoas muscle anterolaterally (M), the femoral vessels anteriorly or anteromedially (F), the pectineal eminence of the pubic bone medially (P), and the joint capsule and labrum posteriorly (*asterisk*).

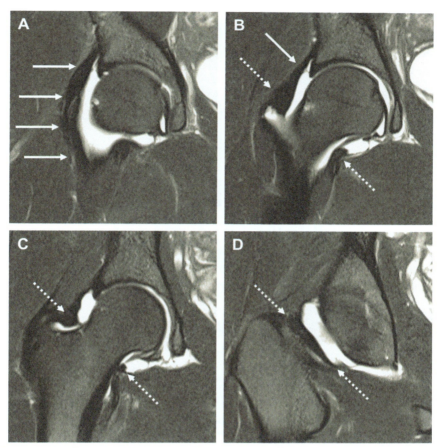

Fig. 12. (*A–D*) Representative coronal T2-weighted fat-suppressed MR images after the injection of intra-articular dilute gadopentetate dimeglumine from anterior to posterior show the iliofemoral ligament (*solid arrows*), which extends from the anterior inferior iliac spine to the femoral neck, and the zona orbicularis (*dotted arrows*), which encircles the femoral neck.

DDH. The function of the ligamentum teres femoris is not clear, although it may provide some hip stability on external rotation, adduction, and flexion. It also contains nerve endings that help with hip proprioception.[17] Tears of the ligamentum teres femoris, which occur in twisting injuries, can be a source of pain, catching, or instability.[1,9,42]

Like the knee, the hip has plicae (synovial folds or reflections) that can become symptomatic if they are entrapped or impinged during movements of the joint. Improved techniques in hip arthroscopy and MR arthrography have contributed to increasing interest in the hip plicae. In their anatomic study of the hip plicae, Fu and colleagues[43] categorized them by their appearance (flat and villous) and by their location (along the femoral neck, adjacent to the ligamentum teres femoris (see **Fig. 7**A), and at the medial surface of the inferomedial aspect of the labrum). The femoral neck plicae were originally described

by Weitbrecht in 1742 and thus are referred to in the anatomic literature as the retinacula of Weitbrecht. There are anterior, medial, and lateral retinacula, and they are significant because arteries that supply the femoral neck traverse the retinacula.[44] The medial femoral neck retinaculum or plica is also known as the pectinofoveal fold (of Amantini). It arises from the medial aspect of the femoral neck near the edge of the articular cartilage, travels inferolaterally, and inserts on the hip joint capsule near its attachment to the lesser trochanter of the femur (**Fig. 16**).[45] This fold has not been shown to cause symptoms and can be seen in 95% of MR arthrography of the hip.[17,46]

LABRUM

The labrum is a low signal intensity fibrocartilaginous structure that is attached to the acetabular rim. The sensitivity of MR arthrography for the

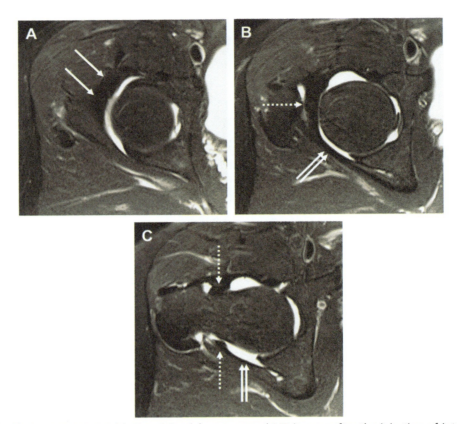

Fig. 13. (*A–C*) Representative axial T2-weighted fat-suppressed MR images after the injection of intra-articular dilute gadopentetate dimeglumine from superior to inferior (same patient as in **Fig. 12**) show the merged iliofemoral ligament and zona orbicularis (*solid arrows*), the zona orbicularis proper (*dotted arrows*) encircling the femoral neck, and the ischiofemoral ligament (*double arrows*) extending from the ischial margin of the acetabulum to the base of the greater trochanter of the femur.

detection of labral tears is at least 90%,[24,42,47] and its accuracy is 91%,[6] compared with conventional noncontrast MR imaging, where the sensitivity and accuracy are 30% and 36%, respectively.[6] Byrd and Jones[42] found a lower sensitivity (66%) of MR arthrography caused by overinterpretation of labral abnormalities. The specificity of MR arthrography for labral tear approaches 100%.[47]

Evaluation of the labrum is challenging because of its inherently curved morphology. In addition to using the standard coronal, axial, and sagittal imaging planes, the authors also use an oblique axial imaging plane (see **Fig. 1**) to evaluate for labral tears, because it has been shown to be the best individual plane for detecting them.[48] The sagittal plane is also very good for visualizing anterior superior labral tears and detachments.[22,48] Some authors use radial imaging of the labrum or generate radial reconstructions of the labrum perpendicular to the acetabular rim.[49–51] Plötz and colleagues[51] achieved 80% sensitivity and

100% specificity for labral pathology on cadaveric specimens using radial reconstructions. Imaging with 3-T scanners is comparable to imaging with 1.5-T scanners, although 3-T scanners may detect a few additional lesions.[52]

The acetabular labrum attaches to the acetabular rim in a similar fashion that the glenoid labrum attaches to the glenoid rim (**Fig. 17**). However, unlike the glenoid labrum, the acetabular labrum only surrounds approximately 270 degrees of the acetabular rim circumference, and its functional importance in stabilizing the femoral head within the acetabulum is questionable.[10] Inferiorly, the labrum blends with the fibers of the transverse acetabular ligament at the acetabular margins. At this junction, there is a cleft, which can be misread as a labral tear (**Fig. 18**).[53] Occasionally, the labrum attaches directly to cartilage instead of to bone (**Fig. 19**). Cartilage can also "undercut" the labrum at its attachment to the acetabulum. This is seen as a smooth focus of intermediately

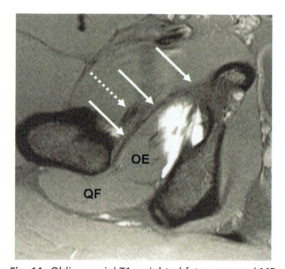

Fig. 14. Oblique axial T1-weighted fat-suppressed MR image after the injection of intra-articular dilute gadopentetate dimeglumine shows the pubofemoral ligament as a low signal intensity linear structure (*solid arrows*) that arises from the pectineal eminence of the pubic bone and travels inferiorly and posteriorly before attaching to the proximal femur near the lesser trochanter. The iliopsoas tendon (*dotted arrow*) is seen anterior to the pubofemoral ligament. OE, obturator externus; QF, quadratus femoris.

increased signal intensity, isointense to cartilage, which is minimally interposed between the labrum and the acetabulum (see **Fig. 17**).

The joint capsule inserts approximately at the level of the labral base, which creates a normal perilabral recess between the peripheral surface of the labrum and the joint capsule. This finding should not be mistaken for extra-articular leak of contrast on MR arthrography (**Fig. 20**). Absence or abnormality of the perilabral recess indicates an abnormality of the adjacent labrum.[6]

The labrum exhibits a range of morphologies. Most asymptomatic labra have a triangular cross section (66%–80%); the remainder have round, flat, or irregular contours.[10,49,54] The posterosuperior labrum is slightly thicker.[4] The labrum may be hypertrophic in DDH.[21] The labrum may also be absent or hypoplastic.[17,49,54] This should be considered abnormal until more work to support or refute this finding as a normal variant has been performed.[17] Regardless, the clinical significance of an absent labrum is unknown.[9]

The labrum also exhibits a spectrum of signal intensities. Only approximately half (56%) of asymptomatic labra are homogeneously low in signal intensity.[49] Increased labral intrasubstance signal intensity can be globular, linear, or curvilinear and can even extend to the capsular or articular surfaces and mimic a labral tear. This finding is most often seen in the superior labrum.[17] The labrum tends to decrease in signal intensity from anterior to posterior and to increase in signal intensity with age.[49]

The existence of a sublabral sulcus or foramen has been a subject of debate. Initial studies comparing surgical findings against MR arthrography concluded that there are no sublabral sulci.[4,6,9] Later studies reported the existences of posteroinferior and anteroinferior sublabral sulci.[53,55] One study even found anteroinferior, anterosuperior, posterosuperior, and posteroinferior sublabral sulci.[56]

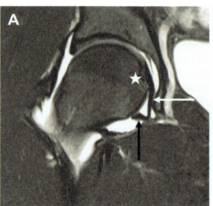
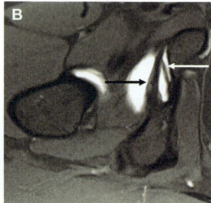

Fig. 15. (*A*) Coronal T2-weighted fat-suppressed and (*B*) oblique axial T1-weighted fat-suppressed MR images after the injection of intra-articular dilute gadopentetate dimeglumine show the ligamentum teres femoris as a linear low signal intensity structure (*white arrow*) that arises from the fovea of the femoral head proximally (*asterisk*) and attaches to the transverse acetabular ligament distally (*black arrow*).

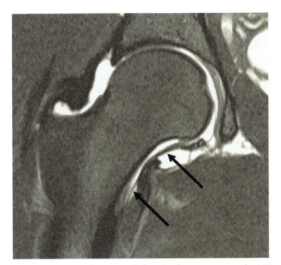

Fig. 16. Coronal T2-weighted fat-suppressed MR image after the injection of intra-articular dilute gadopentetate dimeglumine shows the pectinofoveal fold (*arrows*) as a curvilinear low signal intensity structure in the inferomedial aspect of the hip joint that arises from the medial aspect of the femoral neck, travels inferolaterally, and attaches near the lesser trochanter of the femur.

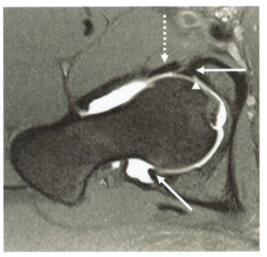

Fig. 17. Oblique axial T1-weighted fat-suppressed MR image after the injection of intra-articular dilute gadopentetate dimeglumine shows the labrum as a low signal intensity structure attached to the acetabular rim (*solid arrows*). The free margin of the anterior labrum is sharp, whereas that of the posterior labrum is somewhat more rounded in this case. Note the normal intermediate signal intensity linear interface between the anterior labrum and the crossing iliopsoas tendon (*dotted arrow*), which should not be misinterpreted as a labral tear. Additionally, there is minimal cartilage (*arrowhead*) interposed between, or "undercutting," the labrum and the acetabulum, which also should not be misinterpreted as a labral tear.

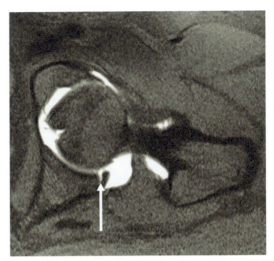

Fig. 18. Oblique axial T1-weighted fat-suppressed MR image after the injection of intra-articular dilute gadopentetate dimeglumine near the inferior margin of the acetabulum shows a normal linear high signal intensity cleft where the transverse acetabular ligament attaches to the posterior inferior aspect of the acetabulum, simulating a labral tear (*arrow*).

Distinguishing a sublabral sulcus from a labral tear can be difficult. Studler and colleagues[55] characterized a sublabral sulcus as a focus of linear high signal intensity interposed between the base of the labrum and the adjacent acetabulum that extends only partially through the thickness of the labrum and is not accompanied by any paralabral abnormalities, such as cartilage loss, osseous changes, or paralabral cysts (**Fig. 21**). The location of these linear high signal intensity foci also helps to distinguish sulci from tears. Abnormally increased signal intensity at the anterosuperior labrum-cartilage junction is more likely to represent a tear because tears outnumber sulci in this location.[55] However, abnormally increased signal intensity at the posteroinferior labrum-cartilage junction is more likely to be a sublabral sulcus or a foramen, because tears are rare in this location.[4,9,17,55] A total of 92% of labral tears are located in the anterior or anterosuperior aspect of the labrum.[53] There is no significant difference between the longitudinal extent of sulci and tears.[55]

NERVES

On MR imaging, nerves appear round or oval in cross section with a stippled or honeycombed appearance. The stippling represents individual nerve fascicles separated by variable amounts of fat; this appearance is also called a "fascicular pattern." The fascicles are of similar or slightly

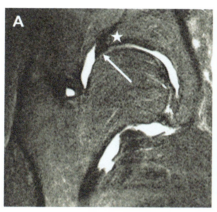
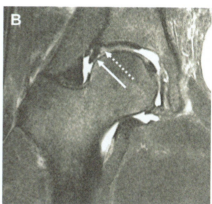

Fig. 19. Coronal T2-weighted fat-suppressed MR images after the injection of intra-articular dilute gadopentetate dimeglumine in two different patients show that the labrum (*solid arrows*) sometimes attaches (*A*) directly to the acetabulum (*Asterisk*) and sometimes (*B*) directly to intermediate signal intensity articular cartilage (*dotted arrow*).

higher signal intensity compared with skeletal muscle on T2-weighted MR images, are uniform in size, and give larger nerves, such as the sciatic nerve, a striated appearance when imaged longitudinally.[27]

The largest nerves in the hip and thigh are the sciatic nerve, which originates from L2 to S3; the femoral nerve, which originates from L2 to L4; and the obturator nerve, which originates from L2 to L4. The sciatic nerve pierces the piriformis; exits posteriorly through the sciatic notch; courses deep to the gluteus maximus; innervates the posterior muscles of the thigh and the muscles of the leg; and provides cutaneous sensation to the posterior thigh, the leg, and the foot (**Fig. 22**).[41,57] The sciatic nerve bifurcates into the tibial and common peroneal nerves usually around the distal third of the thigh.

The femoral nerve lies anterior to the iliopsoas; exits the pelvis through the femoral canal;

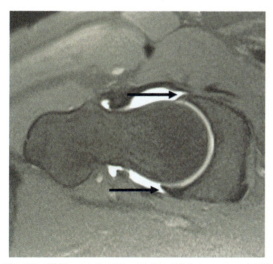

Fig. 20. Oblique axial T1-weighted fat-suppressed MR image after the injection of intra-articular dilute gadopentetate dimeglumine shows normal anterior and posterior perilabral recesses (*arrows*), formed because of the joint capsule attaching to the acetabulum at approximately the level of the labral base.

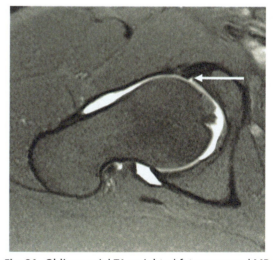

Fig. 21. Oblique axial T1-weighted fat-suppressed MR image after the injection of intra-articular dilute gadopentetate dimeglumine shows minimal linear contrast interposed between the anterior inferior labrum and the adjacent acetabulum without any accompanying cartilage or bony abnormalities. The contrast does not extend through the base of the labrum. The finding is consistent with a sublabral sulcus (*arrow*).

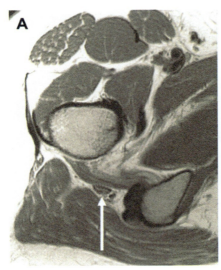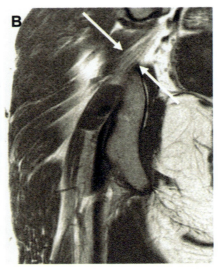

Fig. 22. (*A*) Axial proton density weighted MR image shows the normal stippled appearance of the sciatic nerve in cross section (*arrow*) lateral to the origin of the hamstring tendons. (*B*) Coronal T1-weighted MR image shows the normal striated appearance of the sciatic nerve in longitudinal section (between the two *arrows*) as it passes through the sciatic foramen.

innervates the quadriceps muscles (rectus femoris, vastus lateralis, vastus intermedius, and vastus medius); and provides cutaneous sensation to the anterior thigh (**Fig. 23**).[57]

The obturator nerve also lies anterior to the iliopsoas; passes posterior to the common iliac arteries; travels along the lateral wall of the pelvis; and exits the pelvis through the obturator canal, where it innervates the obturator externus, the adductors (longus, brevis, and magnus), the gracilis, and the pectineus (**Fig. 24**).[57]

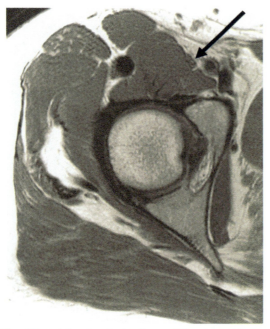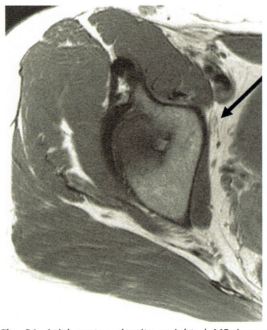

Fig. 23. Axial proton density weighted MR image shows the normal stippled appearance of the femoral nerve in cross section (*arrow*) on the surface of the iliopsoas muscle and lateral to the femoral vessels.

Fig. 24. Axial proton density weighted MR image shows the normal striated appearance of the obturator nerve in longitudinal section (*arrow*) coursing posterior to the femoral vessels along the lateral aspect of the pelvic sidewall.

VESSELS

The external iliac artery and vein exit the pelvis with the femoral nerve and become the femoral artery and vein at the level of the inguinal ligament; at the level of the femoral heads, the neurovascular structures from lateral to medial are the femoral nerve, the femoral artery, the femoral vein, and the lymphatics. The femoral artery divides into the superficial femoral artery and the profunda femoris artery as it exits the femoral triangle, approximately 2 to 5 cm below the inguinal ligament. The profunda femoris artery supplies blood to the thigh muscles; the superficial femoral artery continues to the knee to supply the lower leg and foot. The internal iliac artery gives branches, which supply the gluteal muscles.[36]

SUMMARY

Imaging evaluation of the hip presents many challenges because of its intrinsically complex biomechanics and multiple anatomic structures, which constitute and surround the hip joint. In addition, there are developmental variations and anatomic variants that can be mistaken for pathology. Awareness of these entities helps the radiologist to make the appropriate diagnosis.

REFERENCES

1. Tibor LM, Sekiya JK. Differential diagnosis of pain around the hip joint. Arthroscopy 2008;24(12): 1407–21.
2. Tönnis D, Heinecke A. Acetabular and femoral anteversion: relationship with osteoarthritis of the hip. J Bone Joint Surg Am 1999;81(12): 1747–70.
3. Tönnis D. Normal values of the hip joint for the evaluation of X-rays in children and adults. Clin Orthop Relat Res 1976;119:39–47.
4. Czerny C, Hofmann S, Urban M, et al. MR arthrography of the adult acetabular capsular-labral complex: correlation with surgery and anatomy. AJR Am J Roentgenol 1999;173(2):345–9.
5. Leunig M, Werlen S, Ungersböck A, et al. Evaluation of the acetabular labrum by MR arthrography. J Bone Joint Surg Br 1997;79(2):230–4.
6. Czerny C, Hofmann S, Neuhold A, et al. Lesions of the acetabular labrum: accuracy of MR imaging and MR arthrography in detection and staging. Radiology 1996;200(1):225–30.
7. Nötzli HP, Wyss TF, Stoecklin CH, et al. The contour of the femoral head-neck junction as a predictor for the risk of anterior impingement. J Bone Joint Surg Br 2002;84(4):556–60.
8. Bencardino JT, Palmer WE. Imaging of hip disorders in athletes. Radiol Clin North Am 2002;40(2):267–87, vi–vii.
9. Petersilge CA. From the RSNA Refresher Courses. Radiological Society of North America. Chronic adult hip pain: MR arthrography of the hip. Radiographics 2000;20(Spec No):S43–52.
10. Hong RJ, Hughes TH, Gentili A, et al. Magnetic resonance imaging of the hip. J Magn Reson Imaging 2008;27(3):435–45.
11. Khoury NJ, Birjawi GA, Chaaya M, et al. Use of limited MR protocol (coronal STIR) in the evaluation of patients with hip pain. Skeletal Radiol 2003; 32(10):567–74.
12. Khurana B, Okanobo H, Ossiani M, et al. Abbreviated MRI for patients presenting to the emergency department with hip pain. AJR Am J Roentgenol 2012;198(6):W581–8.
13. Browning WH, Rosenkrantz H, Tarquinio T. Computed tomography in congenital hip dislocation. The role of acetabular anteversion. J Bone Joint Surg Am 1982;64(1):27–31.
14. Conway WF, Totty WG, McEnery KW. CT and MR imaging of the hip. Radiology 1996;198(2): 297–307.
15. Vogler JB III, Murphy WA. Bone marrow imaging. Radiology 1988;168(3):679–93.
16. Chatha DS, Arora R. MR imaging of the normal hip. Magn Reson Imaging Clin N Am 2005;13(4): 605–15.
17. DuBois DF, Omar IM. MR imaging of the hip: normal anatomic variants and imaging pitfalls. Magn Reson Imaging Clin N Am 2010;18(4):663–74.
18. Hergan K, Oser W, Moriggl B. Acetabular ossicles: normal variant or disease entity? Eur Radiol 2000; 10(4):624–8.
19. Lien LC, Hunter JC, Chan YS. Tubular acetabular intraosseous contrast tracking in MR arthrography of the hip: prevalence, clinical significance, and mechanisms of development. AJR Am J Roentgenol 2006; 187(3):807–10.
20. Dietrich TJ, Suter A, Pfirrmann CW, et al. Supraacetabular fossa (pseudodefect of acetabular cartilage): frequency at MR arthrography and comparison of findings at MR arthrography and arthroscopy. Radiology 2012;263(2):484–91.
21. Stoller DW. Stoller's atlas of orthopaedics and sports medicine. Philadelphia: Lippincott Williams & Wilkins; 2008.
22. Stoller DW. Magnetic resonance imaging in orthopaedics and sports medicine. 3rd edition. Philadelphia: Lippincott Williams & Wilkins; 2007.
23. Schmid MR, Nötzli HP, Zanetti M, et al. Cartilage lesions in the hip: diagnostic effectiveness of MR arthrography. Radiology 2003;226(2):382–6.
24. Freedman BA, Potter BK, Dinauer PA, et al. Prognostic value of magnetic resonance arthrography

for Czerny stage II and III acetabular labral tears. Arthroscopy 2006;22(7):742–7.

25. Nishii T, Tanaka H, Nakanishi K, et al. Fat-suppressed 3D spoiled gradient-echo MRI and MDCT arthrography of articular cartilage in patients with hip dysplasia. AJR Am J Roentgenol 2005;185(2): 379–85.

26. Nakanishi K, Tanaka H, Nishii T, et al. MR evaluation of the articular cartilage of the femoral head during traction. Correlation with resected femoral head. Acta Radiol 1999;40(1):60–3.

27. Kaplan PA, Helms C, Dussault R, et al. Musculoskeletal MRI. 2nd edition. Philadelphia: W.B. Saunders Company; 2001.

28. May DA, Disler DG, Jones EA, et al. Abnormal signal intensity in skeletal muscle at MR imaging: patterns, pearls, and pitfalls. Radiographics 2000;20(Spec No):S295–315.

29. Kassarjian A, Rodrigo RM, Santisteban JM. Current concepts in MRI of rectus femoris musculotendinous (myotendinous) and myofascial injuries in elite athletes. Eur J Radiol 2011. Available at: http://www.ncbi.nlm.nih.gov/pubmed/21514758. Accessed July 31, 2012.

30. Bencardino JT, Mellado JM. Hamstring injuries of the hip. Magn Reson Imaging Clin N Am 2005;13(4): 677–90, vi.

31. Moeller TB, Reif E. Atlas of sectional anatomy: the musculoskeletal system. New York: Georg Theime Verlag; 2009.

32. Koulouris G, Connell D. Hamstring muscle complex: an imaging review. Radiographics 2005; 25(3):571–86.

33. Bordalo-Rodrigues M, Rosenberg ZS. MR imaging of the proximal rectus femoris musculotendinous unit. Magn Reson Imaging Clin N Am 2005;13(4): 717–25.

34. Gyftopoulos S, Rosenberg ZS, Schweitzer ME, et al. Normal anatomy and strains of the deep musculotendinous junction of the proximal rectus femoris: MRI features. AJR Am J Roentgenol 2008;190(3): W182–6.

35. Dwek J, Pfirrmann C, Stanley A, et al. MR imaging of the hip abductors: normal anatomy and commonly encountered pathology at the greater trochanter. Magn Reson Imaging Clin N Am 2005;13(4): 691–704, vii.

36. Standring S. Gray's anatomy: the anatomical basis of clinical practice, expert consult. 40th edition. Madrid, Spain: Churchill Livingstone; 2008.

37. Tatu L, Parratte B, Vuillier F, et al. Descriptive anatomy of the femoral portion of the iliopsoas muscle. Anatomical basis of anterior snapping of the hip. Surg Radiol Anat 2001;23(6):371–4.

38. D'Costa S, Ramanathan LA, Madhyastha S, et al. An accessory iliacus muscle: a case report. Rom J Morphol Embryol 2008;49(3):407–9.

39. Varma DG, Richli WR, Charnsangavej C, et al. MR appearance of the distended iliopsoas bursa. AJR Am J Roentgenol 1991;156(5):1025–8.

40. Byrd JW, editor. Operative hip arthroscopy. 2nd edition. New York: Springer Science + Business Media; 2005.

41. Callaghan JJ, Rosenberg AG, Rubash HE. The adult hip. 2nd edition. New York: Lippincott Williams & Wilkins; 2007.

42. Byrd JW, Jones KS. Diagnostic accuracy of clinical assessment, magnetic resonance imaging, magnetic resonance arthrography, and intra-articular injection in hip arthroscopy patients. Am J Sports Med 2004; 32(7):1668–74.

43. Fu Z, Peng M, Peng Q. Anatomical study of the synovial plicae of the hip joint. Clin Anat 1997; 10(4):235–8.

44. Gojda J, Bartoníček J. The retinacula of Weitbrecht in the adult hip. Surg Radiol Anat 2012; 34(1):31–8.

45. Bencardino JT, Kassarjian A, Vieira RL, et al. Synovial plicae of the hip: evaluation using MR arthrography in patients with hip pain. Skeletal Radiol 2011; 40(4):415–21.

46. Blankenbaker DG, Davis KW, De Smet AA, et al. MRI appearance of the pectinofoveal fold. AJR Am J Roentgenol 2009;192(1):93–5.

47. Toomayan GA, Holman WR, Major NM, et al. Sensitivity of MR arthrography in the evaluation of acetabular labral tears. AJR Am J Roentgenol 2006;186(2): 449–53.

48. Ziegert AJ, Blankenbaker DG, De Smet AA, et al. Comparison of standard hip MR arthrographic imaging planes and sequences for detection of arthroscopically proven labral tear. AJR Am J Roentgenol 2009;192(5):1397–400.

49. Abe I, Harada Y, Oinuma K, et al. Acetabular labrum: abnormal findings at MR imaging in asymptomatic hips. Radiology 2000;216(2):576–81.

50. Kubo T, Horii M, Harada Y, et al. Radial-sequence magnetic resonance imaging in evaluation of acetabular labrum. J Orthop Sci 1999;4(5):328–32.

51. Plötz GM, Brossmann J, von Knoch M, et al. Magnetic resonance arthrography of the acetabular labrum: value of radial reconstructions. Arch Orthop Trauma Surg 2001;121(8):450–7.

52. Sundberg TP, Toomayan GA, Major NM. Evaluation of the acetabular labrum at 3.0-T MR imaging compared with 1.5-T MR arthrography: preliminary experience. Radiology 2006;238(2):706–11.

53. Dinauer PA, Murphy KP, Carroll JF. Sublabral sulcus at the posteroinferior acetabulum: a potential pitfall in MR arthrography diagnosis of acetabular labral tears. AJR Am J Roentgenol 2004;183(6): 1745–53.

54. Lecouvet FE, Vande Berg BC, Malghem J, et al. MR imaging of the acetabular labrum: variations in 200

asymptomatic hips. AJR Am J Roentgenol 1996; 167(4):1025–8.

55. Studler U, Kalberer F, Leunig M, et al. MR arthrography of the hip: differentiation between an anterior sublabral recess as a normal variant and a labral tear. Radiology 2008;249(3): 947–54.

56. Saddik D, Troupis J, Tirman P, et al. Prevalence and location of acetabular sublabral sulci at hip arthroscopy with retrospective MRI review. AJR Am J Roentgenol 2006;187(5):W507–11.

57. Moore KL, Agur AM, Dalley AF. Essential clinical anatomy. 4th edition. Baltimore (MD): Lippincott Williams & Wilkins; 2011.

Acetabular Labrum

Donna G. Blankenbaker, MD*, Michael J. Tuite, MD

KEYWORDS

• MR • MR arthrography • Hip • Labrum • Sublabral sulcus

KEY POINTS

- MR arthrography is the imaging technique of choice for evaluation of labral pathology.
- Intra-articular anesthetic injection at the time of MR arthrography is key to many ordering providers in determining if hip pain is related to an intra-articular cause and helps guide treatment.
- Using all MR imaging planes aids in detection of labral tears.

INTRODUCTION

The acetabular labrum is an important structure within the hip that is believed to provide joint stability,[1] although the exact role of the labrum continues to be studied. Labral pathology is a known cause of hip pain in the active population. Labral abnormalities are associated with femoroacetabular impingement and are a significant factor in the development and progression of degenerative joint disease. Those patients with labral abnormalities may have acute or chronic symptoms of widely ranging intensities, locations, and duration. Clinical findings are highly variable, and numerous regional anatomic structures can make the clinical evaluation difficult. Demands for improved diagnosis of hip conditions continue with several advanced imaging techniques, including MR imaging, MR arthrography, CT arthrography, and sonography (**Box 1**). This article reviews the normal anatomy, imaging techniques, imaging findings, pathology, and pitfalls in the assessment of the acetabular labrum.

NORMAL ANATOMY

The acetabular labrum is a fibrocartilagenous structure that is located circumferentially around the acetabular perimeter and attaches to the transverse acetabular ligament posteriorly and anteriorly. The acetabular labrum is attached to the perimeter of the acetabular hyaline cartilage.[2,3] The appearance of a cleft or sulcus can often be seen between the labrum and transverse ligament where they join.[4] The labrum is primarily composed of circumferential type I collagen fibers.[5] The labrum is triangular in cross-section, with a base approximately 4.7 mm wide at the osseous attachment by approximately 4.7 mm tall.[6] The medial extent of the labrum from the acetabular rim varies by subject and location within the acetabulum.[6,7]

The labrum is innervated by nerves that play a role in proprioception and pain production.[8] The vascular supply to the labrum is from capsular blood vessels that are derived from the obturator, superior gluteal, and inferior gluteal arteries.[5,9,10] The labral substance blood supply is from small vessels along the capsular side of the labrum. The vessels do not penetrate deeply, which limits the blood supply such that the majority of the labrum is avascular and, therefore, an injured labrum has limited potential to heal.[5,6,10–12] The healing potential is greatest at the peripheral capsulolabral junction, where the blood supply is greatest, an important factor when considering whether a labral tear is repairable.[9]

The labrum is believed to have several important functions, including the containment of the femoral head during acetabular formation and stabilization

Department of Radiology, University of Wisconsin School of Medicine and Public Health, E3/366 Clinical Science Center, 600 Highland Avenue, Madison, WI 53792-3252, USA

* Corresponding author. University of Wisconsin School of Medicine and Public Health, Department of Radiology, E3/366 Clinical Science Center, 600 Highland Avenue, Madison, WI 53792-3252.

E-mail address: dblankenbaker@uwhealth.org

Magn Reson Imaging Clin N Am 21 (2013) 21–33
http://dx.doi.org/10.1016/j.mric.2012.09.006
1064-9689/13/$ – see front matter © 2013 Elsevier Inc. All rights reserved.

of the hip by deepening the acetabulum[13,14] and maintaining hip joint congruity. The hip joint is subject to a large transmitted load. The acetabular labrum is placed under undue stress in conditions where the morphology of the hip is abnormal, such as in developmental dysplasia and femoroacetabular impingement. Biomechanical studies have shown that the labrum aids in sealing the hip joint and preventing the expression of fluid when the joint is stressed.[1] This sealing effect is believed to offer cartilage protection within the hip joint.[1,15] The labrum is not designed to withstand significant weight-bearing forces; when subjected to such forces, it eventually degenerates and tears.

The normal anatomy of the hip has been reviewed earlier within this issue by Chang and Huang. The relationship of the joint capsule and the iliopsoas tendon with the acetabular labrum is discussed in this article. The proximal attachment of the capsule of the hip joint is along the osseous rim of the acetabulum. Typically, the capsule inserts near the base of the labrum, creating the perilabral recess.[2,16] Anteriorly and posteriorly, the capsule courses further away from the acetabular margin and the recess is deeper, particularly anteriorly.[2] The capsule attaches distally along the anterior aspect of the femoral neck at the base of the trochanters.[16] A series of ligaments helps reinforce the capsule and the iliofemoral, ischiofemoral, and pubofemoral ligaments. There is also a circular layer of fibers along the deep surface of the joint capsule at the base of the femoral neck, called the zona orbicularis. The iliopsoas tendon is closely related to the anterior aspect of the hip joint and lies adjacent to the anterior aspect of the acetabular labrum at the level of the acetabular rim.

CLINICAL PRESENTATION

Diagnosis of acetabular labral tears can be difficult and they are a known cause of mechanical hip pain. Labral tears can be seen in patients with femoroacetabular impingement (see article by Bredella and colleagues in this issue discussing femoroacetabular impingement), hip dysplasia, slipped capital femoral epiphysis, Legg-Calvé-Perthes disease, osteoarthritis, and trauma. Labral tears often occur in young patients with normal radiographs and no history of prior trauma.[13,17] More recently, iliopsoas impingement has been identified as a cause of labral pathology.[18] Athletic activities that involve repetitive pivoting movements or repetitive hip flexion are recognized as additional causes of acetabular labral injury, and tears of the acetabular labrum have become increasingly recognized disorder in young adult and middle-aged patients.[10,11,17,19,20] Labral tears as the culprit for hip pain may be due to the increasing recognition of changes associated with femoroacetabular impingement. The mechanism of injury is commonly reported as a sudden twisting or pivoting motion, with a pop, click, catching, or locking sensation.[21] More commonly, the symptom presentation is subtle, characterized by dull activity-induced or positional pain that fails to improve over time. Patients may describe a deep discomfort within the anterior groin or lateral hip pain proximal to the greater trochanter or posteriorly.[11,22,23] A clicking mechanical symptom may suggest an acetabular labral tear although other entities, such as snapping iliopsoas tendon, may give a similar presentation.

The impingement test, in which the hip is flexed to 90° with maximum internal rotation and adduction, may produce pain and is associated with intra-articular hip pain; it is useful for diagnosis of femoroacetabular impingement and potentially associated with labral pathologic conditions.[21] The labral stress test, in which the hip is brought into flexion, abduction, and external rotation and then extended as the extremity is adducted and internally rotated, may reproduce pain and/or cause a clunk of a labral tear.[21] Together, the clinical and imaging tests help diagnose labral pathology. Early diagnosis and treatment of acetabular labral tear are important because they not only provides pain relief but may prevent the early onset of osteoarthritis.[10,24]

IMAGING TECHNIQUE

MR imaging remains the imaging technique of choice in the evaluation of the acetabular labrum. Both conventional MR imaging and MR arthrography are commonly used to diagnose internal derangements of the hip joint.[3,25] Hip MR imaging is best performed on 1.5-T or 3-T magnets because higher field strength provides a higher intrinsic signal-to-noise ratio, which is critical for high-resolution imaging. Hip imaging should be performed with either a surface phased array coil or a multiple channel, cardiac coil.

Conventional MR Imaging

Conventional MR imaging of the hip with small field-of-view (14–16 cm) and high-resolution imaging has been shown by some investigators to have similar diagnostic performance to MR arthrography for labral tear detection.[26] Sundberg and colleagues[27] compared acetabular labral tear detection at 3-T conventional MR with 1.5-T MR arthrography. In this study, conventional MR imaging found 4 arthroscopically confirmed labral tears also identified at MR arthrography; however, conventional MR imaging found 1 labral tear that was not visualized at MR arthrography. A limitation of this study was that only 8 patients were studied and only 5 patients underwent arthroscopic surgery. Moderate echo time fast spin-echo sequencing with an effective echo of approximately 34 ms at 1.5 T and 28 ms at 3 T is recommended for conventional MR imaging.[28]

MR Arthrography (Direct)

MR arthrography of the hip is the preferred imaging technique for evaluating the labrum due to joint distention and anesthetic injected at the time of arthrography. The anesthetic portion of the arthrogram is key to many ordering providers because of the potential association between pain relief with anesthetic and intra-articular pathology.[29,30]

The hip joint is usually injected under fluoroscopic guidance using an anterior/anterolateral approach. The standard dilution of gadolinium for joint distention is 0.2 mmol/L to optimize the paramagnetic effect. There are several ways to obtain this concentration, depending on whether iodinated contrast material is mixed with the gadolinium. This mixture is injected until the joint is distended (approximately 12–15 mL), stopping if the patient feels an uncomfortable fullness or a higher pressure impedes injection. Intra-articular administration of anesthetic within this solution is considered standard to determine any relief of pain with intra-articular anesthetic. The authors' injectate consists of 0.1 mL gadolinium, 5 mL iodinated contrast, 5 mL normal saline, 5 mL 0.5% ropivacaine, and 5 mL 1% lidocaine. Patient pain level should be recorded immediately and 2 to 4 hours after injection, and patients should perform activities after the injection that typically produce their pain to determine if there is improvement in pain symptoms.

Imaging should be performed using a surface coil. Because of the spherical nature of the acetabulum, it is important to use at least 3 imaging planes to ensure that all portions of the labrum are assessed. Imaging parameters include a small field of view (14 cm to 16 cm), at least a 256 to 320 × 224 to 256 matrix (512 × 512 matrix, if possible), and section thickness of 3 mm to 4 mm. T1-weighted fast spin-echo with fat-suppression images are obtained in at least 3 imaging planes (**Fig. 1**). The authors obtain T1 fat-suppressed images in the standard coronal, sagittal, and axial oblique planes. A fluid-sensitive sequence, either T2 fat-suppressed or short tau inversion recovery (STIR), should be obtained to assess bone marrow edema or other soft tissue or muscle abnormalities around the hip. The authors perform a coronal T2-weighted sequence. A non–fat-suppressed T1-weighted sequence to assess bone marrow and muscles should be included; the authors obtain axial T1 and have added a sagittal intermediate-weighted sequence for additional assessment of the labrum, cartilage, and hip abductor tendons. Radial imaging may be used for the assessment of labral pathology.[31] Yoon and colleagues,[32] however, found that radial imaging did not reveal any additional labral tears at MR arthrography; however, the morphologic assessment for femoroacetabular impingement changes may be better detected with radial imaging. Some investigators advocate large field-of-view STIR coronal images that include the entire symphysis pubis and the sacrum.

MR arthrography has high diagnostic performance for the detection of labral tears with accuracies greater than 90%.[33–36] Ziegert and colleagues[34] found the axial oblique plane to have the highest detection rate of arthroscopically proved acetabular labral tears and more than 95% of tears were identified with the use of 3 imaging planes. A recent meta-analysis of the literature comparing the diagnostic accuracy of acetabular labral tear detection, using conventional MR imaging and MR arthrography, concluded conventional MR imaging and MR arthrography are both useful imaging techniques in diagnosing labral tears in the adult population.[37] MR arthrography seems, however, superior to conventional MR imaging with higher sensitivity with MR arthrography.[37]

MR Arthrography (Indirect)

There are few data on the diagnostic performance of indirect MR arthrography in the detection of acetabular labral tears. The impetus to use indirect MR arthrography is that it is considered by some investigators less invasive than the direct technique and does not require fluoroscopy or a physician to perform the injection and allows visualization of synovitis and extra-articular enhancement. A main disadvantage compared with direct MR arthrography, however, is the lack of capsular distention. Timing of the scan after intravenous

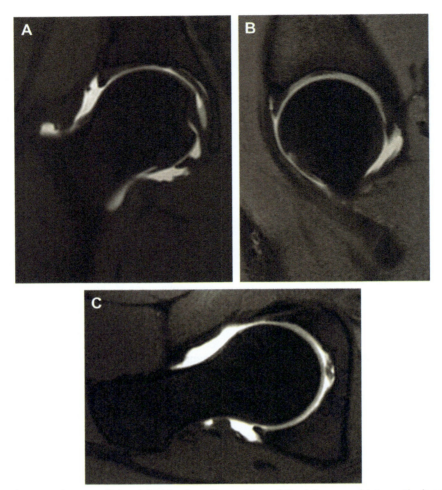

Fig. 1. MR arthrogram images of the right hip show the outline of the labrum and intra-articular structures by gadolinium. Coronal (*A*), sagittal (*B*), and axial oblique (*C*) T1-weighted fat-suppressed images demonstrate the normal triangular appearance of the acetabular labrum.

injection also may be problematic. A recent study by Zlatkin and colleagues[38] found 100% of labral tears at indirect MR arthrography (13 labral tears at arthroscopy), whereas 85% were detected by conventional MR imaging. They did not compare the diagnostic performance in this patient population with direct MR arthrography. They conclude that indirect MR arthrography may be a viable alternative to direct MR arthrography when appropriate. It is these investigators' belief, however, that indirect MR arthrography of the hip is not yet ready for prime time.

CT Arthrography

CT arthrography of the hip may be a useful technique in patients with adjacent metal hardware or in those who are unable to complete the MR examination due to claustrophobia. CT arthrography

with radial reformation was found to have a high sensitivity (97%), specificity (87%), and accuracy (92%) in labral tear detection in patients with hip dysplasia[39] and has been shown to accurately define articular cartilage defects. In the study by Perdikakis and colleagues[35] comparing MR arthrography with multidetector CT arthrography, MR arthrography was found better for the detection of labral tears. The scan parameters should include thin slice thickness (0.5–1.25 mm), small field of view (16 cm), 120 to 140 kV(p), and 140 to 300 mAs.[29,35] Isotropic data acquisition allows multiplanar reformation with 1-mm section thickness in the sagittal, coronal, and axial oblique planes.

Sonography

As with most joints, the role of sonography in the hip is probably best limited to evaluation of 1 or 2 specific questions. For instance, this is a fine technique for evaluating pathology of individual tendons but should not be routinely used to survey the entire hip joint. Sonography can pinpoint suspected bursitis and can demonstrate snapping tendons. It is ideal for performing imaging-guided injections. The acetabular labrum can be visualized at the anterior attachment onto the acetabulum with sonography. The normal fibrocartilage labrum appears hyperechoic and triangle-shaped, whereas a labral tear appears as a hypoechoic cleft (**Fig. 2**). The longitudinal plane allows the best assessment of the anterior labrum. The role of sonography in diagnosis of labral pathology is limited given the incomplete evaluation of the entire labrum and low diagnostic accuracy and sensitivity (44%–82%) compared with MR arthrography.[40,41] A paralabral cyst appears as a hypoechoic multilocular fluid collection adjacent to the acetabular labrum and may aid in the diagnosis of labral tear.

NORMAL IMAGING ANATOMY

Understanding the MR imaging appearance of the normal labrum is important for accurate MR assessment of the labrum. The labrum is generally triangular in cross-section[2,33] because it arises from the rim of the acetabulum (see **Fig. 1**), although it can have a variable shape at MR imaging.[42] These labral shapes include triangular (most common), round, flat, or absent.[42] A

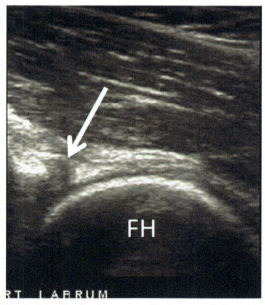

Fig. 2. Longitudinal sonography image of the anterior hip demonstrates an anterior labral tear of the anterior acetabular labrum (*arrow*). FH, femoral head.

previous study by Abe and colleagues[43] showed a triangular labral shape in 96% of patients who are 10 to 19 years old but in only 62% of patients older than 50 years of age. They proposed that the loss of the normal triangular-shaped labrum may be due to degeneration. There is controversy whether an absent labrum is congenital or secondary to degeneration. In middle-aged or elderly patients, an absent labrum is likely due to labral tearing or degeneration. The labrum is thinner anteriorly and thicker posteriorly.[2,33] The labrum is diffusely low signal intensity on all pulse sequences due to the fibrocartilage composition. Intermediate or high signal intensity can be present within the acetabular labrum as seen in asymptomatic individuals.[13] This intermediate to high signal intensity may be due to mucoid degeneration, presence of intralabral fibrovascular bundles, or may be due to magic angle.[3,13] This labral signal may mimic a labral tear on conventional MR imaging.

LABRAL PATHOLOGY AND IMAGING FINDINGS

Labral abnormalities include partial tears of the labrum or labral detachments at the labral-chondral junction, with detachments more common than tears, with up to 90% labral detachments.[16,19,33] The terms, *labral tears* and *detachments*, are often used interchangeably. Labral tears have been classified according to location, etiology, and morphologic features. The most common location for labral tears to occur is anterosuperiorly.[12,14,19] This is the location that would be affected by femoroacetabular impingement.[44] Extension of these tears into other portions of the labrum may be seen.[6,12] The authors commonly see tear extension across quadrants in patients with degenerative labral tears and developmental dysplasia (**Fig. 3**). Posterior labral tears have been described in younger athletic patients that have been shown to be associated with a discrete episode of hip trauma, typically involving impact loading of the extremity, causing the femoral head to be driven posteriorly within the acetabulum.[12,45] Isolated tears of the posterior superior labrum are also most frequently seen after a posterior hip dislocation or in patients with dysplasia.[10] The location of tears can be divided into quadrants—anterior, anterior superior, posterior superior, and posterior—or can be described by the extent of the tear using a clock face.[46] If using the clock face description, discuss with a hip arthroscopist the approach for using this localization terminology to accurately report the tear extent.

The cause of labral tears can be degenerative, dysplastic, traumatic, idiopathic, or impingement.

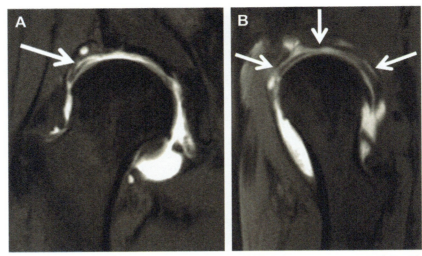

Fig. 3. Coronal (*A*) and sagittal (*B*) T1-weighted fat-suppressed MR arthrogram images in this patient with developmental dysplasia demonstrates an enlarged, thickened, and extensively torn acetabular labrum (*arrows*). Note acetabular and femoral head chondrosis.

Degenerative tears may be related to old trauma, osteoarthritis, or inflammatory arthropathies. The labrum in dysplastic hips is commonly hypertrophied and when torn the tears are often diffuse. Traumatic labral tears are typically isolated to one particular location. Patients who have a traumatic labral tear without dislocation usually have anterior labral tears. These tears occur in the same region as those seen in athletes, femoroacetabular impingement, or mild hip dysplasia.[10,47] There is a strong association between labral abnormalities and cartilage lesions, with 73% of labral lesions accompanied by a cartilaginous lesion.[12] Most cartilage lesions are seen within the anterior aspect of the hip joint where the majority of labral tears occur.[12] Idiopathic tears are those that do not fall into any of these categories.

Morphology of tears has been classified by Lage and colleagues[14] as radial flap, radial fibrillated, longitudinal peripheral, and unstable tears. It is often difficult to subtype labral tears on MR arthrography. Blankenbaker and colleagues[46] evaluated Lage and colleagues' classification[14] for hip labral tears at arthroscopy and found that it did not correlate well with Czerny and colleagues'[33] MR arthrography classification or an MR arthrography modification of Lage and colleagues' classification. Therefore, a more useful classification system for labral tears would be description of these tears as most hip arthroscopists resect or repair the labrum based on other features. This classification by description would include frayed (irregularity of the free edge of the labrum substance), partial-thickness tear (**Fig. 4**), full-thickness tear (**Fig. 5**), and complex tear (**Fig. 6**).

In the assessment of the acetabular labrum for tears, the morphology of the labrum should be evaluated on all imaging planes on MR arthrography. Is the labrum triangular in shape, rounded, thickened, distorted, or irregular? If the labrum is distorted and irregular, this is considered a labral tear. The second assessment is to determine if contrast extends into the labrum, indicating a tear, or if contrast extends between the labrum and acetabulum, indicating labral detachment. Finally, if the signal intensity within the labrum is increased, this may represent mucoid degeneration and not tear. Confirming the diagnosis of labral degeneration, however, based only on signal intensity change is difficult at arthroscopy because of the normal contours of the labrum and intact labral surface.

Tears of the acetabular labrum are identified on MR arthrography by the presence of labral distortion, high signal intensity on T2-weighted imaging, or gadolinium contrast material extending into the labral substance or into the acetabular labral junction. The signal intensity within a labral tear does not have to be equal to gadolinium or fluid to represent a tear (**Fig. 7**).[34] Fraying of the labrum, when the free edge is irregular, is commonly encountered in the middle-aged and elderly population and occurs at all regions of the hip and often coexists with labral tearing. Because of the shape of the acetabulum, no single imaging plane detects all labral tears.[34] Therefore, the labrum should be assessed on all planes, especially when assessing for small labral tears (**Box 2**).

Recognizing a paralabral cyst is helpful in the MR evaluation of the hip and may help confirm

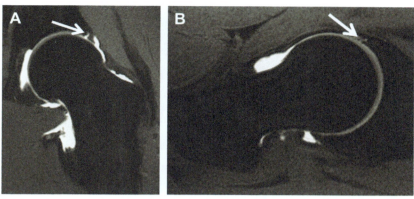

Fig. 4. Coronal (*A*) and axial oblique (*B*) T1-weighted fat-suppressed MR arthrogram images show a partial-thickness acetabular labral tear with gadolinium signal extending into the labral tear (*arrows*).

the diagnosis of a nondisplaced labral tear. Paralabral cysts are typically low to intermediate signal intensity on T1-weighted images and high signal intensity on T2-weighted images (**Fig. 8**). A recent study by Magerkurth and colleagues[48] found paralabral cysts are most commonly anterosuperior in location, multilocular, and often extend superiorly. Paralabral cysts were highly associated with full-thickness labral detachment tears, seen in almost all patients (94%) in their study of 18 patients.[48]

Less commonly, labral disorders occur directly anterior adjacent to the iliopsoas tendon without any osseous abnormalities of femoroacetabular impingement.[49] Labral injury due to iliopsoas impingement is a newly recognized cause of labral pathology.[18,49] These tears occur at the 3-o'clock position. Domb and colleagues[18] explanation for this distinct isolated anterior labral injury, which includes a tight or inflamed iliopsoas tendon, which causes impingement of the anterior labrum with hip extension; the iliopsoas tendon may become scarred or adherent to the anterior capsule-labral complex, which could lead to a repetitive traction injury; or a hyperactive iliocapsularis muscle may cause labral injury by a traction phenomenon. The importance in making this diagnosis is that the treatment would be tenotomy of the iliopsoas tendon at the level of the hip joint, which may be a useful adjunct to débridement or repair of the labrum.[18,49] A recent study evaluating whether labral injuries due to iliopsoas impingement can be diagnosed on MR arthrography found that an isolated acetabular labral tear at the 3-o'clock position suggests a diagnosis of iliopsoas impingement, especially if the tear does not extend above the 2:30-o'clock position.[50]

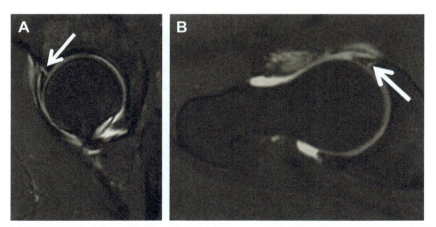

Fig. 5. Sagittal (*A*) and axial oblique (*B*) T1-weighted fat-suppressed MR arthrogram images show gadolinium signal traversing across the acetabular labral base (*arrows*) and adjacent acetabular rim representing a full-thickness labral tear (detachment).

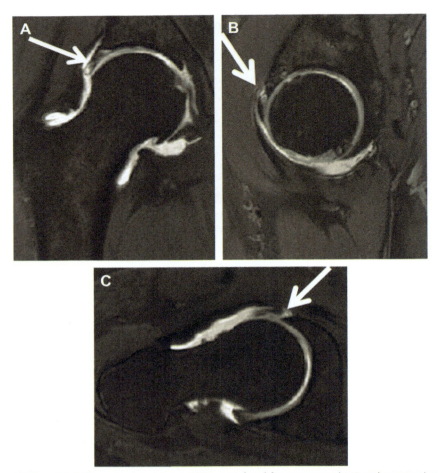

Fig. 6. Coronal (*A*), sagittal (*B*), and axial oblique (*C*) T1-weighted fat-suppressed MR arthrogram images demonstrate a complex degenerative tear of the anterosuperior acetabular labrum (*arrows*). The morphology is abnormal and distorted with gadolinium signal within the labral tear. Note acetabular and femoral head chondrosis.

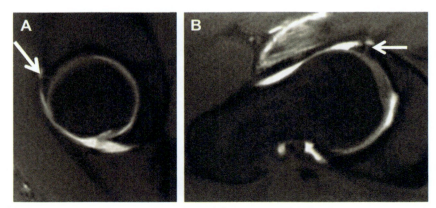

Fig. 7. Sagittal (*A*) and axial oblique (*B*) T1-weighted fat-suppressed MR arthrogram images demonstrate an intermediate signal intensity line traversing the anterior labrum not as bright as gadolinium representing a non-displaced full-thickness labral tear (*arrows*).

PITFALLS IN DIAGNOSING LABRAL TEARS

One pitfall of MR imaging of the labrum is the normal posterior inferior acetabular sulcus or groove (**Box 3**).[4] Dinauer and colleagues[4] defined the presence of a posterior inferior sulcus when labral separation from the articular cartilage was clearly observed on at least 2 MR images in the absence of surgical pathology in the same region of the acetabulum. Posterior labral tears are uncommon in this location, helping to make this distinction. A sulcus or groove at the anterior inferior labral ligamentous junction can also be found. This sulcus or groove is formed at the junction of the transverse ligament with the labrum and may

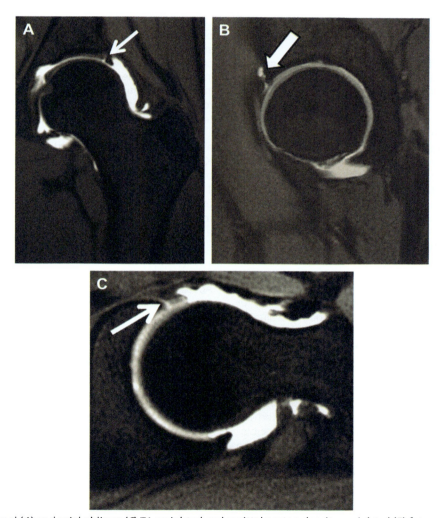

Fig. 8. Coronal (A) and axial oblique (C) T1-weighted and sagittal proton density–weighted (B) fat-suppressed MR arthrogram images of the hip demonstrate a small paralabral cyst adjacent to the anterior labrum (B) (*block arrow*). On initial coronal image, a sublabral sulcus could be considered although other imaging planes better depict the anterior superior labral tear (*thin arrows*). Identification of a paralabral cyst adjacent to the acetabulum/labrum should raise the suspicion for labral tear.

also give the false impression of a labral tear. This should be recognized as a normal variant and should not be interpreted as labral pathology because its location is distinct from most labral tears. Report of a bifid posterior labrum at arthroscopy has been reported in 3 cases and is believed to represent an anatomic variant.[51]

The presence of an anterosuperior sulcus is considered by some investigators a potential pitfall in the diagnosis of labral tears. There is controversy about the existence of the anterosuperior sublabral sulcus. Some studies have found no evidence of labral sulci, whereas others speculate about, suggest, or support its existence.[2,3,13,16,33,42,52–54] A sulcus may be a healing labral tear.[19] In a study by Dinauer and colleagues,[4] they did not find any sublabral sulcus at the anterior or anterosuperior acetabulum, which is the most common sites for labral injury. Saddik and colleagues[53] evaluated the prevalence and location of acetabular sublabral sulci diagnosed at hip arthroscopy. Arthroscopy revealed 30 sulci in 27 of 121 patients. Of those with a single sulcus (25 patients), 11 (44%) were located anterosuperiorly, 12 (48%) posteroinferiorly, 1 (4%) anteroinferiorly, and 1 (4%) posterosuperiorly.[53] A study by Studler and colleagues[54] evaluated the imaging characteristics of surgically proved sublabral recess and labral tears in the anterior portion of the acetabulum at MR arthrography. Ten of 57 (18%) patients had recesses and 44 (77%) of 57 had labral tears. Using the clock position with direct anterior at 9 o'clock in this study, they found 7 recesses at 8 o'clock, 2 recesses at 9 o'clock, and 1 recess at 10 o'clock.[54] MR imaging feature of recesses include a shallow depth (less than one-half labral thickness) and linear shape.[54,55] The mean depth and longitudinal extent of a recess

does not statistically differ between a recess and labral tear (3.2 mm vs 4.9 mm and 15.2 mm vs 14.7 mm).[54] The depth of a labral tear is greater with full-thickness or nearly full-thickness tear, and the shape may be complex, gaping, or linear. The borders of a labral recess should be smooth. The recess occurs at the labral-chondral junction; when contrast material on MR arthrography extends into the labral substance, this is indicative of a labral tear. Additionally, if there is adjacent cartilage or osseous abnormalities or paralabral cyst, a labral tear should be suspected.[54] These investigators believe that sulci occur around the acetabular labral complex; however, it is uncommon to identify an isolated anterosuperior sulcus because this is the common location for labral tears, and, when seen, there is often also a tear. Closely scrutinizing the labrum on all imaging planes improves the diagnostic ability to detect small labral tears by using the stated imaging criteria. Additionally, if a patient gets pain relief after intra-articular anesthetic injection and there are MR imaging findings of subtle changes within the anterosuperior acetabular labrum, this likely is a labral tear.

The obturator externus bursa may also serve as a potential pitfall in diagnosing labral tear pathology. Kassarjian and colleagues[56] found communication of the obturator externus bursa with the hip joint in 11 of 200 (5.5%) hip MR arthrograms. Knowledge of this potential normal communication prevents misinterpretation of gadolinium in the bursa as filling a paralabral cyst or synovial cyst/ganglion.

TREATMENT

Acetabular labral pathology remains the most common indication for arthroscopic hip surgery.[20] The mainstay of treatment is delineating areas of labral degeneration that may be amenable to labral resection or repair.[57] Labral tears can be technically challenging to repair; however, newer suture anchors and knotless anchors have increased the number of tears that are amenable to surgical repair.[57] The results of labral repair seem promising,[58,59] although labral resection remains the treatment of choice for those tears that are impossible to reconstruct.[57]

IMAGING THE POSTOPERATIVE LABRUM

After acetabular labral excision or repair, many patients return to an active lifestyle and may reinjure or develop new hip pain. The question arises whether there may be a labral retear or articular cartilage abnormality that may be the culprit for a patient's hip pain. MR arthrography is often

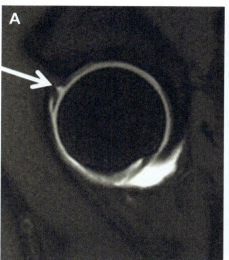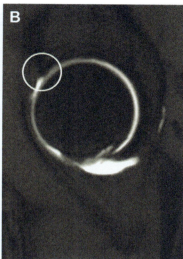

Fig. 9. (*A*) Sagittal T1-weighted fat-suppressed MR arthrogram images demonstrate an anterior labral tear on the initial MR arthrogram (*arrow*). (*B*) MR arthrogram performed after labral resection of the tear for hip pain demonstrates a shorter anterior labrum (*circle*), an expected finding after surgical intervention.

ordered to elucidate the problem. It may be difficult in many cases to determine whether there is postoperative fraying, surgical change, or tearing. The authors have noticed that often the high signal intensity within the labral substance has a similar imaging appearance on MR arthrography after arthroscopic surgery as on the initial MR arthrogram.

A shorter labrum is the common expected finding on MR arthrography after labral resection (**Fig. 9**).[60] Criteria that can be used to diagnose a recurrent labral tear on MR arthrography after labral resection includes a new line to the labral surface, an enlarged and distorted labrum, or a new paralabral cyst (**Fig. 10**).[60] If the labral tip is irregular, this imaging appearance is considered fraying without discrete tear. No studies to date have evaluated the postoperative MR imaging findings after acetabular labral repair. They may be similar to the resected acetabular labrum.

SUMMARY

Hip pain is common with many causes. Tear of the acetabular labrum is one of the many culprits of the painful hip. Conventional MR imaging, MR arthrography, CT arthrography, and ultrasound all offer a role in imaging the painful hip. MR arthrography remains the imaging technique of choice in the assessment of the labrum because many ordering providers gain information from the anesthetic portion of the intra-articular injection. Using a standard approach for evaluating the labrum and remembering the pitfalls can aid the detection of labral tears.

REFERENCES

1. Ferguson SJ, Bryant JT, Ganz R, et al. The influence of the acetabular labrum on hip joint cartilage consolidation: a poroelastic finite element model. J Biomech 2000;33(8):953–60.

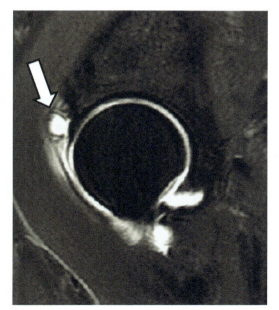

Fig. 10. Sagittal proton density–weighted MR arthrogram image 1 year after labral resection. A new paralabral cyst (*arrow*) is demonstrated adjacent to the anterosuperior acetabulum and a recurrent labral tear was suspected.

2. Keene GS, Villar RN. Arthroscopic anatomy of the hip: an in vivo study. Arthroscopy 1994;10(4):392–9.

3. Hodler J, Yu JS, Goodwin D, et al. MR arthrography of the hip: improved imaging of the acetabular labrum with histologic correlation in cadavers. AJR Am J Roentgenol 1995;165(4):887–91.

4. Dinauer PA, Murphy KP, Carroll JF. Sublabral sulcus at the posteroinferior acetabulum: a potential pitfall in MR arthrography diagnosis of acetabular labral tears. AJR Am J Roentgenol 2004;183(6):1745–53.

5. Petersen W, Petersen F, Tillmann B. Structure and vascularization of the acetabular labrum with regard to the pathogenesis and healing of labral lesions. Arch Orthop Trauma Surg 2003;123(6):283–8.

6. Seldes RM, Tan V, Hunt J, et al. Anatomy, histologic features, and vascularity of the adult acetabular labrum. Clin Orthop Relat Res 2001;(382):232–40.

7. Won YY, Chung IH, Chung NS, et al. Morphological study on the acetabular labrum. Yonsei Med J 2003;44(5):855–62.

8. Kim YT, Azuma H. The nerve endings of the acetabular labrum. Clin Orthop Relat Res 1995;(320):176–81.

9. Kelly BT, Shapiro GS, Digiovanni CW, et al. Vascularity of the hip labrum: a cadaveric investigation. Arthroscopy 2005;21(1):3–11.

10. McCarthy J, Noble P, Aluisio FV, et al. Anatomy, pathologic features, and treatment of acetabular labral tears. Clin Orthop Relat Res 2003;(406):38–47.

11. Mason JB. Acetabular labral tears in the athlete. Clin Sports Med 2001;20(4):779–90.

12. McCarthy JC, Noble PC, Schuck MR, et al. The Otto E. Aufranc Award: the role of labral lesions to development of early degenerative hip disease. Clin Orthop Relat Res 2001;(393):25–37.

13. Cotten A, Boutry N, Demondion X, et al. Acetabular labrum: MRI in asymptomatic volunteers. J Comput Assist Tomogr 1998;22(1):1–7.

14. Lage LA, Patel JV, Villar RN. The acetabular labral tear: an arthroscopic classification. Arthroscopy 1996;12(3):269–72.

15. Ferguson SJ, Bryant JT, Ganz R, et al. The acetabular labrum seal: a poroelastic finite element model. Clin Biomech (Bristol, Avon) 2000;15(6):463–8.

16. Petersilge CA. MR arthrography for evaluation of the acetabular labrum. Skeletal Radiol 2001;30(8):423–30.

17. McCarthy JC, Busconi B. The role of hip arthroscopy in the diagnosis and treatment of hip disease. Orthopedics 1995;18(8):753–6.

18. Domb BG, Shindle MK, McArthur B, et al. Iliopsoas impingement: a newly identified cause of labral pathology in the hip. HSS J 2011;7(2):145–50.

19. Fitzgerald RH Jr. Acetabular labrum tears. Diagnosis and treatment. Clin Orthop Relat Res 1995;(311):60–8.

20. Farjo LA, Glick JM, Sampson TG. Hip arthroscopy for acetabular labral tears. Arthroscopy 1999;15(2):132–7.

21. Freehill MT, Safran MR. The labrum of the hip: diagnosis and rationale for surgical correction. Clin Sports Med 2011;30(2):293–315.

22. Burnett RS, Della Rocca GJ, Prather H, et al. Clinical presentation of patients with tears of the acetabular labrum. J Bone Joint Surg Am 2006;88(7):1448–57.

23. Arnold DR, Keene JS, Blankenbaker DG, et al. Hip pain referral patterns in patients with labral tears: analysis based on intra-articular anesthetic injections, hip arthroscopy, and a new pain "circle" diagram. Phys Sportsmed 2011;39(1):29–35.

24. Altenberg AR. Acetabular labrum tears: a cause of hip pain and degenerative arthritis. South Med J 1977;70(2):174–5.

25. Petersilge CA, Haque MA, Petersilge WJ, et al. Acetabular labral tears: evaluation with MR arthrography. Radiology 1996;200(1):231–5.

26. Mintz DN, Hooper T, Connell D, et al. Magnetic resonance imaging of the hip: detection of labral and chondral abnormalities using noncontrast imaging. Arthroscopy 2005;21(4):385–93.

27. Sundberg TP, Toomayan GA, Major NM. Evaluation of the acetabular labrum at 3.0-T MR imaging compared with 1.5-T MR arthrography: preliminary experience. Radiology 2006;238(2):706–11.

28. Potter HG, Schachar J. High resolution noncontrast MRI of the hip. J Magn Reson Imaging 2010;31(2):268–78.

29. Kivlan BR, Martin RL, Sekiya JK. Response to diagnostic injection in patients with femoroacetabular impingement, labral tears, chondral lesions, and extra-articular pathology. Arthroscopy 2011;27(5):619–27.

30. Byrd JW, Jones KS. Diagnostic accuracy of clinical assessment, magnetic resonance imaging, magnetic resonance arthrography, and intra-articular injection in hip arthroscopy patients. Am J Sports Med 2004;32(7):1668–74.

31. Plotz GM, Brossmann J, von Knoch M, et al. Magnetic resonance arthrography of the acetabular labrum: value of radial reconstructions. Arch Orthop Trauma Surg 2001;121(8):450–7.

32. Yoon LS, Palmer WE, Kassarjian A. Evaluation of radial-sequence imaging in detecting acetabular labral tears at hip MR arthrography. Skeletal Radiol 2007;36(11):1029–33.

33. Czerny C, Hofmann S, Neuhold A, et al. Lesions of the acetabular labrum: accuracy of MR imaging and MR arthrography in detection and staging. Radiology 1996;200(1):225–30.

34. Ziegert AJ, Blankenbaker DG, De Smet AA, et al. Comparison of standard hip MR arthrographic imaging planes and sequences for detection of

arthroscopically proven labral tear. AJR Am J Roentgenol 2009;192(5):1397–400.

35. Perdikakis E, Karachalios T, Katonis P, et al. Comparison of MR-arthrography and MDCT-arthrography for detection of labral and articular cartilage hip pathology. Skeletal Radiol 2011;40(11):1441–7.

36. Toomayan GA, Holman WR, Major NM, et al. Sensitivity of MR arthrography in the evaluation of acetabular labral tears. AJR Am J Roentgenol 2006;186(2):449–53.

37. Smith TO, Hilton G, Toms AP, et al. The diagnostic accuracy of acetabular labral tears using magnetic resonance imaging and magnetic resonance arthrography: a meta-analysis. Eur Radiol 2011;21(4):863–74.

38. Zlatkin MB, Pevsner D, Sanders TG, et al. Acetabular labral tears and cartilage lesions of the hip: indirect MR arthrographic correlation with arthroscopy—a preliminary study. AJR Am J Roentgenol 2010;194(3):709–14.

39. Nishii T, Tanaka H, Sugano N, et al. Disorders of acetabular labrum and articular cartilage in hip dysplasia: evaluation using isotropic high-resolutional CT arthrography with sequential radial reformation. Osteoarthritis Cartilage 2007;15(3):251–7.

40. Troelsen A, Jacobsen S, Bolvig L, et al. Ultrasound versus magnetic resonance arthrography in acetabular labral tear diagnostics: a prospective comparison in 20 dysplastic hips. Acta Radiol 2007;48(9):1004–10.

41. Jin W, Kim KI, Rhyu KH, et al. Sonographic evaluation of anterosuperior hip labral tears with magnetic resonance arthrographic and surgical correlation. J Ultrasound Med 2012;31(3):439–47.

42. Lecouvet FE, Vande Berg BC, Malghem J, et al. MR imaging of the acetabular labrum: variations in 200 asymptomatic hips. AJR Am J Roentgenol 1996;167(4):1025–8.

43. Abe I, Harada Y, Oinuma K, et al. Acetabular labrum: abnormal findings at MR imaging in asymptomatic hips. Radiology 2000;216(2):576–81.

44. Pfirrmann CW, Mengiardi B, Dora C, et al. Cam and pincer femoroacetabular impingement: characteristic MR arthrographic findings in 50 patients. Radiology 2006;240(3):778–85.

45. Ikeda T, Awaya G, Suzuki S, et al. Torn acetabular labrum in young patients. Arthroscopic diagnosis and management. J Bone Joint Surg Br 1988;70(1):13–6.

46. Blankenbaker DG, De Smet AA, Keene JS, et al. Classification and localization of acetabular labral tears. Skeletal Radiol 2007;36(5):391–7.

47. Kassarjian A, Yoon LS, Belzile E, et al. Triad of MR arthrographic findings in patients with cam-type femoroacetabular impingement. Radiology 2005;236(2):588–92.

48. Magerkurth O, Jacobson JA, Girish G, et al. Paralabral cysts in the hip joint: findings at MR arthrography. Skeletal Radiol 2012;41(10):1279–85.

49. Shindle MK, Voos JE, Nho SJ, et al. Arthroscopic management of labral tears in the hip. J Bone Joint Surg Am 2008;90(Suppl 4):2–19.

50. Blankenbaker DG, Tuite MJ, Keene JS, et al. Labral Injuries Due to Iliopsoas Impingement: can they be diagnosed on MR arthrography? AJR Am J Roentgenol 2012;199:894–900.

51. Miller R, Villar RN. The bifid posterior labrum: an anatomic variant of the acetabular labrum. Arthroscopy 2009;25(4):413–5.

52. Byrd JW. Labral lesions: an elusive source of hip pain case reports and literature review. Arthroscopy 1996;12(5):603–12.

53. Saddik D, Troupis J, Tirman P, et al. Prevalence and location of acetabular sublabral sulci at hip arthroscopy with retrospective MRI review. AJR Am J Roentgenol 2006;187(5):W507–11.

54. Studler U, Kalberer F, Leunig M, et al. MR arthrography of the hip: differentiation between an anterior sublabral recess as a normal variant and a labral tear. Radiology 2008;249(3):947–54.

55. Blankenbaker DG, Tuite MJ. The painful hip: new concepts. Skeletal Radiol 2006;35(6):352–70.

56. Kassarjian A, Llopis E, Schwartz RB, et al. Obturator externus bursa: prevalence of communication with the hip joint and associated intra-articular findings in 200 consecutive hip MR arthrograms. Eur Radiol 2009;19(11):2779–82.

57. Griffiths EJ, Khanduja V. Hip arthroscopy: evolution, current practice and future developments. Int Orthop 2012;36(6):1115–21.

58. Larson CM, Giveans MR. Arthroscopic debridement versus refixation of the acetabular labrum associated with femoroacetabular impingement. Arthroscopy 2009;25(4):369–76.

59. Larson CM, Giveans MR, Stone RM. Arthroscopic debridement versus refixation of the acetabular labrum associated with femoroacetabular impingement: mean 3.5-year follow-up. Am J Sports Med 2012;40(5):1015–21.

60. Blankenbaker DG, De Smet AA, Keene JS. MR arthrographic appearance of the postoperative acetabular labrum in patients with suspected recurrent labral tears. AJR Am J Roentgenol 2011;197(6):W1118–22.

Novel Cartilage Imaging Techniques for Hip Disorders

Young-Jo Kim, MD, PhD[a,b,*]

KEYWORDS

- Hip deformity • Acetabular dysplasia • Osteoarthritis • Imaging

KEY POINTS

- Acetabular dysplasia, cam, and pincer deformities are a major cause of premature hip osteoarthritis.
- An early feature of osteoarthritis is loss of the negatively charged proteoglycans in the extracellular matrix.
- Delayed gadolinium-enhanced MR imaging of cartilage (dGEMRIC) and sodium-imaging techniques are highly specific for assessing cartilage charge density.
- T2 and T1rho are noncontrast biochemical imaging techniques that show early cartilage matrix damage in vitro and some clinical studies.
- dGEMRIC is clinically useful in staging early osteoarthritis in patients with acetabular dysplasia.

INTRODUCTION

Increasingly, hip osteoarthritis is thought to be caused by structural deformities, such as acetabular dysplasia and femoroacetabular impingement (FAI). Acetabular dysplasia results in a shallow acetabulum that leads to hip instability, increased mechanical stress on the acetabular cartilage, and eventual joint degeneration. FAI syndrome is a dynamic mechanical phenomenon of the hip in which the femoral head or neck causes damage to the acetabular labrum and/or cartilage from direct collision between the 2 bony structures. Often the hip is predisposed to FAI syndrome because of a femoral and/or acetabular hip deformity. Currently, surgical techniques such as periacetabular osteotomy, femoral head-neck osteoplasty, and acetabular rim osteoplasty are available to correct the deformities that lead to instability or impingement. The surgical results are limited by the extent of articular damage before surgical intervention. Increasingly, high-resolution MR imaging and biochemical cartilage imaging techniques are becoming clinically important in detecting preradiographic cartilage damage. This article outlines the imaging methods to assess hip structural deformities and methods to assess chondral damage using MR imaging. Imaging is becoming critically important in treating patients with these hip disorders; however, as always, careful clinical-radiographic correlation must be performed to determine if the structural deformity seen on imaging studies is responsible for the patient's problem and hence justifies surgical intervention.

PLAIN RADIOGRAPHIC ANALYSIS OF HIP OSTEOARTHRITIS

Plain radiographic analysis is the main method through which hip structural abnormalities are assessed, and is the gold standard for assessing radiographic osteoarthritis. However, by the time clear evidence of radiographic osteoarthritis is seen, often extensive damage is present in the joint, such that most surgeons would see this as a contraindication for joint-preserving surgery.

[a] Harvard Medical School, MA, USA; [b] Child and Adult Hip Program, Boston Children's Hospital, 300 Longwood Avenue, Hunnewell 225, Boston, MA 02115, USA
* Boston Children's Hospital, 300 Longwood Avenue, Hunnewell 225, Boston, MA 02115.
E-mail address: young-jo.kim@childrens.harvard.edu

Magn Reson Imaging Clin N Am 21 (2013) 35–44
http://dx.doi.org/10.1016/j.mric.2012.09.003
1064-9689/13/$ – see front matter © 2013 Elsevier Inc. All rights reserved.

Pelvic Radiograph

The anteroposterior pelvic radiograph is used to assess the presence of radiographic osteoarthritis, determine acetabular coverage and orientation, and increasingly determine femoral head-neck offset.

A properly obtained pelvic radiograph should have the coccyx directly over the pubic symphysis, and the iliac wings, obturator foramina, and acetabular tear drops should be symmetric in appearance (**Fig. 1**). Additionally, if the pelvic inclination is appropriate, the distance between the superior border of the pubic symphysis and the first sacrococcygeal joint should average approximately 32 mm in men and 47 mm in women.[1]

Radiographic osteoarthritis is often graded using the Tönnis classification in hip joint preservation surgery.[2] A more quantitative method of assessing radiographic osteoarthritis is to measure the minimum joint space width (mJSW) of the weight-bearing zone. An mJSW less than 2.5 mm is considered to be definitely pathologic and is associated with poor outcome after FAI surgery.[3] When treating acetabular dysplasia with periacetabular osteotomy, some radiographic osteoarthritis is tolerated as long as the joint space improves and becomes more congruent on abduction internal rotation functional radiographs.[4] However, as a general rule in joint preservation surgery, the presence of Tönnis grade 2 or higher or mJSW less than or equal to 2 mm has been shown to be associated with poor prognosis after surgery.[5]

False Profile Radiograph

For a complete assessment of the acetabular deformity, obtaining a false profile view[6] is recommended (**Fig. 2**). It is a good view to detect early cartilage loss in the superior weight-bearing zone typically seen in cam impingement and acetabular dysplasia. In cases of pincer impingement, the loss of posterior acetabular cartilage can be seen on the false profile view.

In a normal hip, the superior joint space is larger than the posterior joint space on a false profile view (see **Fig. 2**). When this relationship is reversed, it is a sign of significant cartilage loss in the weight-bearing acetabulum. Additionally, in pincer impingement, the counter-coup damage in the posterior acetabulum will be seen as joint space narrowing in this area, subchondral sclerosis, and cyst formation.

MR IMAGING

High-resolution MR imaging is widely used to detect the presence of chondral damage associated with FAI and acetabular dysplasia. MR imaging as a cross-sectional imaging modality also allows assessment of proximal femur and acetabulum morphology. Additionally, MR imaging is useful to rule out other causes of hip pain such as femoral neck stress fracture, benign and malignant tumors, and tendinopathy. True acetabular dysplasia is uncommon; however, cam deformity

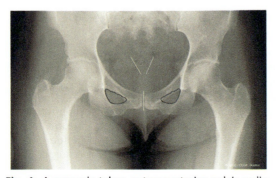

Fig. 1. A properly taken anteroposterior pelvic radiograph should have the coccyx directly over the symphysis and symmetric obturator foramina. Additionally, if the pelvic inclination is appropriate, the distance between the superior border of the pubic symphysis and the first sacrococcygeal joint should average approximately 32 mm in men and 47 mm in women.

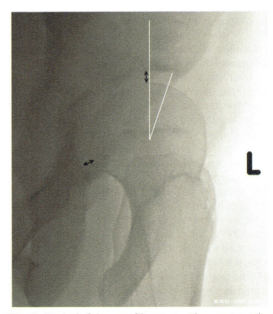

Fig. 2. Typical false profile view. The center-edge angle is measured by drawing a vertical line through the center of the femoral head and a second line through the center of the femoral head to the anterior edge of the sourcil. Typically on a false profile view, the superior joint space is wider than the posterior joint space.

can be present up to 20% of the general population. Hence, a non-FAI cause of hip pain can be mistakenly attributed to the incidentally noted FAI deformity.

To maximally use the MR imaging study, high-resolution dedicated images of the hip are required. Additionally, appropriate sequences are required for accurate detection of the expected intraarticular and nonexpected extra-articular abnormalities.

Chondral Pathology

One of the primary purposes of MR imaging is to detect and stage chondral damage, because the extent of cartilage damage will determine the clinical outcome after surgery. The sensitivity of MR imaging for detecting cartilage damage is highly variable. The reported sensitivities vary from 50% to 90%.[7–11] The detection of chondral flaps is especially difficult, with one report demonstrating sensitivity of only 23%.[8] This finding is because the femoral and acetabular cartilage layers are in close approximation and hence very little contrast would penetrate into the potential space between the delaminated cartilage and bone. However, MR imaging is useful in identifying cases of minimal radiographic evidence of osteoarthritis but extensive local damage seen on MR imaging. These cases should be excluded from surgical interventions.

Many normal variants in labral and acetabular morphology may be mistaken for labral tears or cartilage defects. The supraacetabular fossa (**Fig. 3**) is a common (10%) finding on MR arthrograms that may be mistaken for a cartilage defect.[12] The supraacetabular fossa is a distinct structure separate from the acetabular notch that may (8.9%) or may not (1.6%) be filled with cartilage. It is usually located in the acetabular roof

near the 12 o'clock position in the coronal and sagittal imaging planes. This appearance is in contrast to the stellate crease that is a continuation of the acetabular notch.[13]

Bony Abnormalities Associated With Chondral Damage

In early osteoarthritis, secondary changes to the bone and labrum may help diagnose early cartilage damage and lend increased specificity to the detection of labral tears.[14] Bony cyst formation in either the acetabulum or femoral head is usually associated with underlying cartilage damage. Additionally, osteophyte formation is a sign of early osteoarthritis.

Screening MR Imaging

A major benefit of MR imaging is its ability to screen for unexpected bony and soft tissue abnormalities. Because FAI deformity is highly prevalent in the asymptomatic population, one cannot assume that the detection of an FAI deformity is always the source of the patient's symptoms. Having a sequence in the MR protocol designed to detect stress fractures (**Fig. 4**) and tumors (**Fig. 5**) is very useful and may potentially help the surgeon avoid catastrophic complications.

ROLE OF BIOCHEMICAL IMAGING

Biochemical or compositional MR imaging techniques for cartilage hold the promise of detecting cartilage damage before irreversible structural damage occurs. Currently, 5 techniques are designed to probe different macromolecular components of the cartilage matrix. Each technique has its own advantages and challenges to practical clinical application.

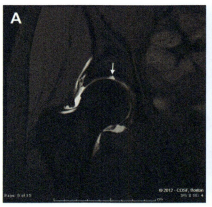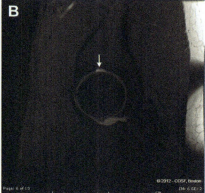

Fig. 3. Supraacetabular fossa (*arrow*) seen on coronal (*A*) and sagittal MR (*B*) arthrogram.

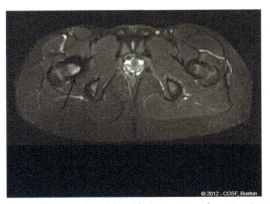

Fig. 4. 16-year-old girl with hip pain after starting track. MR imaging was initially read as having a posterior labral tear, but a screening water-sensitive sequence shows evidence for a right femoral neck stress fracture (*arrow*). On further review, the labral tear in the posterior acetabulum represented a labral sulcus. Pain resolved with rest.

Delayed gadolinium enhanced MR imaging of cartilage (dGEMRIC) is a contrast-based technique designed to specifically detect the loss of sulfated glycosaminoglycan content of articular cartilage. The MR imaging is performed after an intravenous or intraarticular injection of an anionic contrast agent chelate, $Gd-DTPA^{2-}$. This contrast agent is allowed sufficient time to partition into the cartilage before imaging is started. Because the contrast agent is negatively charged, it will partition into the articular cartilage in an inversely proportional manner. Through quantitating the amount of contrast agent in cartilage using MR imaging, the charge density of cartilage can be calculated or inferred. This technique is highly specific for glycosaminoglycan loss in cartilage, mainly because of the use of a negatively charged contrast agent. However, the need for contrast injection poses challenges, including the need for delay between contrast injection and imaging, need for a specific

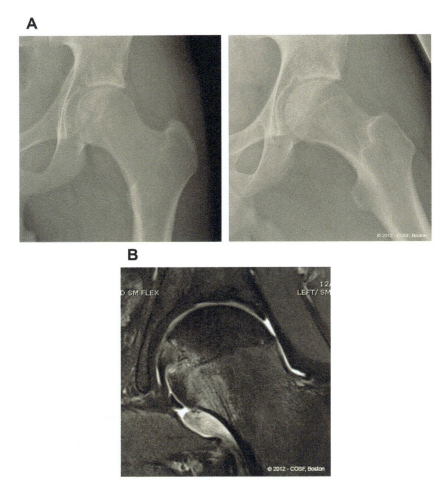

Fig. 5. (*A*) Mild cam deformity in an 18-year-old who presented with mild hip pain. (*B*) MR imaging shows a synovitic reaction in the inferior femoral head with bony edema. CT scan confirmed the presence of an osteoid osteoma, which was treated with radiofrequency ablation.

exercise protocol to facilitate contrast penetration into cartilage, and the risk of contrast reaction. Recently, concern has been raised with the use of contrast agent in patients with poor renal function because of the risk of developing nephrogenic systemic fibrosis, which is a rare and sometimes fatal syndrome. Despite these challenges, if the issues regarding timing of the scan after contrast administration[15] and exercise protocol[16] are respected, reproducible quantitative results can be obtained with root-mean-square average coefficient of variation less than 10%. Additionally, validated fast T1 mapping sequences are available, and therefore imaging times around 5 minutes are now feasible.[17] In addition to the hip studies outlined previously, multiple clinical studies have been performed using dGEMRIC, showing the effect of exercise on knee cartilage,[18] reconstitution of a more normal cartilage after autologous chondrocyte transplantation,[19] and perhaps preservation of cartilage after high tibial osteotomy for knee osteoarthritis.[20]

Currently, the most validated and commonly used technique for the hip is dGEMRIC. dGEMRIC has been validated against histology in vitro and ex vivo and clinically in hips and knees.[21–29] dGEMRIC index has been shown to correlate with hip pain and degree of hip dysplasia.[24] Similar findings were also seen in patients with FAI, in whom dGEMRIC correlated with pain and alpha angle.[30–32] Additionally, dGEMRIC mapping of hips with a history of slipped capital femoral epiphysis showed differences between hips with normal and severe offsets.[33] In FAI, comparison of MR imaging against surgical assessment of articular cartilage suggests that morphologic imaging correlates well with surgical findings. dGEMRIC findings did not correlate as well as morphologic MR imaging findings; however, dGEMRIC detected more areas of abnormal cartilage than both gross surgical inspection and morphologic imaging, perhaps suggesting that dGEMRIC is detecting morphologically normal but biochemically abnormal cartilage.[34]

The cartilage matrix will modulate its charge density in response to mechanical loading. Presumably, because the mechanical load distribution in the hip joint is uneven, the charge density and hence the T1 value on 3-dimensional dGEMRIC scans are higher in the superior weight-bearing zone compared with the anterior or posterior aspect of the joint.[35] In disease states such as acetabular dysplasia, the alteration in T1 value with progression of osteoarthritis seems to be much more diffuse throughout the joint than for FAI.[35] Hence, the authors were able to demonstrate even with thick-section coronal slice dGEMRIC scans the predictive value of dGEMRIC in early clinical outcome after periacetabular osteotomy for acetabular dysplasia.[23] In FAI, because the changes seen on dGEMRIC are often focal, normalizing the values at the labral chondral junction against the central dGEMRIC values seem to increase the ability to detect early disease.[36]

Currently, dGEMRIC is used to increase the reliability in detecting chondral lesions in patients with FAI. Sagittal, oblique axial, or radial cuts can be used to confirm areas of chondral damage seen on standard morphologic sequences using the dGEMRIC data in the corresponding region. The authors do not rely solely on the dGEMRIC data in FAI cases but rather use it as additional quantitative data that may assist in the subjective image interpretation. **Fig. 6** illustrates an example of a patient with FAI. Radiographs show minimal osteoarthritis, but on the dGEMRIC images the acetabular cartilage at the labral-chondral junction is clearly abnormal, especially compared with the normal femoral head cartilage.

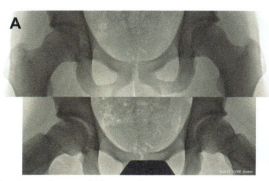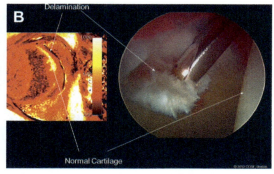

Fig. 6. A 16-year-old boy with symptomatic right hip cam impingement on radiographs (*A*). (*B*) dGEMRIC scan (*left*) shows areas of low T1 (*dark red/black areas*) in the acetabular cartilage, whereas the femoral head cartilage appeared normal. Arthroscopy (*right*) confirms the chondral damage on the acetabular side and normal femoral head cartilage.

In acetabular dysplasia, the authors use the quantitative dGEMRIC data to determine whether a patient is a candidate for periacetabular osteotomy. **Fig. 7** shows a 33-year-old woman with acetabular dysplasia. The left hip is symptomatic and has mild joint space narrowing on the radiograph. Based on radiographic criteria, she would be a candidate for a periacetabular osteotomy. The morphologic MR image shows some signal heterogeneity in the articular cartilage; however, on the dGEMRIC scan, the average T1 value is 319 ms. Based on the dGEMRIC value, she would be a poor candidate for joint preservation treatment. In acetabular dysplasia, the authors would use biochemical imaging data to aid in clinical decision making.

The main advantage of dGEMRIC is its specificity for assessing cartilage charge density. It can provide similar specificity as sodium MR imaging, but without the need for contrast injection. In sodium MR imaging, sodium itself rather than gadolinium is used as the probe to measure charge density. Unlike the typical proton MR imaging, the nuclear spin momentum of the positively charged sodium ions is used to generate the MR imaging signal. However, because there are far fewer sodium atoms in the body than water, sodium MR imaging requires a minimum of 3T or higher field strength magnets, specialized hardware, and radiofrequency coils. Its use is currently limited to strictly research purposes, although its use at 7T was recently published and correlated with dGEMRIC after matrix-associated autologous chondrocyte transplantation.[37] In the future, widespread availability of high-field scanners may make this technique practical.

Some of the other noncontrast MR imaging techniques include diffusion-weighted MR imaging, which measures the diffusion characteristics of water molecules in tissue. The diffusivity of water is affected by intracellular and extracellular barriers and is most commonly used to detect early central nervous system cell necrosis. It can also provide information regarding the macromolecular environment, which includes glycosaminoglycan and collagen, and tissue ultrastructure. It is

A

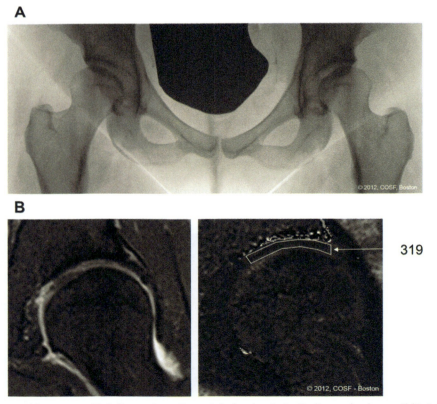

B

319

Fig. 7. A 33-year-old woman with left symptomatic acetabular dysplasia. Radiographs show mild joint space narrowing (*A*). Based on radiographic criteria, she would still be a candidate for periacetabular osteotomy. The morphologic MR images suggest articular cartilage abnormalities and dGEMRIC scan show average T1 value of 319 ms (*B*). Based on the MR imaging finding, she would be a poor surgical candidate.

an attractive technique in the clinical setting because images can be obtained without contrast injection and scan times are quick. However, it is sensitive to motion artifacts, and it is demanding to get absolute quantitative measurements. It has been used to evaluate patients after matrix-associated autologous chondrocyte transplantation to show distinction between healthy cartilage and cartilage repair tissue, but it has had limited use in other clinical settings to evaluate cartilage.[38,39]

T2 mapping, like diffusion-weighted imaging, does not require contrast injection, and scan times are short. It assesses interaction between water and collagen fibers to quantify water content and collagen anisotropy.[40] High anisotropy of highly organized collagen will lead to shortened T2 relaxation times. Hence, T2 relaxation times vary from low in the deep layers to higher values in the transitional layers of cartilage because of anisotropy of collagen fibers, which in the deep layers is high with dense collagen matrix and low in the transitional layers.[41,42] Additionally, disruption of collagen fiber matrices and increase in water content as a result of cartilage damage will increase T2 relaxation times.[43,44] Areas of high T2 relaxation times in osteoarthritic knees correlate with findings on arthroscopy.[45] However, concerns have been raised that no linear relationship exists between T2 mapping and severity of osteoarthritis.[46] Nishii and colleagues[47] compared T2 values and distribution in normal volunteers and patients with hip dysplasia using graded plain radiographs into normal, prearthritic, and mild-arthritic hips and found no difference in T2 relaxation times between the different radiographic grades. T2 mapping is also sensitive to the loading state of the joint, which may alter T2 signal independent of cartilage damage if joint unloading before scanning is not controlled.[48–51] Finally, T2 values are sensitive to the orientation of the collagen fibers relative to the B0 magnetic field because of the magic angle effect. In a spherical structure such as the hip joint, this will need to be taken into account when interpreting the T2 mapping data.

T1rho MR imaging is a noncontrast technique that detects low-frequency interactions between water molecules and macromolecular protons. This may allow T1rho maps in cartilage to be more specific than T2 to assess glycosaminoglycan loss; however, debate and conflicting data exist regarding this characteristic of T1rho measurement in cartilage. Some studies have shown that T1rho is sensitive to proteoglycan and collagen content.[52–54] T1rho relaxation times have been shown in vivo to correlate with the severity of radiographic and MR grading of

osteoarthritis.[55] Although other studies have shown that T1rho is specific to glycosaminoglycan loss,[56–58] the most recent study by Keenan and colleagues[59] found that T2 and T1rho values correlated and, when T2 effects were isolated by looking at tissue only with T2 within normal range, T1rho correlated with glycosaminoglycan content. They concluded that T2 relaxation time should be incorporated into a predictive model when using T1rho data to estimate glycosaminoglycan content. Comparing T1rho with T2 mapping, Regatte and colleagues[60] suggested that T1rho had higher dynamic range, which allowed greater accuracy than T2 mapping. Disadvantages of T1rho mapping include the length of time required to obtain the multiple data sets and that the requirement for the spin lock pulse may increase the specific absorption rate. Although to a lesser extent than in T2 mapping, magic angle effect is also observed in T1rho.[58]

Currently, many of these biochemical MR imaging techniques hold the promise of improving diagnostics and patient management for clinical problems. Although each technique has its own challenges and limitations, the true value of these techniques will not be known until well-conducted clinical studies demonstrate this in the clinical setting.

SUMMARY

Careful assessment of the hip deformity using radiographs and advanced cross-sectional imaging such as with MR imaging or CT is essential for accurately diagnosing the cause of hip pain and surgical planning for joint preservation surgery. Understanding the various measures of hip structure is important; however, it is more important to keep in mind that good clinical-radiographic correlation is essential to identify the right patient with the right bony abnormality that will benefit from surgical treatment. High-resolution MR imaging of the hip and increasingly biochemical imaging techniques for cartilage are becoming clinically important in detecting preradiographic cartilage damage. Chondral damage has direct relevance to clinical outcome after joint preservation surgeries and hence will continue to play an important role in advancing this new field of orthopedic surgery.

REFERENCES

1. Siebenrock KA, Kalbermatten DF, Ganz R. Effect of pelvic tilt on acetabular retroversion: a study of pelves from cadavers. Clin Orthop Relat Res 2003;(407):241–8.

2. Tonnis D. Congenital dysplasia and dislocation of the hip in children and adults. New York: Springer; 1987.

3. Philippon MJ, Schroder ES, Briggs KK. Hip arthroscopy for femoroacetabular impingement in patients aged 50 years or older. Arthroscopy 2012;28(1):59–65.

4. Murphy S, Deshmukh R. Periacetabular osteotomy: preoperative radiographic predictors of outcome. Clin Orthop Relat Res 2002;(405):168–74.

5. Beck M, Leunig M, Parvizi J, et al. Anterior femoroacetabular impingement: part II. Midterm results of surgical treatment. Clin Orthop Relat Res 2004;(418): 67–73.

6. Lequesne M, de Seze S. False profile of the pelvis. A new radiographic incidence for the study of the hip. Its use in dysplasias and different coxopathies. Rev Rhum Mal Osteoartic 1961;28:643–52 [in French].

7. Edwards DJ, Lomas D, Villar RN. Diagnosis of the painful hip by magnetic resonance imaging and arthroscopy. J Bone Joint Surg Br 1995;77(3):374–6.

8. Anderson LA, Peters CL, Park BB, et al. Acetabular cartilage delamination in femoroacetabular impingement. Risk factors and magnetic resonance imaging diagnosis. J Bone Joint Surg Am 2009;91(2):305–13.

9. Neumann G, Mendicuti AD, Zou KH, et al. Prevalence of labral tears and cartilage loss in patients with mechanical symptoms of the hip: evaluation using MR arthrography. Osteoarthritis Cartilage 2007;15(8):909–17.

10. Keeney JA, Peelle MW, Jackson J, et al. Magnetic resonance arthrography versus arthroscopy in the evaluation of articular hip pathology. Clin Orthop Relat Res 2004;(429):163–9.

11. Mintz DN, Hooper T, Connell D, et al. Magnetic resonance imaging of the hip: detection of labral and chondral abnormalities using noncontrast imaging. Arthroscopy 2005;21(4):385–93.

12. Dietrich TJ, Suter A, Pfirrmann CW, et al. Supraacetabular fossa (pseudodefect of acetabular cartilage): frequency at MR arthrography and comparison of findings at MR arthrography and arthroscopy. Radiology 2012;263(2):484–91.

13. Keene GS, Villar RN. Arthroscopic anatomy of the hip: an in vivo study. Arthroscopy 1994;10(4):392–9.

14. Stelzeneder D, Mamisch TC, Kress I, et al. Patterns of joint damage seen on MRI in early hip osteoarthritis due to structural hip deformities. Osteoarthritis Cartilage 2012;20(7):661–9.

15. Tiderius CJ, Jessel R, Kim YJ, et al. Hip dGEMRIC in asymptomatic volunteers and patients with early osteoarthritis: the influence of timing after contrast injection. Magn Reson Med 2007;57(4):803–5.

16. Multanen J, Rauvala E, Lammentausta E, et al. Reproducibility of imaging human knee cartilage by delayed gadolinium-enhanced MRI of cartilage (dGEMRIC) at 1.5 Tesla. Osteoarthritis Cartilage 2009;17(5):559–64.

17. Mamisch TC, Dudda M, Hughes T, et al. Comparison of delayed gadolinium enhanced MRI of cartilage (dGEMRIC) using inversion recovery and fast T1 mapping sequences. Magn Reson Med 2008; 60(4):768–73.

18. Tiderius CJ, Svensson J, Leander P, et al. dGEMRIC (delayed gadolinium-enhanced MRI of cartilage) indicates adaptive capacity of human knee cartilage. Magn Reson Med 2004;51(2):286–90.

19. Gillis A, Bashir A, McKeon B, et al. Magnetic resonance imaging of relative glycosaminoglycan distribution in patients with autologous chondrocyte transplants. Invest Radiol 2001;36(12):743–8.

20. Parker DA, Beatty KT, Giuffre B, et al. Articular cartilage changes in patients with osteoarthritis after osteotomy. Am J Sports Med 2011;39(5):1039–45.

21. Bashir A, Gray ML, Hartke J, et al. Nondestructive imaging of human cartilage glycosaminoglycan concentration by MRI. Magn Reson Med 1999; 41(5):857–65.

22. Burstein D, Velyvis J, Scott KT, et al. Protocol issues for delayed Gd(DTPA)(2-)-enhanced MRI (dGEMRIC) for clinical evaluation of articular cartilage. Magn Reson Med 2001;45(1):36–41.

23. Cunningham T, Jessel R, Zurakowski D, et al. Delayed gadolinium-enhanced magnetic resonance imaging of cartilage to predict early failure of Bernese periacetabular osteotomy for hip dysplasia. J Bone Joint Surg Am 2006;88(7):1540–8.

24. Kim YJ, Jaramillo D, Millis MB, et al. Assessment of early osteoarthritis in hip dysplasia with delayed gadolinium-enhanced magnetic resonance imaging of cartilage. J Bone Joint Surg Am 2003;85(10): 1987–92.

25. McKenzie CA, Williams A, Prasad PV, et al. Three-dimensional delayed gadolinium-enhanced MRI of cartilage (dGEMRIC) at 1.5T and 3.0T. J Magn Reson Imaging 2006;24(4):928–33.

26. Neuman P, Tjornstrand J, Svensson J, et al. Longitudinal assessment of femoral knee cartilage quality using contrast enhanced MRI (dGEMRIC) in patients with anterior cruciate ligament injury–comparison with asymptomatic volunteers. Osteoarthritis Cartilage 2011;19(8):977–83.

27. Nieminen MT, Rieppo J, Silvennoinen J, et al. Spatial assessment of articular cartilage proteoglycans with Gd-DTPA-enhanced T1 imaging. Magn Reson Med 2002;48(4):640–8.

28. Roos EM, Dahlberg L. Positive effects of moderate exercise on glycosaminoglycan content in knee cartilage: a four-month, randomized, controlled trial in patients at risk of osteoarthritis. Arthritis Rheum 2005;52(11):3507–14.

29. Tiderius CJ, Olsson LE, Leander P, et al. Delayed gadolinium-enhanced MRI of cartilage (dGEMRIC) in early knee osteoarthritis. Magn Reson Med 2003;49(3):488–92.

30. Jessel RH, Zilkens C, Tiderius C, et al. Assessment of osteoarthritis in hips with femoroacetabular impingement using delayed gadolinium enhanced MRI of cartilage. J Magn Reson Imaging 2009; 30(5):1110–5.

31. Pollard TC, McNally EG, Wilson DC, et al. Localized cartilage assessment with three-dimensional dGEMRIC in asymptomatic hips with normal morphology and cam deformity. J Bone Joint Surg Am 2010; 92(15):2557–69.

32. Mamisch TC, Kain MS, Bittersohl B, et al. Delayed gadolinium-enhanced magnetic resonance imaging of cartilage (dGEMRIC) in femoacetabular impingement. J Orthop Res 2011;29(9):1305–11.

33. Zilkens C, Miese F, Bittersohl B, et al. Delayed gadolinium-enhanced magnetic resonance imaging of cartilage (dGEMRIC), after slipped capital femoral epiphysis. Eur J Radiol 2011;79(3):400–6.

34. Bittersohl B, Hosalkar HS, Apprich S, et al. Comparison of pre-operative dGEMRIC imaging with intra-operative findings in femoroacetabular impingement: preliminary findings. Skeletal Radiol 2011; 40(5):553–61.

35. Domayer SE, Mamisch TC, Kress I, et al. Radial dGEMRIC in developmental dysplasia of the hip and in femoroacetabular impingement: preliminary results. Osteoarthritis Cartilage 2010;18(11):1421–8.

36. Lattanzi R, Petchprapa C, Glaser C, et al. A new method to analyze dGEMRIC measurements in femoroacetabular impingement: preliminary validation against arthroscopic findings. Osteoarthritis Cartilage 2012;20(10):1127–33.

37. Trattnig S, Welsch GH, Juras V, et al. 23Na MR imaging at 7 T after knee matrix-associated autologous chondrocyte transplantation preliminary results. Radiology 2010;257(1):175–84.

38. Mamisch TC, Menzel MI, Welsch GH, et al. Steady-state diffusion imaging for MR in-vivo evaluation of reparative cartilage after matrix-associated autologous chondrocyte transplantation at 3 tesla–preliminary results. Eur J Radiol 2008;65(1):72–9.

39. Welsch GH, Trattnig S, Domayer S, et al. Multimodal approach in the use of clinical scoring, morphological MRI and biochemical T2-mapping and diffusion-weighted imaging in their ability to assess differences between cartilage repair tissue after microfracture therapy and matrix-associated autologous chondrocyte transplantation: a pilot study. Osteoarthritis Cartilage 2009;17(9):1219–27.

40. Mosher TJ, Dardzinski BJ. Cartilage MRI T2 relaxation time mapping: overview and applications. Semin Musculoskelet Radiol 2004;8(4):355–68.

41. Mosher TJ, Dardzinski BJ, Smith MB. Human articular cartilage: influence of aging and early symptomatic degeneration on the spatial variation of T2–preliminary findings at 3 T. Radiology 2000; 214(1):259–66.

42. Smith HE, Mosher TJ, Dardzinski BJ, et al. Spatial variation in cartilage T2 of the knee. J Magn Reson Imaging 2001;14(1):50–5.

43. Dunn TC, Lu Y, Jin H, et al. T2 relaxation time of cartilage at MR imaging: comparison with severity of knee osteoarthritis. Radiology 2004;232(2):592–8.

44. Gold GE, Thedens DR, Pauly JM, et al. MR imaging of articular cartilage of the knee: new methods using ultrashort TEs. AJR Am J Roentgenol 1998;170(5): 1223–6.

45. Broderick LS, Turner DA, Renfrew DL, et al. Severity of articular cartilage abnormality in patients with osteoarthritis: evaluation with fast spin-echo MR vs arthroscopy. AJR Am J Roentgenol 1994;162(1): 99–103.

46. Koff MF, Amrami KK, Kaufman KR. Clinical evaluation of T2 values of patellar cartilage in patients with osteoarthritis. Osteoarthritis Cartilage 2007; 15(2):198–204.

47. Nishii T, Tanaka H, Sugano N, et al. Evaluation of cartilage matrix disorders by T2 relaxation time in patients with hip dysplasia. Osteoarthritis Cartilage 2008;16(2):227–33.

48. Apprich S, Mamisch TC, Welsch GH, et al. Quantitative T2 mapping of the patella at 3.0T is sensitive to early cartilage degeneration, but also to loading of the knee. Eur J Radiol 2012;81(4):e438–43.

49. Mamisch TC, Trattnig S, Quirbach S, et al. Quantitative T2 mapping of knee cartilage: differentiation of healthy control cartilage and cartilage repair tissue in the knee with unloading–initial results. Radiology 2010;254(3):818–26.

50. Nag D, Liney GP, Gillespie P, et al. Quantification of T(2) relaxation changes in articular cartilage with in situ mechanical loading of the knee. J Magn Reson Imaging 2004;19(3):317–22.

51. Nishii T, Kuroda K, Matsuoka Y, et al. Change in knee cartilage T2 in response to mechanical loading. J Magn Reson Imaging 2008;28(1):175–80.

52. Akella SV, Regatte RR, Gougoutas AJ, et al. Proteoglycan-induced changes in T1rho-relaxation of articular cartilage at 4T. Magn Reson Med 2001;46(3): 419–23.

53. Duvvuri U, Reddy R, Patel SD, et al. T1rho-relaxation in articular cartilage: effects of enzymatic degradation. Magn Reson Med 1997;38(6):863–7.

54. Menezes NM, Gray ML, Hartke JR, et al. T2 and T1rho MRI in articular cartilage systems. Magn Reson Med 2004;51(3):503–9.

55. Li X, Benjamin Ma C, Link TM, et al. In vivo T(1rho) and T(2) mapping of articular cartilage in osteoarthritis of the knee using 3 T MRI. Osteoarthritis Cartilage 2007;15(7):789–97.

56. Regatte RR, Akella SV, Borthakur A, et al. Proteoglycan depletion-induced changes in transverse relaxation maps of cartilage: comparison of T2 and T1rho. Acad Radiol 2002;9(12):1388–94.

57. Wheaton AJ, Casey FL, Gougoutas AJ, et al. Correlation of T1rho with fixed charge density in cartilage. J Magn Reson Imaging 2004;20(3):519–25.

58. Li X, Cheng J, Lin K, et al. Quantitative MRI using T1rho and T2 in human osteoarthritic cartilage specimens: correlation with biochemical measurements and histology. Magn Reson Imaging 2011;29(3): 324–34.

59. Keenan KE, Besier TF, Pauly JM, et al. Prediction of glycosaminoglycan content in human cartilage by age, T1rho and T2 MRI. Osteoarthritis Cartilage 2011;19(2):171–9.

60. Regatte RR, Akella SV, Lonner JH, et al. T1rho relaxation mapping in human osteoarthritis (OA) cartilage: comparison of T1rho with T2. J Magn Reson Imaging 2006;23(4):547–53.

Femoroacetabular Impingement

Miriam A. Bredella, MD[a],*, Erika J. Ulbrich, MD[b],
David W. Stoller, MD[c,d], Suzanne E. Anderson, MD[e]

KEYWORDS

- Femoroacetabular impingement - Hip - Imaging - Magnetic resonance imaging - Radiographs

KEY POINTS

- Femoroacetabular impingement (FAI) is a common cause of osteoarthritis of the hip in young adults.
- Impingement can be due to femoral abnormalities (cam impingement) or acetabular abnormalities (pincer impingement), or a combination of both (mixed type).
- FAI occurs as a result of abnormal contact between the proximal femur and acetabular rim, causing degeneration and avulsion of the acetabular labrum and cartilage damage.
- Early diagnosis of FAI is important for awareness, to initiate appropriate therapy and to delay the onset of osteoarthritis.
- The role of imaging in FAI is to make/confirm the diagnosis of FAI; depict and quantify morphologic osseous abnormalities of the femoral head and acetabular rim; define the exact location, extent, and severity of cartilage and labral damage; and to exclude advanced osteoarthritis and other diagnoses.

INTRODUCTION

Femoroacetabular impingement (FAI) is increasingly recognized as a pathomechanical process that can lead to hip pain and osteoarthritis in young adults.[1–4] FAI occurs as a result of abnormal contact between the proximal femur and acetabular rim caused by morphologic abnormalities affecting the femoral head-neck junction or the acetabulum. In most cases a combination of femoral and acetabular abnormalities is identified.[5] In addition, hypermobility of the hip can lead to FAI even in the setting of only minor osseous abnormalities,[1] and reduced femoral antetorsion, impairing internal rotation, has recently been described as a cause of FAI.[6] Repetitive microtrauma from impingement of the femoral head against the acetabulum causes degeneration and avulsion/tearing of the acetabular labrum, as well as progressive damage to the adjacent articular cartilage, leading to osteoarthritis of the hip.[3,7–11] Through the development of hip arthroscopy, FAI can now be better treated, with fewer complications and shorter recovery time.[12–14] Early diagnosis of FAI, before significant cartilage loss is evident, is therefore of paramount importance in initiating appropriate therapy and thereby reducing or delaying the onset of osteoarthritis. Unfortunately, the diagnostic accuracy of clinical tests for diagnosing FAI has been found to be too low to provide a conclusive recommendation.[15] Therefore, imaging plays a crucial role in identifying morphologic abnormalities associated with FAI, and has become an important predictor of outcome and surgical success in patients with FAI.

Disclosure: The authors have nothing to disclose.
[a] Division of Musculoskeletal Radiology and Interventions, Department of Radiology, Massachusetts General Hospital, Harvard Medical School, 55 Fruit Street, Yawkey building 6400, Boston, MA 02114, USA; [b] Department of Diagnostic and Interventional Radiology, University Hospital Zurich, Raemistrasse 100, Zurich 8091, Switzerland; [c] National Orthopaedics Imaging Associates and MRI at California Pacific Medical Center, San Francisco, 3700 California Street, CA, USA; [d] Department of Radiology, Johns Hopkins University School of Medicine, 601 N. Caroline street, Baltimore, MD 21287, USA; [e] School of Medicine Sydney, The University of Notre Dame Australia, 160 Oxford Street, Darlinghurst 2010, Sydney, New South Wales, Australia
* Corresponding author.
E-mail address: mbredella@partners.org

Magn Reson Imaging Clin N Am 21 (2013) 45–64
http://dx.doi.org/10.1016/j.mric.2012.08.012
1064-9689/13/$ – see front matter © 2013 Elsevier Inc. All rights reserved.

mri.theclinics.com

CLINICAL SYMPTOMS

Patients with FAI are usually young and physically active, and present with slow or more acute onset of anterior hip or groin pain and pain with hip rotation, particularly flexion and internal rotation.[1–3,15,16] The prevalence of FAI is estimated to be between 10% and 15%.[17] Sports activities such as soccer, football, kickboxing, hockey, or volleyball, which require hip flexion with variable torque or axial loading, may aggravate symptoms and are all associated with FAI.[14,18,19] The pain in FAI often occurs after mild trauma or minor repetitive sports-related trauma, or occasionally without specific preceding trauma. Pain resulting from FAI has been described as being worse when significant stress is placed on the hip, when climbing stairs, or after prolonged periods of sitting.[20] Patients with FAI and acetabular labral avulsion may report mechanical symptoms such as painful clicking or locking. The pain can also be located over the trochanters or be referred to the knee.[2] Clinical and imaging review for potential referred pain from greater trochanteric enthesopathy, with gluteus minimus and medius tendon insertional partial-thickness or full-thickness tears, and of the lumbar spine for radiculopathy associated with disc hernia, may be required. Morphologic FAI abnormalities are often bilateral, but patients frequently present with unilateral symptoms.[21] During physical examination, patients typically present with restricted internal rotation in hip flexion. Multiple clinical tests to diagnose FAI have been described. For example, the impingement sign (pain with flexion-internal rotation), the anterior hip impingement test (pain with flexion-adduction-internal rotation), or the FABER test (pain/decreased range of motion with Flexion and ABduction-External Rotation) are commonly positive in cam-type FAI, while posterior impingement tests with pain during forced external rotation in maximal extension can be positive in pincer-type FAI. However, these tests often have a low diagnostic accuracy and there can be overlap with other entities.[15,22] Clinical experience is also influential (**Box 1**).

ETIOLOGY OF FEMOROACETABULAR IMPINGEMENT

Hip impingement has been described after total hip arthroplasty in patients with abnormal hip anatomy, such as developmental hip dysplasia (DDH), slipped capital femoral epiphysis (SCFE), Legg-Calve-Perthes disease, or posttraumatic deformity whereby there is a mismatch between the femoral head-neck junction and the acetabulum.[10,23–29]

A conceptual mechanism for the etiology of FAI and features associated with FAI has been described by Ganz and colleagues.[3,7,9,30] This conceptual discussion allowed for some subdivision of potential causes of osteoarthritis instead of a general indiscriminant grouping of all hip joint forms being associated with "idiopathic osteoarthritis." The etiology of FAI in patients without preexisting hip disease with subtle morphologic anatomic variations or abnormalities of the femoral head-neck junction or acetabulum continues to evolve. An osseous bony excrescence or "bony bump" at the femoral head-neck junction (cam deformity) may be the result of a subclinical SCFE during adolescence in some cases.[31] Abnormal lateral extension of the physeal scar (**Fig. 1**) caused by delayed separation of the common femoral head and greater trochanteric physis, or eccentric closure of the femoral head epiphysis, suggests

---

Box 1
Clinical symptoms

- Young active individuals with increasing intensity of anterior hip and groin pain
- Activity-dependent pain
- Pain with flexion-internal rotation, climbing stairs, prolonged sitting
- Restricted range of hip motion compared with contralateral side, and/or compared with known clinical range of hip motion
- Painful clicking, locking
- Positive impingement tests

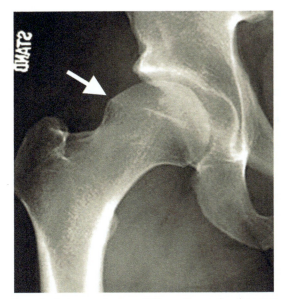

Fig. 1. Anteroposterior (AP) radiograph showing abnormal lateral extension of the common physis, terminating in a bony excrescence, pistol-grip deformity (*arrow*), in a patient with cam-type impingement.

an epiphyseal growth abnormality as the underlying cause for the decreased femoral head-neck junction.[32,33] Congenitally reduced femoral antetorsion/anteversion can also impair internal rotation of the hip, leading to FAI.[6,34–36] Genetic factors in the etiology of FAI have been proposed in a sibling study, which demonstrated an increased risk of siblings with FAI to have cam or pincer deformities.[37] Putting a name to the impingement mechanism in young people allowed for potential treatment (eg, offset surgery and arthroscopic offset interventions) and being able to continue with sports and activities, instead of complete hip replacements at a young age or cessation of sports activities.

However, not all individuals with abnormal femoral and acetabular morphology develop symptoms, and morphologic findings of FAI-like appearances have been reported in asymptomatic subjects.[38–41] These findings support the notion that additional factors, such as activity type and especially intensity of sporting or other activity, and vulnerability of the labrum and articular cartilage to injury, are important factors in determining whether the abnormal morphology will potentially result in symptoms.[42]

In addition, in a study of asymptomatic male Swiss army recruits, magnetic resonance imaging (MRI) findings suggestive of cam impingement were seen in 24% of asymptomatic subjects, and the prevalence increased with decreasing internal rotation to 48%.[43] In the same cohort, MRI findings of cam-type FAI were associated with labral lesions and cartilage thinning, which are precursors of osteoarthritis.[44] This demonstrates that in so-called asymptomatic subjects, restriction in range of hip motion and morphologic MRI abnormalities of labral and cartilage damage can be evident (**Box 2**).

PATHOGENESIS OF FEMOROACETABULAR IMPINGEMENT

The normal anatomy of the hip joint allows for a wide range of motion. The morphologic abnormalities of the femoral head or acetabular rim that predispose a patient to FAI result in decreased joint clearance

---

Box 2
Potential etiology of FAI

- Subclinical SCFE
- Growth abnormality of capital physis
- Growth variation of acetabulum
- Decreased femoral antetorsion
- Genetic factors
- Activity type and intensity

---

between the femoral head and acetabulum.[3,11,35] In cam-type FAI, mechanical impingement of the femoral neck against the acetabulum and labrum occurs during terminal motion of the hip, leading to "outside-in" abrasions of the articular cartilage and damage to the adjacent labrum. Linear impact between a local (acetabular retroversion) or general (coxa profunda/protrusio) overcoverage of the acetabulum and a normal femoral-head morphology leads to pincer-type FAI, which first leads to acetabular damage (**Fig. 2**).[11,24,45,46] Reduced femoral antetorsion or anteversion can also impair internal rotation of the hip, leading to decreased joint clearance during flexion–internal rotation (**Fig. 3**).[35,36] Reduced femoral antetorsion has been reported in patients with FAI in comparison with controls.[9] The detection of subtle anatomic and alignment abnormalities of the femoral head-neck junction and acetabulum is important for surgical planning, because arthroscopic labral or chondral debridement alone addresses only the site of secondary damage attributable to FAI and does not alter the underlying cause. Lack of treating the underlying osseous abnormality can lead to progression of the early labral and chondral lesions to osteoarthritis.[3,7,10,32,45–48]

MECHANISMS OF FEMOROACETABULAR IMPINGEMENT: CAM AND PINCER IMPINGEMENT

Two types of FAI can be distinguished. Impingement can be due to femoral abnormalities (cam impingement) or acetabular abnormalities (pincer impingement); however, in the majority of cases a combination of both (mixed type) exists.[5]

Cam impingement is caused by abutment of an aspherical femoral head against the acetabulum during hip motion.[3,7–10,46] The cam deformity refers to an osseous excrescence at the femoral head-neck junction or the aspherical portion of the femoral head.[10,23–29] Posterior placement of the femoral head on the femoral neck with inadequate anterior femoral head-neck offset results in abnormal contact and mechanical impingement between the femoral head and acetabular rim when the hip is flexed and/or internally rotated. This process causes abnormal forces to act on the acetabular cartilage and subchondral bone in the anterosuperior acetabular rim area, which leads to damage to the labrum and articular cartilage.[3,9–11,24,25,27,32,49,50] Cam impingement is more frequently seen in young athletic males.[3,7]

Pincer impingement is the result of abnormal contact between the acetabular rim and the femoral neck as a result of acetabular abnormalities, such as acetabular retroversion, coxa

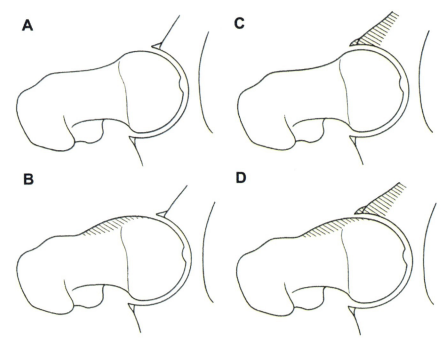

Fig. 2. Pathomechanisms of femoroacetabular impingement. Reduced clearance during joint motion leads to repetitive abutment between the proximal femur and anterior acetabular rim. (*A*) Normal clearance of the hip. (*B*) Reduced femoral head-neck offset. (*C*) Excessive overcoverage of the femoral head by the acetabulum. (*D*) Combination of reduced head-neck offset and excessive anterior overcoverage. (*From* Lavigne M, Parvizi J, Beck M, et al. Anterior femoroacetabular impingement. Part 1. Techniques of joint preserving surgery. Clin Orthop 2004;418:62; with permission.)

profunda, or protrusio acetabuli, leading to anterior overcoverage of the femoral head.[3,46,51–53] Acetabular retroversion refers to a posteriorly oriented acetabulum whereby the anterior acetabular roof edge lies lateral to the posterior edge.[30,53] Abutment of the femoral head against the acetabulum results in degeneration and avulsion of the labrum with ganglion formation or ossification of the acetabular rim, which then further deepens the acetabulum, leading to worsening of the overcoverage.[3,30,53] Persistent anterior abutment of the femoral head against the acetabulum can result

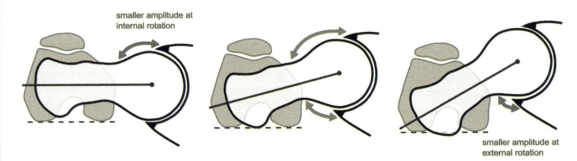

Fig. 3. Diagrams of the right femur and acetabulum show the contribution of abnormal femoral antetorsion to the development of FAI. (*Left*) Markedly reduced femoral antetorsion with smaller amplitude at internal rotation, which may lead to increased mechanical impact at the anterior acetabular rim during internal rotation. (*Middle*) Normal femoral antetorsion with physiologic amplitude for internal and external rotation. (*Right*) Markedly increased femoral antetorsion with smaller amplitude at external rotation, which may lead to an increased mechanical impact at the posterior acetabular rim during external rotation. (*From* Sutter R, Dietrich TJ, Zingg PO, et al. Femoral antetorsion: comparing asymptomatic volunteers and patients with femoroacetabular impingement. Radiology 2012;263:477; with permission.)

in chondral injury of the femoral head, in the "contre-coup" area of the posteroinferior acetabulum. Pincer impingement is more frequently seen in middle-aged women (**Box 3**).[3,7]

IMAGING OF FEMOROACETABULAR IMPINGEMENT
Role of Imaging in Femoroacetabular Impingement

The role of imaging in FAI is to make or confirm the diagnosis of FAI and to depict and quantify the morphologic osseous abnormalities of the femoral head-neck junction and acetabular rim. Imaging is also central in defining the exact location, extent, and severity of articular cartilage and labral damage, and in excluding advanced osteoarthritis, which has a poor surgical outcome, and other diagnoses such as DDH, avascular necrosis, or stress fractures (**Box 4**).

RADIOGRAPHIC IMAGING

Radiographic evaluation in patients with FAI includes a true anteroposterior (AP) pelvic view and an axial cross-table view of the proximal femur.[3] Alternatively, an elongated femoral neck view (Dunn view) obtained in 45° flexion, which depicts the anterior femoral head-neck junction, can

---

Box 3
Mechanisms of FAI

- Cam impingement
  - Decreased femoral head-neck offset/ aspherical femoral head
  - Abnormal contact between femoral head-neck junction and acetabular rim
  - Early cartilage damage at the junction of labrum and cartilage (acetabular > femoral), late extensive labral tears
  - Young males
- Pincer impingement
  - Acetabular overcoverage due to acetabular retroversion, coxa profunda, protrusio acetabuli
  - Abnormal abutment between femoral head against acetabulum
  - Early labral tears, secondary small chondral lesions near the labral defect
  - Middle-aged women
- Mixed type
  - Most common

Box 4
Role of imaging in FAI

- Make or confirm clinical diagnosis of FAI
- Depict morphologic abnormalities of femoral head-neck junction, acetabulum
- Define extent of cartilage and labral damage
- Exclude advanced osteoarthritis
- Exclude other lesions that can mimic FAI (eg, DDH, avascular necrosis, stress fracture)

---

be obtained.[54] It is important to follow standardized techniques for patient positioning to decrease the likelihood of incorrect diagnosis (**Fig. 4**).[21] Acetabular retroversion should only be diagnosed on an AP view of the pelvis to ensure satisfactory pelvic position without rotation or pelvic tilt, which can falsely create or obscure acetabular retroversion.[21] Radiographic findings of cam impingement include an osseous excrescence at the anterolateral femoral head (see **Fig. 4**) and reduced offset of the femoral head-neck junction (**Fig. 5**).

Acetabular retroversion can be diagnosed on AP radiographs by the "crossover" or "figure-of-8" signs and the "posterior wall" sign.[30,53] The crossover sign in acetabular retroversion is created by the anterior acetabular rim being more laterally located than the posterior aspect of the acetabulum. The anterior aspect of the acetabular rim is directed more horizontally and medially, thereby crossing over the more straight and vertical posterior aspect of the acetabular rim (**Fig. 6**).[30,53] Prominence of the ischial spine, whereby the ischial spine projects into the pelvic cavity on AP radiographs of the pelvis (**Fig. 7**), has been described in pincer impingement and acetabular retroversion.[55]

Findings that can be seen with both cam and pincer FAI include synovial herniation pits, also known as fibrocystic change, at the femoral head-neck junction (**Fig. 8**),[56] and os acetabuli/fragmentation of the acetabular rim (**Fig. 9**).[57,58] This finding remains contentious in some circles (**Box 5**).

MAGNETIC RESONANCE IMAGING

Dedicated MRI and magnetic resonance arthrography (MRA) of the hip are the modalities of choice to evaluate the acetabular labrum and articular cartilage. Correlation with standardized radiographic series is performed routinely in well-established centers. Anatomic abnormalities of the femoral head and acetabulum, in addition to labral avulsion and chondral injuries, and associated osseous and soft-tissue findings can be

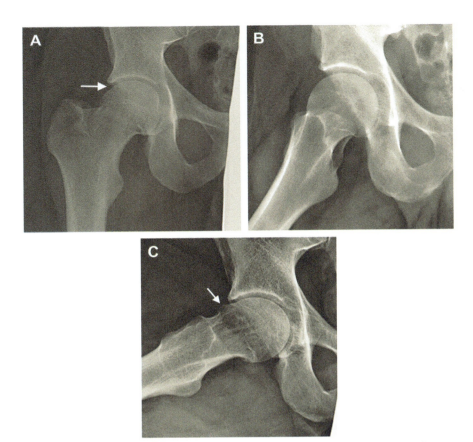

Fig. 4. (*A*) AP radiograph of the hip in a 19-year-old professional hockey player with hip pain demonstrating joint space narrowing (*arrow*). (*B*) Frog-leg lateral view obscures the femoral head-neck junction. (*C*) Elongated femoral neck view demonstrates osseous excrescence at the femoral neck (*arrow*), consistent with a cam deformity.

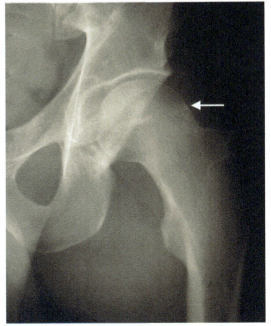

Fig. 5. AP radiograph demonstrates nonspherical femoral head resulting in decreased femoral head-neck offset (*arrow*) in a patient with cam-type impingement.

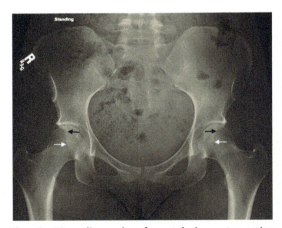

Fig. 6. AP radiograph of acetabular retroversion demonstrating positive crossover sign, where the anterior rim (*black arrow*) crosses over the posterior rim (*white arrow*). Acetabular version should only be assessed on radiographs of the pelvis to confirm correct positioning.

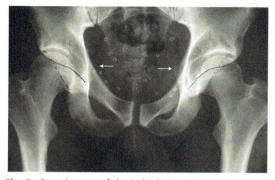

Fig. 7. Prominence of the ischial spine in a patient with acetabular retroversion and pincer-type impingement. AP radiograph with positive crossover sign demonstrates ischial spine projecting into the pelvic cavity (*arrows*).

visualized on MRI in patients with FAI.[8,9,23,30,48,59,60]

Magnetic Resonance Imaging Protocol

Dedicated imaging of the symptomatic hip with a small field of view (FOV) and a dedicated surface coil is important to achieve adequate spatial resolution and high signal-to-noise ratio. The authors' nonarthrographic hip protocol includes a large FOV coronal STIR (short-tau inversion recovery) survey of the pelvis. A large FOV overview of both hips is helpful, as morphologic abnormalities of FAI are often bilateral, but symptoms are usually unilateral at presentation. Higher-resolution MR images of the hip in question are then obtained by placing a local surface coil (eg, body matrix

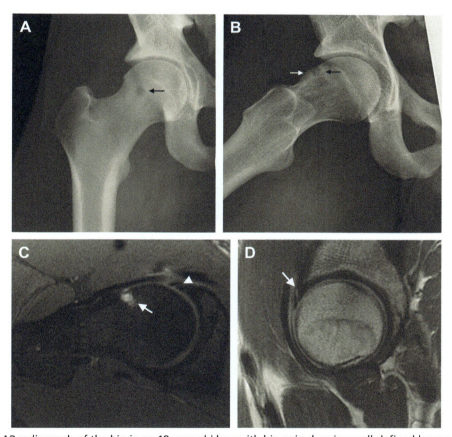

Fig. 8. (*A*) AP radiograph of the hip in an 18-year-old boy with hip pain showing well-defined lucency involving the femoral head (*arrow*), consistent with fibrocystic change. (*B*) Elongated femoral neck view demonstrates osseous excrescence (*white arrow*) adjacent to fibrocystic change (*black arrow*), consistent with a cam deformity. (*C*) Oblique axial fat-saturated (FS) proton density (PD)-weighted image demonstrates fibrocystic change in the anterior femoral head with mild surrounding edema (*white arrow*). Anterior labral avulsion is present (*arrowhead*). (*D*) Sagittal PD-weighted image demonstrates anterosuperior labral avulsion (*arrow*).

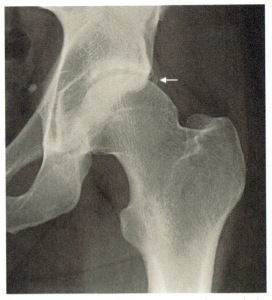

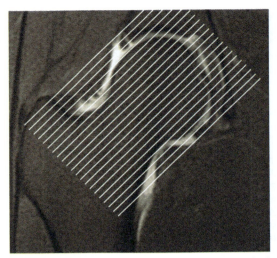

Fig. 10. Prescription of the oblique axial plane, which is obtained along the long axis of the femoral neck.

Fig. 9. AP radiograph in a patient with acetabular retroversion and pincer-type impingement demonstrates periacetabular ossicle (*arrow*).

coil, dedicated hip coil) over the symptomatic hip and using a small FOV (16–20 cm). Sequences include: coronal fat-saturated (FS) T2 fast spin-echo (FSE), coronal T1 FSE, sagittal proton density (PD) FSE, axial PD FSE, and FS oblique axial PD FSE, prescribed along the long axis of the femoral neck (**Fig. 10**). This plane is important in the assessment of the femoral head-neck junction and acetabular retroversion.

Direct MRA is the modality of choice in evaluating patients with FAI at 1.5 T. For direct MRA, approximately 10 to 12 mL of diluted (1:250) MR contrast (gadopentetate dimeglumine, Magnevist; Berlex Laboratories, Wayne, NJ, USA) is injected into the hip joint to achieve capsular distension. A surface coil is positioned over the hip to decrease the FOV and improve spatial resolution. The authors' protocol for MRA includes the same coronal, sagittal, axial, and oblique axial imaging planes as used in conventional MRI of the hip, and sequences include FS T1 FSE, T1 FSE, and FS PD FSE. It is important to always include an FS fluid-sensitive sequence in the MRA protocol to detect stress fractures or paralabral cysts and to exclude other pathology such as crystal deposition (eg, hydroxyapatite deposition disease).

The use of radial sequences, obtained perpendicular to the femoral axis, has been found useful in detecting anatomic abnormalities of the femoral head and acetabular rim, especially for measurement of the alpha angle in different locations, as well as in detecting labral and cartilage tears.[58,61–63] In this regard, 3-dimensional sequences, which can be reformatted in any plane, are useful. These sequences are being increasingly used at 3 T.

Femoral antetorsion has recently been described as a predisposing factor of FAI.[6] Femoral antetorsion can be quickly assessed on MRI by obtaining 2 axial images, 1 through the femoral head and neck, and 1 through the femoral condyles, just above the knee joint (**Fig. 11**).[6]

Box 5
Radiographic findings of femoroacetabular impingement

- Pistol-grip deformity, profunda femora
- Abnormal lateral physeal extension
- Osseous excrescence at anterolateral femoral head, decreased femoral head-neck offset
- Acetabular overcoverage, positive crossover, figure-of-8 sign
- Protrusio acetabuli
- Prominence of the ischial spine
- Synovial herniation pits/fibrocystic change
- Os acetabuli, fragmentation of acetabular rim

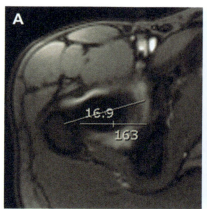
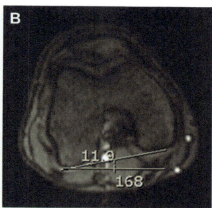

Fig. 11. Measurement of femoral antetorsion in a 15-year-old girl with pincer impingement. Axial T2-weighted fast spin-echo images of the proximal femur (*A*) and distal femur (*B*) are obtained with the patient in supine position, with symmetric positioning of the pelvis and lower extremities and full knee extension. The femoral antetorsion angle is the angle between the reference line along the center of the femoral head/neck and a reference line along the dorsal borders of the two femoral condyles. In this case the femoral head/neck angle (referred to a horizontal line) is 16.9° and that of the two femoral condyles (referred to a horizontal line) is 11.9°, which results in a femoral antetorsion of 5° according to Tomczak and colleagues.[88] The femoral antetorsion angle is calculated depending on the degree of knee rotation by either subtraction (with external knee rotation) or addition (with internal knee rotation) of the 2 angles. (*Courtesy of* Balgrist Hospital, Zurich, Switzerland.)

Several studies have shown that the integrity of the articular cartilage is one of the most important predictors of FAI surgery outcome.[64] The use of 3-T MRI and several novel cartilage imaging techniques of the hip have been described; delayed gadolinium-enhanced MRI of cartilage, which detects glycosaminoglycan content of articular cartilage, has been found to be a good predictor of surgical success in FAI.[65–70]

Magnetic Resonance Imaging Findings of Femoroacetabular Impingement

Cam impingement

Decreased offset of the femoral head-neck junction can be seen on MRI as a prominent lateral extension of the femoral head at the step-off to the adjacent femoral neck.[9,23] The bony femoral excrescence is located lateral (directly lateral, superolateral, or inferolateral) to the physeal scar of the femoral head-neck junction. This feature can be best seen on coronal (**Fig. 12**A) or oblique axial images (see **Fig. 12**B).

Notzli and colleagues[48] described a method using MRI to quantify the concavity of the femoral head-neck junction by measuring the alpha angle.[48] The alpha angle can be measured from an oblique axial image through the center of the femoral neck. A circle is drawn around the femoral head, including the articular cartilage. Then a line is drawn along the long axis of the femoral neck, bisecting the circle. The alpha angle is the angle between this line and the line from the center of the circle to the point at which the femoral head protrudes anterior out of the circle (**Fig. 13**A). An alpha angle of greater than 55° is considered abnormal (see **Fig. 13**B) and is associated with FAI.[48] However, there is a range and overlap in patients with FAI and in asymptomatic patients with normal hip morphology. Quantification of the alpha angle on radial images in the anterosuperior segment and a cutoff of greater than 60° has recently been shown to have high sensitivity and specificity in discriminating symptomatic subjects with cam FAI from asymptomatic controls.[63]

Juxta-articular fibrocystic change or synovial herniation pits can be visualized in the anterosuperior femoral head-neck junction, at the site of the dysplastic femoral excrescence[56] (see **Fig. 8**). Fibrocystic change is best seen on FS T2 on PD-weighted images as T2 hyperintense lesions at the anterior femoral head, and can have associated marrow edema (see **Fig. 8**C). These cystic changes occur at the site of impingement on the femur and therefore are likely not a normal variation of synovial herniations.[56]

The assessment of the articular cartilage is of paramount importance in evaluating patients with FAI. Advanced cartilage loss and signs of osteoarthritis have poor surgical outcome, and the integrity of the articular cartilage is considered to be one of the most important predictors of surgical success. Osteoarthritis is a contraindication for offset interventional therapies. Articular cartilage

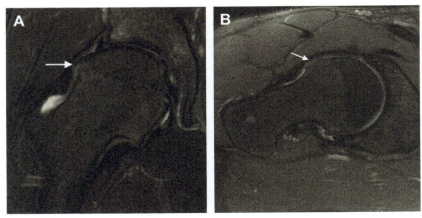

Fig. 12. (*A*) Coronal FS PD-weighted image in a patient with cam-type impingement demonstrates an osseous excrescence involving the lateral femoral head (*arrow*). (*B*) Oblique axial FS PD-weighted image demonstrates osseous excrescence (*arrow*).

lesions in cam-type FAI typically involve the anterosuperior quadrant.[57,62,71,72] MRA is useful in detecting early cartilage damage (**Fig. 14**). Cartilage lesions in cam-type FAI are usually focal and larger than in pincer-type FAI, and can measure approximately 10 mm in width.[62] Advanced cartilage damage can be demonstrated on FS fluid-sensitive sequences as areas of full-thickness cartilage loss with associated marrow changes and subchondral cyst/geode formation (**Fig. 15A**). Osteophyte formation, marrow edema, and subchondral cyst formation are indicators of osteoarthritis. T1 or PD-weighted images are helpful in showing bony proliferative change and the femoral excrescence (see **Fig. 15B**). Cartilage delamination is frequently seen in cam-type FAI,[5] with flap size ranging between 2 and 30 mm and a mean flip size of 7.6 mm in one study.[58] The detection of cartilage delamination can be challenging on MRI. MRA can show contrast intersecting between the

bone-cartilage interface (**Fig. 16**). Hypointense and hyperintense linear areas in the acetabular cartilage on FS intermediate-weighted images have been reported in delamination (**Fig. 17**).[58] It is important to detect the presence of cartilage delamination, especially if joint-preserving surgery is planned, because in patients with advanced delamination of the acetabular cartilage joint-preserving surgery may no longer be possible.

Acetabular labral damage in cam-type FAI typically involves the anterosuperior quadrant[57,62,71–74] Labral avulsion is diagnosed by linear fluid signal or contrast extending through or undercutting the labrum with or without detachment and, in some cases, paralabral cyst formation.[57,74] Most commonly the avulsion occurs at the labral-cartilage interface.[8] The oblique axial and sagittal planes are most helpful in detecting labral abnormality (**Fig. 18**). Injury to the labrochondral transition zone in the anterosuperior

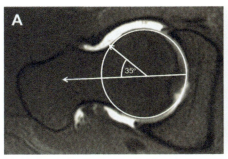
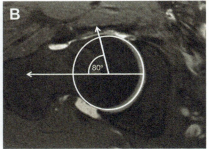

Fig. 13. (*A*) Construction of the alpha angle to evaluate the femoral head-neck junction. A circle is drawn around the femoral head. Then a line is drawn along the long axis of the femoral neck, bisecting the circle. The alpha angle is measured as the angle between this line and the line from the center of the circle to the point at which the femoral head protrudes anteriorly out of the circle. (*B*) Alpha-angle measurement in a patient with abnormal femoral head-neck junction, resulting in increased alpha angle.

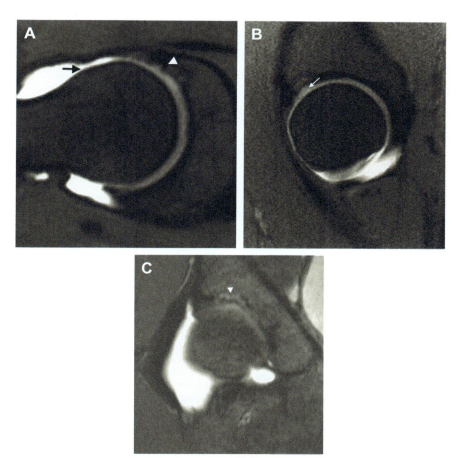

Fig. 14. Cartilage loss and early changes of osteoarthritis in a 16-year-old girl with cam-type impingement. (*A*) Oblique axial FS T1-weighted image from an MR arthrogram demonstrates subtle cam deformity of the femoral head (*black arrow*). Subchondral cystic change of the acetabulum (*arrowhead*) indicates high-grade cartilage loss. (*B*) Sagittal FS T1-weighted image demonstrates subtle cartilage thinning of the anterosuperior acetabulum (*arrow*). (*C*) Anterior coronal FS PD-weighted image demonstrates hyperintense subchondral cystic change involving the acetabulum (*arrowhead*), which indicates high-grade cartilage loss.

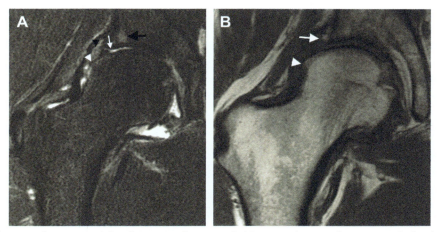

Fig. 15. (*A*) Coronal FS PD-weighted image of osteoarthritis secondary to femoroacetabular impingement demonstrates full-thickness cartilage defect of the acetabular rim (*white arrow*) with underlying subchondral edema (*black arrow*). Femoral head/neck asphericity demonstrates mild edema (*white arrowhead*). There is degeneration of the acetabular labrum (*black arrowhead*). (*B*) Coronal T1-weighted image clearly shows bony proliferative change along the acetabular rim (*arrow*) and femoral head (*arrowhead*).

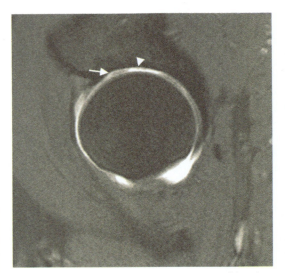

Fig. 16. Cartilage delamination in a 24-year-old patient with cam impingement. Sagittal FS T1-weighted image from an MR arthrogram demonstrates cartilage delamination with contrast extending between the bone-cartilage interface (*arrow*). There is a full-thickness cartilage defect (*arrowhead*).

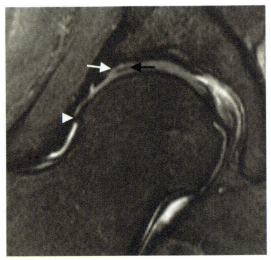

Fig. 17. Coronal FS PD-weighted image from an MR arthrogram in a patient with a cam deformity and cartilage delamination demonstrates hyperintense signal at the bone-cartilage interface (*white arrow*). Hypointense linear signal abnormality in the articular cartilage (*black arrow*) is a sign that has been shown to indicate cartilage delamination. Osseous excrescence involves lateral femoral head (*arrowhead*).

quadrant then predisposes the adjacent articular cartilage to degeneration with softening, fraying, and separation, and ultimately detachment (**Figs. 19** and **20**).[72]

Bony abnormalities involving the acetabular rim, such as an os acetabuli, or periacetabular ossicle, are thought to represent stress changes/fractures from repetitive microtrauma from impingement, and can be best seen on coronal or sagittal images (**Fig. 21**). Subchondral marrow edema at site of impingement can involve the acetabular rim and femoral head (see **Fig. 20**B), and indicates osteoarthritis with cartilage loss.

Pincer impingement
Anterior overcoverage of the acetabulum with a retroverted acetabulum is common in patients with pincer-type FAI.[30] Overcoverage can be focal or diffuse[21] and can be associated with a deep acetabular fossa.[58] Acetabular overcoverage can be seen on coronal images (**Fig. 22**A). A retroverted acetabulum can be detected on axial MR images when the anterior rim of the acetabulum is located lateral to the posterior rim on the most cranial image that includes the femoral head

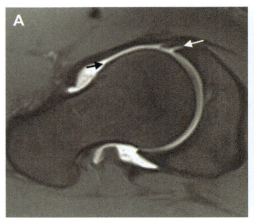

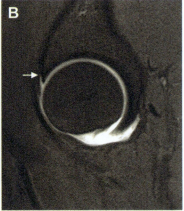

Fig. 18. Labral avulsion in a patient with cam deformity. (*A*) Oblique axial and (*B*) sagittal FS T1-weighted images from an MR arthrogram demonstrates contrast undercutting the anterior labrum (*white arrows*) consistent with labral avulsion. Bony excrescence involves femoral head-neck junction (*black arrow*).

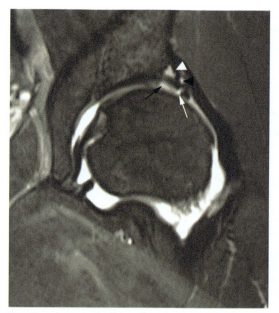

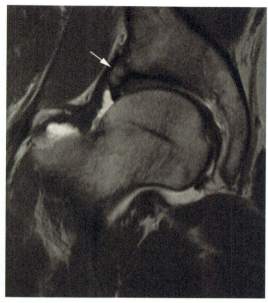

Fig. 19. Injury to the labrochondral transition zone in cam impingement. Coronal FS PD-weighted image from an MR arthrogram demonstrates cartilage defect (*black arrow*) and labral tear (*white arrow*) involving the anterosuperior quadrant with small paralabral cyst formation (*black arrowhead*). Marrow edema involves adjacent acetabular rim (*white arrowhead*), consistent with osteoarthritic change.

Fig. 21. Coronal T1-weighted image from an MR arthrogram demonstrates bony proliferative change (*arrow*) in a patient with femoroacetabular impingement.

(**Fig. 22**B)[53] Acetabular depth, which is increased in pincer-type FAI, can be assessed on oblique axial images through the center of the femoral neck, by drawing a line connecting the anterior to the posterior acetabular rims. The distance between the center of the femoral neck and this line defines the acetabular depth. Increased acetabular depth is present if the center of the femoral neck lies lateral to the line connecting the acetabular rims.[62]

Acetabular labral abnormalities in pincer-type FAI include degeneration and avulsion, and commonly involve the anterosuperior quadrant

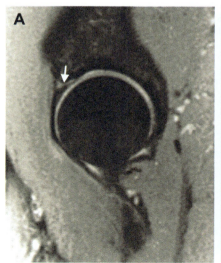

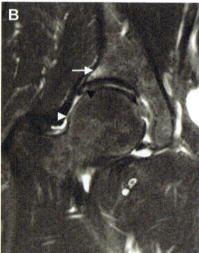

Fig. 20. (*A*) Sagittal FS PD-weighted image demonstrates linear signal abnormality involving labrochondral junction (*arrow*). (*B*) Coronal FS T2-weighted image shows subtle signal abnormality of the lateral labrum (*black arrowhead*). Bony excrescence (*white arrowhead*) is present. Subchondral acetabular edema (*white arrow*) indicates osteoarthritis.

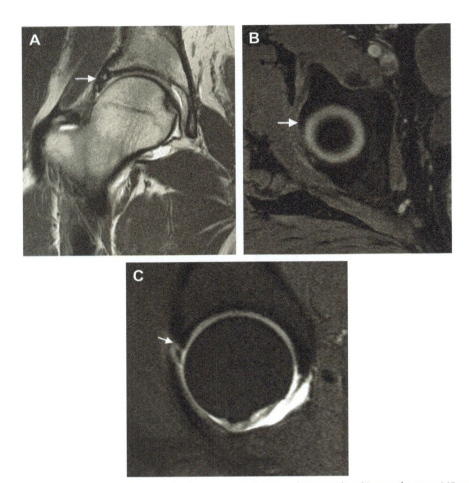

Fig. 22. Acetabular overcoverage in pincer impingement. (*A*) Coronal T1-weighted image from an MR arthrogram demonstrates bony proliferative changes and osseous fragmentation of the acetabular rim (*arrow*), resulting in femoral overcoverage. (*B*) Axial gradient-echo image obtained at the cranial acetabular opening demonstrates anterior acetabular overcoverage (*arrow*). (*C*) Sagittal FS T1-weighted image demonstrates contrast undercutting the anterior labrum (*arrow*) consistent with labral avulsion.

(see **Fig. 22**C)[58] and can also involve the posterior labrum. The labrum can be ossified, and ossification of the labral-acetabular junction can be seen (see **Fig. 22**A). Labral tears predispose to extraosseous ganglia formation with splitting of the labrum and acetabular cartilage, which allows penetration of synovial fluid into subchondral bone, leading to subchondral cyst formation (see **Fig. 23**).[30,53]

Cartilage lesions in pincer-type FAI usually involve a longer thinner area than in cam-type FAI. These lesions involve the superior or posteroinferior quadrant and may be associated with a contrecoup lesion of the posteroinferior margin. It is therefore important to evaluate the posteroinferior quadrant, as damage in this area is associated with a worse outcome.[62]

In later stages of FAI there may be evidence of damage from impingement, and even fragmentation of the bony margin of the prominent anterior acetabular edge. Fibrocystic change at the anterosuperior[62] femoral head can be seen with pincer-type FAI, although it has been more commonly described with camtype FAI (**Box 6**).

TREATMENT

Nonoperative treatment has been shown to have limited success and includes activity modification, nonsteroidal anti-inflammatory medications, and intra-articular injections.[75,76] Some individual patients may benefit from intra-articular injections, and this may be a useful option for a trial.

The goal of surgical treatment of FAI is to allow for a sufficient impingement-free range of motion and to delay the onset of hip osteoarthritis. Surgical treatment includes removal of the aspherical

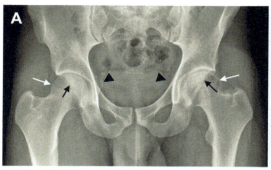
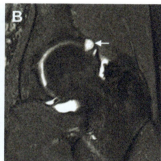
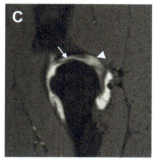

Fig. 23. A 20-year-old male patient with mixed cam and pincer FAI. (*A*) AP radiograph demonstrates bilateral anterolateral femoral bony excrescence (cam deformity) (*white arrows*) and acetabular retroversion (pincer deformity) with positive crossover sign (*black arrows*) and prominence of the ischial spine (*arrowheads*). (*B*) Coronal FS PD-weighted image from an MR arthrogram in the same patient demonstrates posterior labral tear with paralabral cyst formation extending posterior-superiorly (*arrow*). (*C*) Sagittal FS PD-weighted image demonstrates diffuse labral degeneration (*arrow*) with posterior extension and posterior-superior paralabral cyst formation (*arrowhead*). (*Courtesy of* Balgrist Hospital, Zurich, Switzerland.)

portions of the femoral head (femoroplasty) (**Fig. 24**) and reduction of anterior acetabular over-coverage by excising bony prominence at the acetabular rim with debridement of the labral and cartilage damage, including microfracture of acetabular cartilage damage. Surgery can be performed in an open fashion with femoral head dislocation, arthroscopically, or using a combined open and arthroscopic approach.[7,14,30,50,77–80]

Box 6
MRI findings of femoroacetabular impingement

- Decreased femoral head-neck offset, increased alpha angle
- Acetabular retroversion, deep acetabular fossa
- Labral avulsion, chondrolabral separation
- Cartilage damage, delamination
- Fibrocystic change of femoral head-neck junction
- Os acetabuli, osseous fragmentation of acetabular rim

Improvement in symptoms, functionality, and quality of life has been described in small longitudinal studies.[7,64,81–83] However, there are no available prospective long-term data on the natural history of the disease or the long-term outcomes of patients who undergo surgery in comparison with those who do not.[84] Complications of FAI surgery include nerve damage, adhesions (see **Fig. 24**F), fracture, trochanteric nonunion, avascular necrosis, and prolonged pain,[84] requiring conversion to total hip replacement in some patients.[64] Conversion to total hip replacement is more likely to occur when osteoarthritis is already present. These factors highlight the importance of a precise indication for FAI surgery.[63]

PITFALLS

It is important to be aware that the morphologic abnormalities with FAI-like features may be frequently seen in asymptomatic individuals,[38–41,85] and not all subjects with decreased femoral head offset or acetabular retroversion have FAI (ie, restricted range of hip motion, pain, and positive impingement testing) and require surgical correction. Therefore, it is important to remember

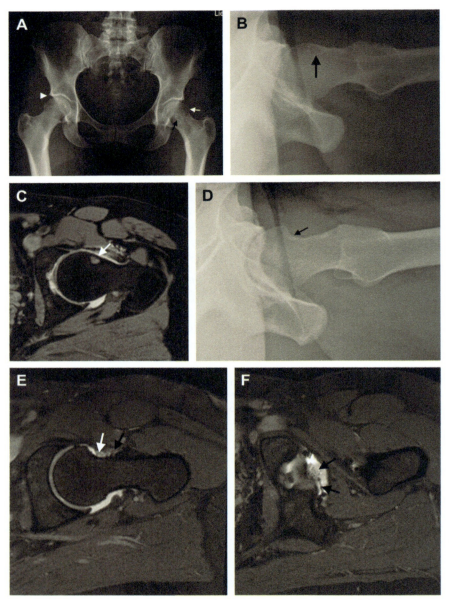

Fig. 24. Postoperative appearance of cam-type FAI in a 42-year-old woman. (*A*) AP radiograph demonstrates femoral bony excrescence (*white arrow*) and fibrocystic change (*black arrow*) of the left femur. A periacetabular ossicle is present on the right (*arrowhead*). (*B*) Lateral radiograph demonstrates preoperative appearance of the left proximal femur. Note fibrocystic change involving anterior femoral head-neck junction (*black arrow*). (*C*) Preoperative oblique axial PD-weighted image from an MR arthrogram demonstrates fibrocystic change and decreased femoral head-neck offset (*white arrow*). (*D*) Postoperative radiograph following femoroplasty demonstrates improved femoral head-neck offset (*black arrow*). (*E*) Postoperative oblique axial PD-weighted image demonstrates improved femoral head-neck offset (*white arrow*) following anterior femoroplasty. Thickening of the anterior capsule with adhesions is demonstrated (*black arrow*). (*F*) Postoperative adhesions and synovitis (*black arrows*) on axial FS PD-weighted image following anterior femoroplasty. (*Courtesy of* Balgrist Hospital, Zurich, Switzerland.)

that the diagnosis of FAI depends on both clinical and imaging findings, and a good history is crucial in making the correct diagnosis and providing useful information to the referring clinician.[86]

Recent articles on so-called asymptomatic young men with cam deformity have shown restricted internal rotation and MRI findings of labral and cartilage damage, which shows that when evaluated by an experienced orthopedic surgeon, clinical symptoms of restricted internal rotation can be elicited and that there is an association with morphologic hip damage, even at the asymptomatic stage.[43,44] Other pitfalls include the presence of adult DDH, which should be excluded on radiographs or MRI by assessing acetabular morphology and positioning of the femoral head in relation to the acetabulum.[21,87] Offset surgery may be catastrophic in this setting, potentially further increasing the lateralization of a DDH hip, and be problematic to solve, requiring, for example, periacetabular osteotomy. Ankylosing spondylitis or diffuse idiopathic skeletal hyperostosis of the hip joint can cause acetabular overcoverage or deepening of the acetabular fossa, thereby mimicking pincer impingement. Careful evaluation of radiographs and MRI for signs of sacroiliitis is advised to arrive at the correct diagnosis.[21,71]

SUMMARY

FAI is a common cause of premature osteoarthritis of the hip. It can be caused by decreased offset of the femoral head-neck junction (cam impingement) or acetabular overcoverage (pincer impingement), causing abutment of the femoral head against the acetabular rim during terminal hip motion. This repetitive microtrauma to the hip joint causes mechanical wear of the labrum and articular cartilage, and if left untreated causes pain, labral avulsion, and cartilage damage, leading to progressive osteoarthritis of the hip. The identification of FAI as a cause of osteoarthritis allows appropriate therapy early, and thus delays or prevents end-stage arthritis.

MRI and MRA are accurate noninvasive imaging modalities able to demonstrate acetabular labral trauma and adjacent cartilage damage associated with impingement. In addition, MRI is able to detect underlying subtle anatomic variations of the femoral head-neck junction and acetabulum associated with FAI.

REFERENCES

1. Leunig M, Beaule PE, Ganz R. The concept of femoroacetabular impingement: current status and future perspectives. Clin Orthop Relat Res 2009; 467(3):616–22.
2. Hart ES, Metkar US, Rebello GN, et al. Femoroacetabular impingement in adolescents and young adults. Orthop Nurs 2009;28(3):117–24 [quiz: 125–6].
3. Ganz R, Parvizi J, Beck M, et al. Femoroacetabular impingement: a cause for osteoarthritis of the hip. Clin Orthop 2003;(417):112–20.
4. Anderson SE, Siebenrock KA, Tannast M. Femoroacetabular impingement: evidence of an established hip abnormality. Radiology 2010;257(1):8–13.
5. Beck M, Kalhor M, Leunig M, et al. Hip morphology influences the pattern of damage to the acetabular cartilage: femoroacetabular impingement as a cause of early osteoarthritis of the hip. J Bone Joint Surg Br 2005;87(7):1012–8.
6. Sutter R, Dietrich TJ, Zingg PO, et al. Femoral antetorsion: comparing asymptomatic volunteers and patients with femoroacetabular impingement. Radiology 2012;263(2):475–83.
7. Beck M, Leunig M, Parvizi J, et al. Anterior femoroacetabular impingement: part II. Midterm results of surgical treatment. Clin Orthop 2004;(418):67–73.
8. Ito K, Leunig M, Ganz R. Histopathologic features of the acetabular labrum in femoroacetabular impingement. Clin Orthop 2004;(429):262–71.
9. Ito K, Minka MA 2nd, Leunig M, et al. Femoroacetabular impingement and the cam-effect. A MRI-based quantitative anatomical study of the femoral head-neck offset. J Bone Joint Surg Br 2001;83(2): 171–6.
10. Jager M, Wild A, Westhoff B, et al. Femoroacetabular impingement caused by a femoral osseous head-neck bump deformity: clinical, radiological, and experimental results. J Orthop Sci 2004;9(3): 256–63.
11. Tanzer M, Noiseux N. Osseous abnormalities and early osteoarthritis: the role of hip impingement. Clin Orthop 2004;(429):170–7.
12. Botser IB, Smith TW Jr, Nasser R, et al. Open surgical dislocation versus arthroscopy for femoroacetabular impingement: a comparison of clinical outcomes. Arthroscopy 2011;27(2):270–8.
13. Guanche CA, Bare AA. Arthroscopic treatment of femoroacetabular impingement. Arthroscopy 2006; 22(1):95–106.
14. Philippon MJ, Schenker ML. Arthroscopy for the treatment of femoroacetabular impingement in the athlete. Clin Sports Med 2006;25(2):299–308, ix.
15. Tijssen M, van Cingel R, Willemsen L, et al. Diagnostics of femoroacetabular impingement and labral pathology of the hip: a systematic review of the accuracy and validity of physical tests. Arthroscopy 2011;28(6):860–71.
16. Samora JB, Ng VY, Ellis TJ. Femoroacetabular impingement: a common cause of hip pain in young adults. Clin J Sport Med 2011;21(1):51–6.
17. Leunig M, Ganz R. Femoroacetabular impingement. A common cause of hip complaints leading to arthrosis. Unfallchirurg 2005;108(1):9–10, 12–7. [in German].
18. Nepple JJ, Brophy RH, Matava MJ, et al. Radiographic findings of femoroacetabular impingement in National Football League combine athletes undergoing radiographs for previous hip or groin pain. Arthroscopy. 2012;28(10):1396–403. http://dx.doi.org/10.1016/j.arthro.2012.03.005. Epub June 13, 2012.

19. Philippon M, Schenker M, Briggs K, et al. Femoroacetabular impingement in 45 professional athletes: associated pathologies and return to sport following arthroscopic decompression. Knee Surg Sports Traumatol Arthrosc 2007;15(7):908–14.

20. Banerjee P, McLean CR. Femoroacetabular impingement: a review of diagnosis and management. Curr Rev Musculoskelet Med 2011;4(1):23–32.

21. Tannast M, Siebenrock KA, Anderson SE. Femoroacetabular impingement: radiographic diagnosis—what the radiologist should know. AJR Am J Roentgenol 2007;188(6):1540–52.

22. Martin RL, Kelly BT, Leunig M, et al. Reliability of clinical diagnosis in intraarticular hip diseases. Knee Surg Sports Traumatol Arthrosc 2010;18(5):685–90.

23. Leunig M, Beck M, Woo A, et al. Acetabular rim degeneration: a constant finding in the aged hip. Clin Orthop 2003;(413):201–7.

24. Beck M, Leunig M, Clarke E, et al. Femoroacetabular impingement as a factor in the development of nonunion of the femoral neck: a report of three cases. J Orthop Trauma 2004;18(7):425–30.

25. Eijer H, Myers SR, Ganz R. Anterior femoroacetabular impingement after femoral neck fractures. J Orthop Trauma 2001;15(7):475–81.

26. Klaue K, Durnin CW, Ganz R. The acetabular rim syndrome. A clinical presentation of dysplasia of the hip. J Bone Joint Surg Br 1991;73(3):423–9.

27. Leunig M, Casillas MM, Hamlet M, et al. Slipped capital femoral epiphysis: early mechanical damage to the acetabular cartilage by a prominent femoral metaphysis. Acta Orthop Scand 2000;71(4):370–5.

28. Myers SR, Eijer H, Ganz R. Anterior femoroacetabular impingement after periacetabular osteotomy. Clin Orthop 1999;(363):93–9.

29. Pitto RP, Klaue K, Ganz R, et al. Acetabular rim pathology secondary to congenital hip dysplasia in the adult. A radiographic study. Chir Organi Mov 1995;80(4):361–8.

30. Siebenrock KA, Schoeniger R, Ganz R. Anterior femoro-acetabular impingement due to acetabular retroversion. Treatment with periacetabular osteotomy. J Bone Joint Surg Am 2003;85(2):278–86.

31. Goodman DA, Feighan JE, Smith AD, et al. Subclinical slipped capital femoral epiphysis. Relationship to osteoarthrosis of the hip. J Bone Joint Surg Am 1997;79(10):1489–97.

32. Siebenrock KA, Wahab KH, Werlen S, et al. Abnormal extension of the femoral head epiphysis as a cause of cam impingement. Clin Orthop 2004;(418):54–60.

33. Morgan JD, Somerville EW. Normal and abnormal growth at the upper end of the femur. J Bone Joint Surg Br 1960;42:264–72.

34. Schaeffeler C, Eiber M, Holzapfel K, et al. The epiphyseal torsion angle in MR arthrography of the hip: diagnostic utility in patients with femoroacetabular impingement syndrome. AJR Am J Roentgenol 2012;198(3):W237–43.

35. Tonnis D, Heinecke A. Acetabular and femoral anteversion: relationship with osteoarthritis of the hip. J Bone Joint Surg Am 1999;81(12):1747–70.

36. Tonnis D, Heinecke A. Diminished femoral antetorsion syndrome: a cause of pain and osteoarthritis. J Pediatr Orthop 1991;11(4):419–31.

37. Pollard TC, Villar RN, Norton MR, et al. Genetic influences in the aetiology of femoroacetabular impingement: a sibling study. J Bone Joint Surg Br 2010;92(2):209–16.

38. Gosvig KK, Jacobsen S, Sonne-Holm S, et al. The prevalence of cam-type deformity of the hip joint: a survey of 4151 subjects of the Copenhagen Osteoarthritis Study. Acta Radiol 2008;49(4):436–41.

39. Hack K, Di Primio G, Rakhra K, et al. Prevalence of cam-type femoroacetabular impingement morphology in asymptomatic volunteers. J Bone Joint Surg Am 2010;92(14):2436–44.

40. Laborie LB, Lehmann TG, Engesaeter IO, et al. Prevalence of radiographic findings thought to be associated with femoroacetabular impingement in a population-based cohort of 2081 healthy young adults. Radiology 2011;260(2):494–502.

41. Pollard TC, Villar RN, Norton MR, et al. Femoroacetabular impingement and classification of the cam deformity: the reference interval in normal hips. Acta Orthop 2010;81(1):134–41.

42. Pollard TC. A perspective on femoroacetabular impingement. Skeletal Radiol 2011;40(7):815–8.

43. Reichenbach S, Juni P, Werlen S, et al. Prevalence of cam-type deformity on hip magnetic resonance imaging in young males: a cross-sectional study. Arthritis Care Res (Hoboken) 2010;62(9):1319–27.

44. Reichenbach S, Leunig M, Werlen S, et al. Association between cam-type deformities and magnetic resonance imaging-detected structural hip damage: a cross-sectional study in young men. Arthritis Rheum 2011;63(12):4023–30.

45. Leunig M, Podeszwa D, Beck M, et al. Magnetic resonance arthrography of labral disorders in hips with dysplasia and impingement. Clin Orthop 2004;(418):74–80.

46. Lavigne M, Parvizi J, Beck M, et al. Anterior femoroacetabular impingement: part I. Techniques of joint preserving surgery. Clin Orthop 2004;(418):61–6.

47. Chell J, Flowers MJ. Is diagnostic arthroscopy of the hip worthwhile? J Bone Joint Surg Br 2000;82(2):306.

48. Notzli HP, Wyss TF, Stoecklin CH, et al. The contour of the femoral head-neck junction as a predictor for the risk of anterior impingement. J Bone Joint Surg Br 2002;84(4):556–60.

49. Crowninshield RD, Maloney WJ, Wentz DH, et al. Biomechanics of large femoral heads: what they do and don't do. Clin Orthop 2004;(429):102–7.

50. Murphy S, Tannast M, Kim YJ, et al. Debridement of the adult hip for femoroacetabular impingement: indications and preliminary clinical results. Clin Orthop Relat Res 2004;(429):178–81.

51. Ferguson SJ, Bryant JT, Ganz R, et al. The acetabular labrum seal: a poroelastic finite element model. Clin Biomech (Bristol, Avon) 2000;15(6):463–8.

52. Ferguson SJ, Bryant JT, Ganz R, et al. An in vitro investigation of the acetabular labral seal in hip joint mechanics. J Biomech 2003;36(2):171–8.

53. Reynolds D, Lucas J, Klaue K. Retroversion of the acetabulum. A cause of hip pain. J Bone Joint Surg Br 1999;81(2):281–8.

54. Meyer DC, Beck M, Ellis T, et al. Comparison of six radiographic projections to assess femoral head/neck asphericity. Clin Orthop Relat Res 2006;445:181–5.

55. Kalberer F, Sierra RJ, Madan SS, et al. Ischial spine projection into the pelvis: a new sign for acetabular retroversion. Clin Orthop Relat Res 2008;466(3):677–83.

56. Leunig M, Beck M, Kalhor M, et al. Fibrocystic changes at anterosuperior femoral neck: prevalence in hips with femoroacetabular impingement. Radiology 2005;236(1):237–46.

57. Kassarjian A, Yoon LS, Belzile E, et al. Triad of MR arthrographic findings in patients with cam-type femoroacetabular impingement. Radiology 2005;236(2):588–92.

58. Pfirrmann CW, Duc SR, Zanetti M, et al. MR arthrography of acetabular cartilage delamination in femoroacetabular cam impingement. Radiology 2008;249(1):236–41.

59. Leunig M, Werlen S, Ungersbock A, et al. Evaluation of the acetabular labrum by MR arthrography. J Bone Joint Surg Br 1997;79(2):230–4.

60. Schmid MR, Notzli HP, Zanetti M, et al. Cartilage lesions in the hip: diagnostic effectiveness of MR arthrography. Radiology 2003;226(2):382–6.

61. Dudda M, Albers C, Mamisch TC, et al. Do normal radiographs exclude asphericity of the femoral head-neck junction? Clin Orthop Relat Res 2009;467(3):651–9.

62. Pfirrmann CW, Mengiardi B, Dora C, et al. Cam and pincer femoroacetabular impingement: characteristic MR arthrographic findings in 50 patients. Radiology 2006;240(3):778–85.

63. Sutter R, Dietrich TJ, Zingg PO, et al. How useful is the alpha angle for discriminating between symptomatic patients with cam-type femoroacetabular impingement and asymptomatic volunteers? Radiology 2012;264(2):514–21.

64. Philippon MJ, Briggs KK, Yen YM, et al. Outcomes following hip arthroscopy for femoroacetabular impingement with associated chondrolabral dysfunction: minimum two-year follow-up. J Bone Joint Surg Br 2009;91(1):16–23.

65. Apprich S, Mamisch TC, Welsch GH, et al. Evaluation of articular cartilage in patients with femoroacetabular impingement (FAI) using T2* mapping at different time points at 3.0 Tesla MRI: a feasibility study. Skeletal Radiol 2012;41(8):987–95.

66. Bittersohl B, Hosalkar HS, Apprich S, et al. Comparison of pre-operative dGEMRIC imaging with intra-operative findings in femoroacetabular impingement: preliminary findings. Skeletal Radiol 2011;40(5):553–61.

67. Bittersohl B, Hosalkar HS, Kim YJ, et al. Delayed gadolinium-enhanced magnetic resonance imaging (dGEMRIC) of hip joint cartilage in femoroacetabular impingement (FAI): are pre- and postcontrast imaging both necessary? Magn Reson Med 2009;62(6):1362–7.

68. Bittersohl B, Hosalkar HS, Werlen S, et al. Intravenous versus intra-articular delayed gadolinium-enhanced magnetic resonance imaging in the hip joint: a comparative analysis. Invest Radiol 2010;45(9):538–42.

69. Jessel RH, Zilkens C, Tiderius C, et al. Assessment of osteoarthritis in hips with femoroacetabular impingement using delayed gadolinium enhanced MRI of cartilage. J Magn Reson Imaging 2009;30(5):1110–5.

70. Mamisch TC, Kain MS, Bittersohl B, et al. Delayed gadolinium-enhanced magnetic resonance imaging of cartilage (dGEMRIC) in femoroacetabular impingement. J Orthop Res 2011;29(9):1305–11.

71. Anderson SE, Siebenrock KA, Mamisch TC, et al. Femoroacetabular impingement magnetic resonance imaging. Top Magn Reson Imaging 2009;20(3):123–8.

72. James SL, Ali K, Malara F, et al. MRI findings of femoroacetabular impingement. AJR Am J Roentgenol 2006;187(6):1412–9.

73. Fadul DA, Carrino JA. Imaging of femoroacetabular impingement. J Bone Joint Surg Am 2009;91(Suppl 1):138–43.

74. Kassarjian A, Brisson M, Palmer WE. Femoroacetabular impingement. Eur J Radiol 2007;63(1):29–35.

75. Kivlan BR, Martin RL, Sekiya JK. Response to diagnostic injection in patients with femoroacetabular impingement, labral tears, chondral lesions, and extra-articular pathology. Arthroscopy 2011;27(5):619–27.

76. Zebala LP, Schoenecker PL, Clohisy JC. Anterior femoroacetabular impingement: a diverse disease with evolving treatment options. Iowa Orthop J 2007;27:71–81.

77. Espinosa N, Rothenfluh DA, Beck M, et al. Treatment of femoro-acetabular impingement: preliminary

results of labral refixation. J Bone Joint Surg Am 2006;88(5):925–35.

78. Laude F, Sariali E, Nogier A. Femoroacetabular impingement treatment using arthroscopy and anterior approach. Clin Orthop Relat Res 2009;467(3): 747–52.

79. Lincoln M, Johnston K, Muldoon M, et al. Combined arthroscopic and modified open approach for cam femoroacetabular impingement: a preliminary experience. Arthroscopy 2009;25(4):392–9.

80. Philippon MJ, Schenker ML. A new method for acetabular rim trimming and labral repair. Clin Sports Med 2006;25(2):293–7, ix.

81. Beaule PE, Le Duff MJ, Zaragoza E. Quality of life following femoral head-neck osteochondroplasty for femoroacetabular impingement. J Bone Joint Surg Am 2007;89(4):773–9.

82. Khanduja V, Villar RN. The arthroscopic management of femoroacetabular impingement. Knee Surg Sports Traumatol Arthrosc 2007;15(8):1035–40.

83. Peters CL, Erickson JA. Treatment of femoroacetabular impingement with surgical dislocation and debridement in young adults. J Bone Joint Surg Am 2006;88(8):1735–41.

84. Standaert CJ, Manner PA, Herring SA. Expert opinion and controversies in musculoskeletal and sports medicine: femoroacetabular impingement. Arch Phys Med Rehabil 2008;89(5):890–3.

85. Kang AC, Gooding AJ, Coates MH, et al. Computed tomography assessment of hip joints in asymptomatic individuals in relation to femoroacetabular impingement. Am J Sports Med 2010;38(6):1160–5.

86. Palmer WE. Femoroacetabular impingement: caution is warranted in making imaging-based assumptions and diagnoses. Radiology 2010;257(1):4–7.

87. Steppacher SD, Tannast M, Werlen S, et al. Femoral morphology differs between deficient and excessive acetabular coverage. Clin Orthop Relat Res 2008; 466(4):782–90.

88. Tomczak RJ, Guenther KP, Rieber A, et al. MR imaging measurement of the femoral antetorsional angle as a new technique: comparison with CT in children and adults. AJR Am J Roentgenol 1997; 168(3):791–4.

Ischiofemoral Impingement

Atul K. Taneja, MD, Miriam A. Bredella, MD, Martin Torriani, MD, MSc*

KEYWORDS

- Hip pain • Ischiofemoral impingement • Quadratus femoris • Ischium • Lesser trochanter

KEY POINTS

- Ischiofemoral impingement syndrome is defined by hip pain related to narrowing of the space between the ischial tuberosity and lesser trochanter, with abnormalities of the quadratus femoris muscle.
- Narrowing of the ischiofemoral space may be positional, congenital, or acquired.
- Plain radiographs may show chronic osseous changes of impaction between lesser trochanter and ischium. Magnetic resonance imaging is the standard imaging method to diagnose ischiofemoral impingement, showing edema and deformity of the quadratus femoris muscle belly at the site of maximal narrowing. In patients with long-standing impingement, quadratus femoris muscle fatty infiltration and atrophy may be present.
- Associated findings include abnormalities of the hamstring tendons, iliopsoas tendon insertion, and bursalike formations.

INTRODUCTION

Ischiofemoral impingement (IFI) syndrome is defined by hip pain related to narrowing of the space between the ischial tuberosity and lesser trochanter with abnormal morphology and/or magnetic resonance (MR) imaging signal intensity of the quadratus femoris muscle (QFM).[1]

Ischiofemoral narrowing was first described by Johnson in 1977[2] in 3 patients with persistent hip pain after surgery, 2 of them after hip arthroplasty and 1 of them after proximal femoral osteotomy. In all cases, pain and narrowing of ischiofemoral space (IFS) were relieved after a lesser trochanter resection.

More recently, hip pain related to narrowing of IFS on cross-sectional imaging and abnormalities of QFM were reported in patients without history of surgery or trauma,[3,4] supporting IFI as an entity that clinicians, orthopedic surgeons, and radiologists should be aware of.

IFI has been reported to be bilateral in 25% to 40% of cases.[1,5] It is more frequent in women[1,5] and affects all ages, ranging from 11 to 77 years.[1,6] Nonspecific hip pain is a frequent symptom, with duration varying between months and several years.[1]

ANATOMY

The QFM is a flat and quadrilateral muscle, situated along the posterior aspect of the hip joint. It originates at the anterior portion of the ischial tuberosity and inserts on the posteromedial aspect of the proximal femur. The QFM is bordered by the obturator externus muscle anteriorly, sciatic nerve posteriorly, inferior gemellus superiorly and adductor magnus inferiorly.[7,8] The main role of the QFM is to assist in external rotation and adduction of the hip.[9]

As suggested by Torriani and colleagues,[1] ischiofemoral narrowing can be evaluated by measuring the following spaces (**Fig. 1**):

Disclosure: No conflicts of interests.
Musculoskeletal Imaging and Intervention, Massachusetts General Hospital, Harvard Medical School, 55 Fruit Street, Boston, MA 02114, USA
* Corresponding author.
E-mail address: mtorriani@hms.harvard.edu

Magn Reson Imaging Clin N Am 21 (2013) 65–73
http://dx.doi.org/10.1016/j.mric.2012.08.005
1064-9689/13/$ – see front matter © 2013 Elsevier Inc. All rights reserved.

mri.theclinics.com

- Ischiofemoral space (IFS): the narrowest distance between the lateral cortex of the ischial tuberosity and medial cortex of the lesser trochanter;
- Quadratus femoris space (QFS): the narrowest space for passage of the QFM delimited by the superolateral surface of the hamstring tendons and the posteromedial surface of the iliopsoas tendon or lesser trochanter.

Ischiofemoral narrowing may be positional, congenital, or acquired[7] (**Box 1**):

1. Positional factors that may affect the IFS and QFS include lower extremity internal/external

---

Box 1
Causes of IFS narrowing

- Positional
- Congenital
- Acquired

---

rotation, adduction/abduction, and flexion/extension. Previous studies have controlled for these factors by comparing patients with suspected IFI with controls with similar leg positioning.[1,5]

2. Congenital ischiofemoral narrowing can be caused by a larger cross-section of the femur at the level of the lesser trochanter, a congenital

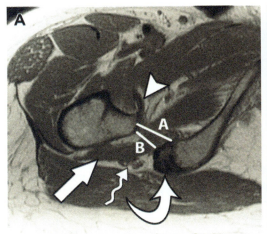
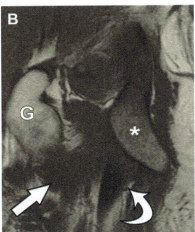
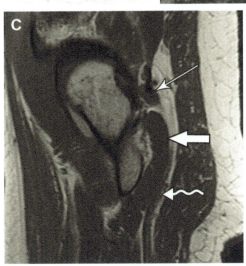

Fig. 1. 54-year-old man with normal IFS and QFS. Axial proton density-weighted (*A*), coronal T1-weighted (*B*) and sagittal proton density-weighted (*C*) MR images of right hip show anatomic relationship of QFM (*straight arrow*), normal IFS (*line A*), normal QFS (*line B*), iliopsoas tendon (*arrowhead*), hamstring tendons (*curved arrow*), greater trochanter (G), ischium (*star*), inferior gemellus muscle (*thin arrow*), and sciatic nerve (*wavy arrow*).

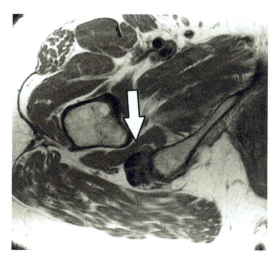

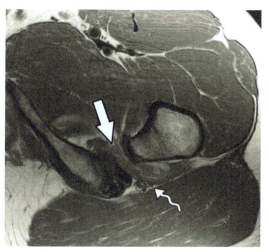

Fig. 2. 56-year-old woman with lower back and right hip pain. Axial proton density-weighted MR image of right hip shows narrowed IFS and QFS with deformity of QFM (*straight arrow*).

Fig. 4. 39-year-old man with shooting pain in the left groin over the hip and exacerbated by bending the leg. Axial proton density-weighted MR image shows IFI with severe edema and mass effect of QFM (*straight arrow*) on sciatic nerve (*wavy arrow*). Because of their close anatomic relationship, this phenomenon may cause distal radiation of pain.

posteromedial position of the femur, lower ischiopubic ramus with an angle closer to the coronal plane, prominence of the lesser trochanter, or configuration of the female pelvic bony anatomy, which shows greater width and lesser anteroposterior dimensions when compared with males (**Fig. 2**).[1,5]

3. Acquired ischiofemoral narrowing may be seen as a result of fractures involving the lesser trochanter, valgus-producing intertrochanteric osteotomy, osteoarthritis leading to superior and medial migration of the femur in older patients,[2] enthesopathy of the proximal hamstring insertion, or expansile bone lesions (eg, osteochondroma) (**Fig. 3**).[3]

CLINICAL PRESENTATION

Patients with IFI present with chronic pain in the groin or buttock, usually without a precipitating injury.[10] The pain may radiate distally to the lower extremity, because of the proximity of QFM with pressure effect on the sciatic nerve (**Fig. 4**),[1,3] and can be related to other symptoms such as snapping, crepitation, or locking.[5]

There is no specific diagnostic clinical test for IFI, but clinicians should keep this diagnosis in mind when pain is reproduced during specific

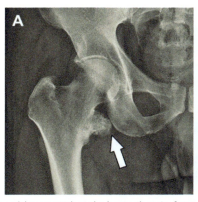

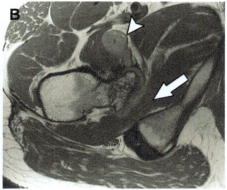

Fig. 3. 41-year-old man with right buttock pain for 5 months precipitated by sitting. Anteroposterior radiograph (*A*) and axial proton density-weighted MR image (*B*) show osteochondroma of lesser trochanter (*arrow* in *A*) leading to secondary IFS narrowing and direct compression of QFM (*arrow* in *B*). Lobular extension of the cartilage cap is seen anteriorly (*arrowhead* in *B*), abutting the distal iliopsoas muscle.

Box 2
Clinical presentation of IFI

- Symptoms: chronic pain in the groin or buttock (which may radiate distally), snapping, crepitation, or locking of the hip
- Clinical examination: no specific diagnostic test; exacerbation with wide range of hip positions, including flexion, abduction, and internal rotation, as well as extension, adduction, and external rotation

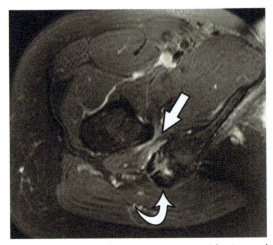

Fig. 6. 48-year-old female swimmer with 4-month history of right buttock pain. Axial T2-weighted fat-suppressed MR image of right hip shows IFI with moderate diffuse edema and deformity of QFM (*straight arrow*). Tendinopathy of hamstring tendons is also noted (*curved arrow*).

maneuvers. Pain symptoms have been described in patients with IFI in response to a wide range of hip positions, including flexion, abduction, or internal rotation,[5] as well as extension, adduction, and external rotation[10] (**Box 2**).

IMAGING PROTOCOL

Radiographs of the hip should include standard anteroposterior view and frog-leg lateral view, which allow for detection of osseous changes from chronic IFI.

A typical routine pelvis or hip MR imaging protocol is sufficient to detect and evaluate IFI. In our institution, the MR imaging protocol for pelvis and hip includes positioning the feet in internal rotation secured by adhesive taping. Pelvic MR imaging performed on a 1.5-T or 3.0-T scanner uses a selection of phased array coils covering symptomatic or both hips, and the following pulses sequences: coronal T1-weighted, axial fast spin echo (FSE) proton density-weighted,

axial FSE fat-suppressed T2-weighted, coronal FSE short-tau inversion recovery, and sagittal FSE fat-suppressed T2-weighted. Contrast-enhanced pulse sequences are not necessary and are performed in select cases excluding other diseases of the hip.

IMAGING FINDINGS

Plain radiographs of the hip are usually normal, although chronic osseous changes such as sclerosis and cystic changes of lesser trochanter and

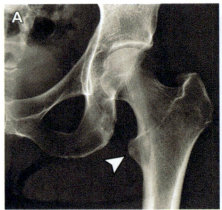
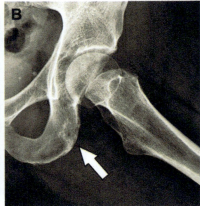

Fig. 5. 47-year-old woman with 2-year history of left posterior hip and thigh pain. Anteroposterior (*A*) and frog-leg lateral (*B*) radiographs show chronic osseous changes of IFI, with subtle sclerosis of lesser trochanter (*arrowhead*) and subcortical cystic changes of ischium (*straight arrow*).

ischium may be present (**Fig. 5**).[3] Radiographs are also useful to diagnose osseous abnormalities that may cause acquired IFI (see **Fig. 3**) or even to depict other causes of hip pain.

MR imaging is the standard method to diagnose IFI, shown by reduced IFS and QFS with concurrent edema centered in the QFM belly at the site of maximal impingement, with crowding of muscle fibers,[1,8] which may be unilateral (**Fig. 6**) or bilateral. Findings of IFI are best seen on axial images, which are optimal to assess the relationship between the affected QFM and structures responsible for impingement, as well as the degree of deformity and tears.[8] Coronal and sagittal images may provide additional information regarding the QFM and surrounding structures (**Box 3**, **Fig. 7**).

With the hip in adduction, external rotation and extension, the lesser trochanter and ischial

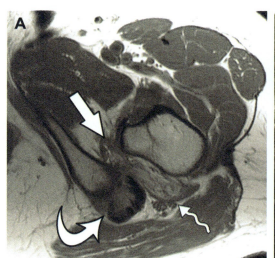
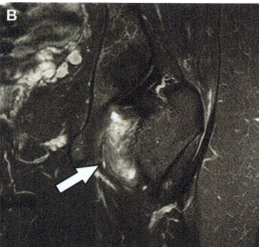
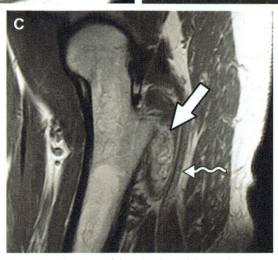

Fig. 7. 51-year-old woman with 3-year history of low back and buttock pain radiating distally to posterior aspect of the leg. Axial proton density-weighted (*A*), coronal T2-weighted fat-suppressed (*B*) and sagittal proton density-weighted (*C*) MR images of left hip show IFI with severe diffuse edema and tear of QFM (*straight arrow*). Mass effect of QFM on sciatic nerve (*wavy arrow*) and tear of hamstring tendons are also noted (*curved arrow*).

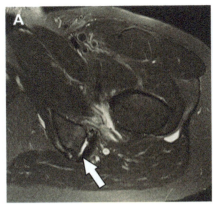
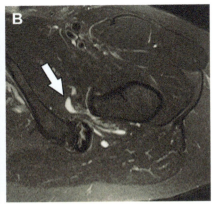

Fig. 8. 47-year-old woman (same patient as Fig. 5). Axial T2-weighted MR images (*A, B*) show IFI with QFM tear, edema surrounding hamstring tendons with partial tear at the attachment (*straight arrow* in *A*), and bursalike formation (*straight arrow* in *B*).

tuberosity are about 2.0 cm apart.[2] Two studies have shown significant reduction of the IFS and QFS when comparing patients with abnormal QFM with control individuals, regardless of the lower leg being in internal rotation or neutral position. With the lower leg in internal rotation, measures of the IFS of 13 ± 5 mm and QFS of 7 ± 3 mm were identified in affected patients.[1] In affected patients with the lower leg in neutral position, IFS measures were on average 12.9 mm and the QFS were on average 6.71 mm.[5]

Additional measurements, such as inclination angle (IA) between the femoral neck and long axis of femoral shaft, hamstring tendon area (HTA), and total QFM volume (TQFMV) have also been reported and may help determine the presence of IFI.[5] In affected patients, TQFMV was significantly lower, whereas HTA and IA measures were significantly higher than controls.[5]

Additional imaging findings present in IFI include[5,9]

- Edema surrounding the iliopsoas tendon insertion
- Edema and tears affecting the hamstring tendons (**Fig. 8**A)
- Bursalike formations (see **Fig. 8**B)
- Reduced muscle volume and fatty infiltration (in patients with long-standing IFI) (**Fig. 9**)

Further studies with dynamic MR imaging may help evaluate the relationship of the QFM and the adjacent osseous, muscle, and fat structures as the hip goes through a full range of motion.[8,11]

DIFFERENTIAL DIAGNOSIS

A wide range of conditions related to hip pain should be considered in the clinical and imaging differential diagnosis for IFI. These conditions include:

- Strain or tear of the QFM without narrowing of the IFS
- Tendinopathy of the iliopsoas or hamstring
- Iliopsoas bursitis
- Denervation

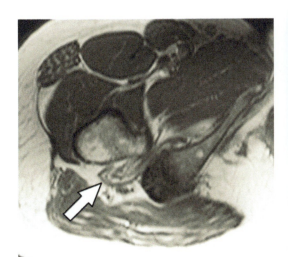

Fig. 9. 48-year-old woman (same patient as Fig. 6). Axial T1-weighted MR image of right hip shows moderate fatty infiltration of QFM (*straight arrow*).

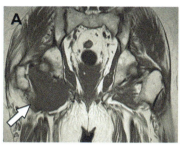
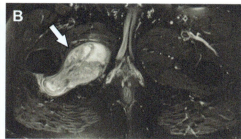

Fig. 10. 65-year-old man with several months of progressive right hip pain. Coronal T1-weighted (*A*) and axial T2-weighted fat-suppressed (*B*) MR images of pelvis show large soft tissue mass (myofibroblastic sarcoma) in posterior right hip (*straight arrow*), occupying the IFS and causing mass effect on the surrounding muscles and with erosion of ischium.

- Delayed-onset muscle soreness
- Mass lesions (**Fig. 10**).[8,9]

It is important to differentiate edema affecting the belly of the QFM (as seen from impingement) from edema at the myotendinous junction, which is most commonly related to tear or strain (**Fig. 11, Table 1**).[8] A potential mechanism for QFM tears is an injury that occurs during eccentric contraction as it tries to control internal hip rotation.[9] In the

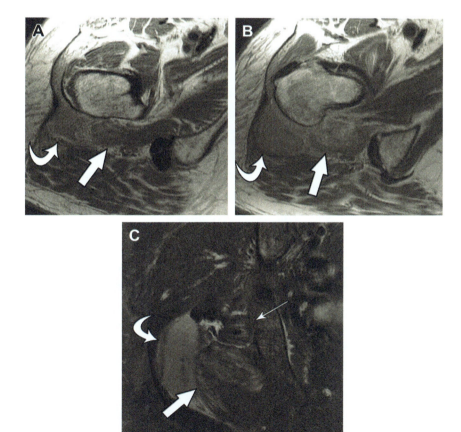

Fig. 11. 75-year-old woman with right hip pain after fall. Axial proton density-weighted (*A, B*) and coronal T2-weighted fat-suppressed (*C*) MR images of right hip show edema and tear at the belly and myotendinous junction near femoral attachment of QFM (*straight arrow*), consistent with strain. Associated strain of inferior gemellus muscle (*thin arrow*) and large hematoma deep to iliotibial band (*curved arrow*) are seen. No narrowing of IFS or QFS is present.

Table 1
MR imaging differential features between IFI and quadratus femoris strain/tear

IFI	Quadratus Femoris Strain
Narrowed IFS and QFS	Not related to space narrowing
Edema centered on the belly of QFM	Edema at the myotendinous junction of QFM

Table 2
Treatment options for IFI

1.	Conservative	Rest, activity restriction, nonsteroidal anti-inflammatory drugs and physical therapy
2.	CT-guided injection	Anesthetics and steroids

3.	Surgical
	   a. Open surgery
	   b. Arthroscopic
		Decompression of quadratus femoris with lesser trochanter resection

case of QFM edema, one should also consider other diagnoses besides IFI. QFM edema visible on MR imaging could be the result of numerous conditions, as listed earlier.[10] Because QFM changes may be multifactorial,[1] the diagnosis of IFI should be considered based on clinical history and physical examination, as well as the presence of IFS and QFS narrowing. Follow-up studies may be helpful to determine whether QFM abnormalities are transient[11] or potentially related to ischiofemoral narrowing. Not everyone with ischiofemoral narrowing has clinical symptoms or QFM abnormalities on MR imaging.

TREATMENT

The optimal treatment strategy for IFI remains unclear, but patients may benefit from conservative measures that include rest, activity restriction, nonsteroidal anti-inflammatory drugs, and physical therapy.[3,6]

Computed tomography (CT)-guided injection of anesthetics and steroids into the QFM is a nonsurgical alternative in selected patients (**Fig. 12**);

however it is palliative in scope and provides only temporary relief of symptoms.[1,7]

Results from surgical treatment of IFI are preliminary. Excision of the lesser trochanter may represent an effective treatment by decompressing the IFS.[2,7] In a recent case report, Ali and colleagues[7] described release of the psoas tendon and QFM, followed by excision of the lesser trochanter and reattachment of the psoas to the proximal femur and QFM to the ischium. This approach yielded adequate decompression of IFS on postoperative radiographs and relief of symptoms 10 weeks after surgery.[7] Because open surgical approaches can be related to higher morbidity,[10] arthroscopic decompression of the quadratus femoris has recently been reported as an alternative technique (**Table 2**).[10]

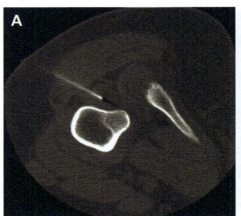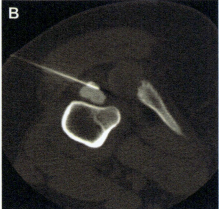

Fig. 12. 51-year-old man (same patient as **Fig. 7**). Left hip CT images with patient in prone position (*A, B*) during CT-guided injection of steroid and anesthetic into QFM.

SUMMARY

IFI is a syndrome defined by hip pain associated with narrowing of the space between the ischial tuberosity and lesser trochanter, which leads to abnormalities of the QFM. Narrowing of IFS may be positional, congenital, or acquired.

Plain radiographs may show chronic osseous changes of impaction between the lesser trochanter and ischium. MR imaging is the standard imaging method to diagnose this entity, showing edema and deformity of the QFM belly at the site of maximal narrowing. In patients with long-standing impingement, fatty infiltration and atrophy may be present. Associated findings include abnormalities of the hamstring tendons, iliopsoas tendon insertion, and bursalike formations.

The ideal treatment approach for IFI is not well defined, and thus a conservative regimen, CT-guided injection (anesthetics and steroids) and surgery (open or arthroscopic) are acceptable options.

REFERENCES

1. Torriani M, Souto SCL, Thomas BJ, et al. Ischiofemoral impingement syndrome: an entity with hip pain and abnormalities of the quadratus femoris muscle. Am J Roentgenol 2009;193(1):186–90.
2. Johnson KA. Impingement of the lesser trochanter on the ischial ramus after total hip arthroplasty. Report of three cases. J Bone Joint Surg Am 1977; 59(2):268–9.
3. Patti JW, Ouellette H, Bredella MA, et al. Impingement of lesser trochanter on ischium as a potential cause for hip pain. Skeletal Radiol 2008;37(10):939–41.
4. Kassarjian A. Signal abnormalities in the quadratus femoris muscle: tear or impingement? Am J Roentgenol 2008;190(6):W379.
5. Tosun O, Algin O, Yalcin N, et al. Ischiofemoral impingement: evaluation with new MRI parameters and assessment of their reliability. Skeletal Radiol 2011;41(5):575–87.
6. Tosun O, Cay N, Bozkurt M, et al. Ischio femoral impingement in an 11-year-old girl. Diagn Interv Radiol 2012. Available at: http://www.ncbi.nlm.nih.gov/pubmed/22684486.
7. Ali AM, Whitwell D, Ostlere SJ. Case report: imaging and surgical treatment of a snapping hip due to ischiofemoral impingement. Skeletal Radiol 2011; 40(5):653–6.
8. Kassarjian A, Tomas X, Cerezal L, et al. MRI of the quadratus femoris muscle: anatomic considerations and pathologic lesions. Am J Roentgenol 2011; 197(1):170–4.
9. O'Brien SD, Bui-Mansfield LT. MRI of quadratus femoris muscle tear: another cause of hip pain. Am J Roentgenol 2007;189(5):1185–9.
10. Stafford GH, Villar RN. Ischiofemoral impingement. J Bone Joint Surg Br 2011;93(10):1300.
11. Bui-Mansfield LT, O'Brien SD. Reply. Am J Roentgenol 2008;190(6):W380–1.

Tendon Injuries of the Hip

Catherine N. Petchprapa, MD*, Jenny T. Bencardino, MD

KEYWORDS

- MR imaging • Hip • Tendon pathology • Overuse injury

KEY POINTS

- History and clinical examination may not reliably stratify those patients with arthritic pain from those with nonarthritic pain.
- MR imaging is an important adjunct to the clinical examination because of its ability to evaluate the joint as well as the periarticular structures, which can be a source of symptoms.
- An anatomy-based search process can facilitate MR imaging interpretation and ensure that both common and less common entities are considered in the differential diagnosis.

INTRODUCTION

One in 164 visits to family physicians[1] is for hip pain. Unfortunately, hip pain can be a vexing clinical problem; symptoms may be protean, referred, and poorly localized. Moreover, history and physical examination have been found unreliable in discriminating between the intra-articular or extra-articular sources of hip pain. In approximately half of the patients studied, Martin and colleagues[2] determined that extra-articular pathology was responsible for patient symptoms despite imaging evidence for labral abnormalities.

Overuse injuries, including tendinopathies, are on the rise.[3] The higher level of performance of competitive and recreational athletes, an emphasis on the health benefits of physical activity leading to greater sports participation in all age groups, and increased longevity of the population probably all contribute to this trend.

These points stress the importance of considering tendon pathology in the differential diagnosis and the need for imaging in the work-up in patients with hip pain. MR imaging augments clinical evaluation by providing information about the hip joint as well as the periarticular structures, which can be a source of symptoms.

Imaging evaluation for extra-articular causes of hip pain necessitates knowledge of normal anatomy and common pathologic tendon conditions in this region.

Hip pain can be characterized as anterior, lateral, or posterior. The content of this review is organized using this anatomic approach (**Fig. 1**):

- Anterior pain (excluding osteoarthritis): enthesial and proximal iliotibial band (ITB) pathology, disorders of the iliopsoas tendon (internal snapping hip and iliopsoas impingement), and disorders of rectus femoris
- Lateral pain: disorders of the hip abductor tendons and external snapping hip syndrome (ESHS)
- Posterior pain: disorders of the hamstring tendons

Disorders of the ischiofemoral space and groin pain are discussed elsewhere in this issue by Torriani and colleagues, and Zoga and colleagues, respectively.

MR IMAGING TECHNIQUE

According to the American College of Radiology, plain radiographs of the pelvis and hip are the most appropriate imaging study for the initial evaluation of chronic hip pain. Radiographs may reveal fractures, osteoarthritis, hydroxyapatite crystal deposition diseases, and other common entities that may explain symptomatology. Initial radiographic findings and clinical information can then

Department of Radiology, NYU Langone Medical Center, Hospital for Joint Diseases, 301 East 17th Street, New York, NY 10003, USA
* Corresponding author.
E-mail address: petchc01@nyumc.org

Magn Reson Imaging Clin N Am 21 (2013) 75–96
http://dx.doi.org/10.1016/j.mric.2012.09.004
1064-9689/13/$ – see front matter © 2013 Elsevier Inc. All rights reserved.

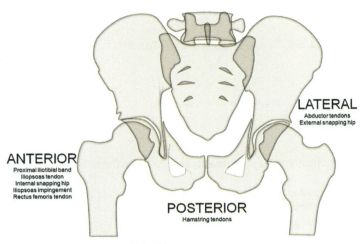

LATERAL
Abductor tendons
External snapping hip

ANTERIOR
Proximal iliotibial band
Iliopsoas tendon
Internal snapping hip
Iliopsoas impingement
Rectus femoris tendon

POSTERIOR
Hamstring tendons

Fig. 1. Overview of tendon pathology around the hip.

guide the choice of more advanced imaging. In cases of suspected musculotendinous etiology, noncontrast MR imaging is the next most commonly performed study because of its ability to diagnose the myriad potential osseous and soft tissue causes of hip pain around the pelvis.[4]

Tendon pathology can be evaluated on standard MR imaging planes. MR imaging protocols can be standardized; the authors use 3 imaging protocols. All start with large field of view (FOV) coronal short tau inversion recovery (STIR) images of the pelvis using the body coil; this provides an overview of the pelvis and allows a radiologist/technologist to modify the imaging protocol to evaluate unexpected pathology if necessary.

The protocol for the bony pelvis continues with large FOV imaging of the pelvis using anatomic (T1 and proton density [PD]) and fluid-sensitive (fat-suppressed T2 or PD) sequences, and a sagittal sequence through the affected side if there is symptom laterality.

In patients younger than 50 years of age (in whom diagnosing intra-articular pathology is relevant to management), axial fat-suppressed T2, axial oblique PD, sagittal fat-suppressed PD, and coronal PD are performed using a high-resolution technique that uses a flexible surface coil wrapped around the affected hip (**Table 1**). The affected hip is positioned closest to isocenter with the surface coil in place at the start of the examination; off-isocenter position optimizes imaging of the affected hip and in the authors' practice does not have a significant impact on the diagnostic quality of the large FOV sequence for the remainder of the pelvis (**Fig. 2**).

For patients over age 50 (in whom marrow abnormalities, including fractures and metastatic disease, may be a concern), the large FOV STIR coronal sequence is followed by a large FOV T1 coronal sequence (Table **2**). Subsequent coronal, sagittal, and axial images are done of the affected hip only.

Skin markers placed in the region of symptoms can help ensure adequate imaging coverage and direct attention to the region of clinical concern during image interpretation.

Table 1
Protocol for routine hip, patients under 50 years old

Sequence	Plane	Slice Thickness	Tr	Te	FOV	Matrix	Comment
STIR	Cor	5 mm	4000	35	350	192 × 256	Cover whole pelvis
PD TSE	Cor	3 mm	3000–3500	34–38	160	192 × 256	Unilateral
PD TSE FS	Sag	3 mm	2900–3000	22–35	160	256 × 256	Unilateral
T2 TSE FS	Ax Straight	3 mm	3500–4500	40	200	224 × 256	Unilateral
PD TSE	Obl Ax	3 mm	2800–3000	33	140–160	224 × 256	Unilateral

Abbreviations: STIR, short tau inversion recovery; PD, proton density; TSE, turbo spin echo; FS, fat suppressed; Cor, coronal; Sag, sagittal; Ax, axial; Obl, oblique; Tr, repetition time; Te, excitation time; FOV, field of view.

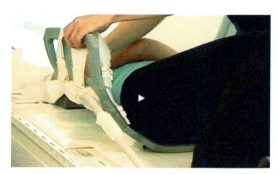

Fig. 2. Patient positioning. The flexible coil is placed over the affected hip and patient positioned with the affected hip closest to isocenter.

GENERAL CONSIDERATIONS/PITFALLS/CAVEATS

Tendons are designed to transmit forces generated from muscle contraction to bone. Their tensile strength is owed in large part to densely packed and aligned collagen fibers. Thus, healthy tendons do not rupture under normal conditions. Repetitive submaximal tendon loading due to chronic overuse, however, results in tendon degeneration; this reduces the tendon's strength and puts it at risk for failure.

Tendons undergo stereotypic changes with aging and injury regardless of their location. This alters their size, signal, and morphology on imaging. Peritendinitis represents the earliest injury, and manifests as increased T2 signal around the tendon (**Fig. 3**).[5] Tendinosis or tendinopathy is the result of mechanical, degenerative, or overuse injuries. Whether the result of myxoid, hypoxic, hyaline, fatty, fibrinoid, or calcific degeneration, structural changes and accumulated degradation byproducts leave the tendon more prone to injury. This is reflected on MR imaging as an increase in size and signal heterogeneity (see **Fig. 3**). Tears within a weakened tendon are identified as fluid-filled defects on PD, T2, or STIR sequences (**Fig. 4B**). Partial thickness tears

may heal over time and leave the tendon thickened, thinned, irregular, or lax. Full-thickness tears are defined as complete fiber discontinuity and can be associated with tendon retraction, fluid gap, and muscle atrophy (**Fig. 5**).

Spuriously increased intratendinous signal may be the result of magic angle phenomenon. Seen on sequences with short echo times, the signal in a tendon may increase as the orientation of the intratendinous collagen is aligned at an angle with the main magnetic field. This is greatest at 55% and can be mitigated with the use of longer echo times (30 ms for gradient echo, 40 ms for spin echo, and 70 ms for fast spin-echo imaging at 1.5 T).[6]

Decreased tendon signal can be related to the deposition of basic calcium phosphate, such as hydroxyapatite, in the setting of calcific tendinitis. This can be clinically silent; symptomatic crystal deposition is most common in patients in their 40s to 60s.[7] The hip is the second most commonly affected joint; calcium deposits are most common around the greater trochanter (hip abductor tendons) and ischial tuberosity (hamstring tendons). They are also seen at the femoral insertion of the gluteus maximus tendon and at the origin of rectus femoris and vastus musculature (**Fig. 6**). Initial patient presentation can be dramatic. The painful inflammatory response can manifest as bone and soft tissue edema[8] and bone erosions, which can mimic infection or malignancy[9,10] both clinically and on MR imaging. Although osseous involvement is rare, when present in the hip, the proximal linea aspera of the femur is most likely affected (see **Fig. 6A, B**). Enthesial calcifications without a discrete soft tissue mass are substantiating evidence for this diagnosis on MR imaging.[11] Plain radiographs and CT may help to confirm soft tissue calcifications when they are not evident on MR imaging (see **Fig. 6**).

"Treat the patient, not the imaging" could not be truer than in musculoskeletal imaging. Imaging-detected pathologic changes in the hip abductor

Table 2							
Protocol for routine hip, patients over 50 years old							
Sequence	Plane	Slice Thickness	Tr	Te	FOV	Matrix	Comment
STIR	Cor	5 mm	4000	35	350	192 × 256	Cover whole pelvis
T1 SE	Cor	5 mm	500–735	12	350	240 × 320	Cover whole pelvis
PD TSE	Cor	3 mm	3000–3500	34–38	160	192 × 256	Unilateral
PD TSE FS	Sag	3 mm	2900–3000	22–35	160	256 × 256	Unilateral
T2 TSE FS	Ax Straight	3 mm	3500–4500	40	200	224 × 256	Unilateral

Abbreviations: STIR, short tau inversion recovery; PD, proton density; TSE, turbo spin echo; FS, fat suppressed; Cor, coronal; Sag, sagittal; Ax, axial; Obl, oblique; Tr, repetition time; Te, excitation time; FOV, field of view.

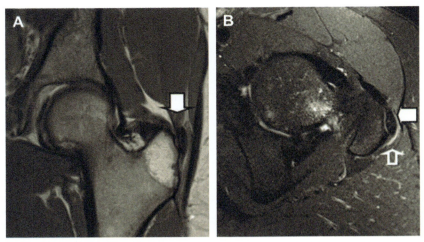

Fig. 3. (A) Coronal PD and (B) axial oblique fat-suppressed PD-weighted images show increased tendon size and signal related to tendinopathy ([A,B] solid arrows) and fluid signal around the tendon ([B] open arrow) related to peritendinitis of the lateral portion of gluteus medius.

tendons[12] and proximal hamstring tendons[13] are common in the asymptomatic population[12] and underscore the point that not all tendinopathy is symptomatic.[3] Imaging findings do not always correlate with clinical symptoms and it is the onus of the clinician to determine their relevance.

ANTERIOR PAIN

- Disorders of the origin of the ITB
- Disorders of the iliopsoas tendon
  - Tendinopathy/tendon tears
  - Internal snapping hip
  - Iliopsoas impingement

- Disorders of the tendon origin of rectus femoris

Abnormalities of the Origin of the Iliotibial Band

As the attachment site of tensor fascia lata as well as the external and internal abdominal oblique, transverse abdominis, and gluteus medius,[14] the iliac crest apophysis is at risk for injury in adolescent athletes. Seen in long distance runners between the ages of 13 and 25 years, iliac crest apophysitis is the result of repetitive submaximal traction of the unfused apophysis.

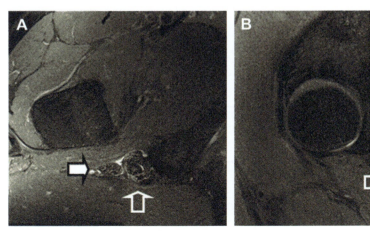

Fig. 4. (A) Axial oblique and (B) sagittal fat-suppressed PD-weighted image in a 51-year-old runner complaining of pain with prolonged sitting and sciatica. Severe tendinopathy ([A,B] open arrows) with superimposed partial tear ([B] white bracket) of the semimembranosus tendon at its insertion. There is also fluid tracking around the sciatic nerve (solid white arrow).

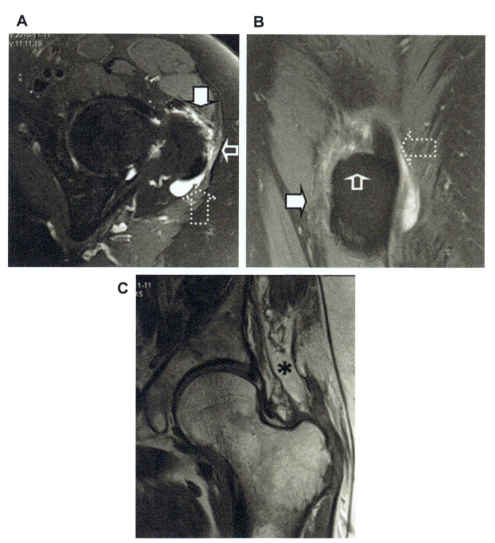

Fig. 5. (*A*) Axial oblique and (*B*) sagittal fat-suppressed intermediate-weighted images and (*C*) coronal PD-weighted image of the left hip. Complete gluteus minimus (*white arrows*) and lateral portion of gluteus medius (*open white arrows*) tear. Both muscles are atrophied ([*C*] *asterisk*); therefore, surgical repair is not an option. The posterior insertion of gluteus medius (*dotted open white arrows*) is intact.

Pathology at origin of the ITB has also been recently reported in a small cohort of adult women[15] from two disparate groups—young athletes and older overweight women.

Anatomy

The ITB represents a thickening of the fascial investiture of tensor fascia lata and gluteus maximus muscles. It originates at the iliac crest apophysis, which appears at approximately age 13 and fuses at age 25. The ITB divides into deep and superficial layers to envelop the tensor fascia lata muscle. At the hip, the ITB receives contributions from gluteus maximus fascia before it continues distally toward its major insertion on the anterolateral tibia at Gerdy tubercle.[16]

The ITB helps stabilize the extended knee and hip,[17] in part through the contraction of gluteus maximus and tensor fascia lata muscles, which tighten it.[16]

Imaging

Adequate coverage is the most important aspect of imaging. The authors' routine large FOV coronal STIR sequence of the pelvis always includes the iliac crest and allows evaluating this region on all

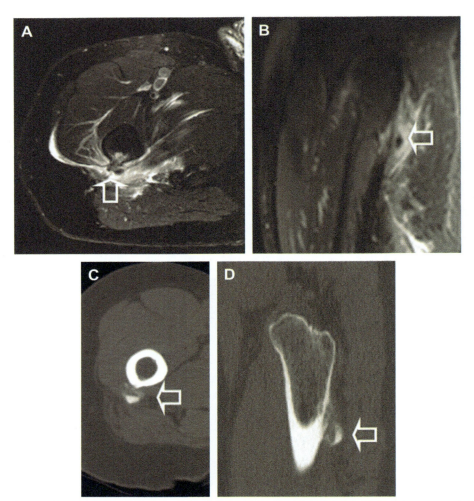

Fig. 6. Calcific tendinitis. (*A*) Axial and (*B*) sagittal fat-suppressed PD-weighted images of the proximal right thigh in 47-year-old man presenting with atraumatic hip and thigh pain. There is exuberant soft tissue edema centered on an ovoid focus of low signal at the femoral insertion of the gluteus maximus tendon (*open white arrow*). The subjacent cortex is thinned and irregular, and there is edema in the marrow space related to intraosseous extension. (*C*) Axial and (*D*) sagittal reformatted CT examination in another patient demonstrates a focal deposit with internal fluid/calcium level (*open white arrow*) adjacent to the linea aspera of the femur.

patients. When pathology in this region is clinically suspected, this region is included in the axial and sagittal imaging FOV and both anatomic and fluid-sensitive sequences are performed.

In skeletally immature individuals, MR imaging findings of apophyseal widening (3–5 mm), physeal signal hyperintensity, and marrow and muscle edema on fluid-sensitive sequences[18] have been reported after injury (**Fig. 7**). Acute injury in adults manifests as edema in/around the ITB and within its iliac enthesis on fluid-sensitive sequences (**Fig. 8**). Thickening of the proximal ITB can be seen on both anatomic and fluid-sensitive sequences in the chronic setting.

Abnormalities Related to the Iliopsoas Tendon

The iliopsoas tendon represents the distal termination of the psoas major and iliacus muscles. Together, these muscles flex the thigh, participate in lateral hip rotation, and contribute to pelvic stability when seated.[19] Abnormalities related to the iliopsoas tendon include tendinopathy, tendon tears, internal snapping hip, and iliopsoas tendon impingement.

Anatomy

The iliopsoas compartment is an elongated extraperitoneal space that extends from the

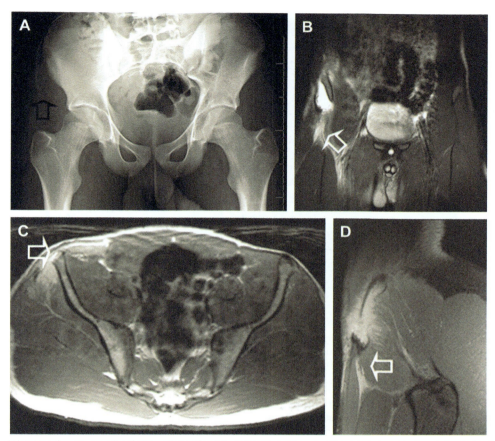

Fig. 7. (*A*) Frontal radiograph of the pelvis of a 14-year-old runner on the track team who experienced a pop while running. The iliac crest apophysis is avulsed and displaced on the right (*open black arrow*). (*B*) Coronal and (*C*) axial fat-suppressed intermediate-weighted and (*D*) sagittal fat-suppressed PD-weighted images show the avulsed cortical fragment ([*C*] *open white arrow*) with attached tensor fascia lata ([*D*] *open arrow*).

posterior mediastinum to the hip joint. It is roofed by the iliopsoas fascia and contains the psoas major and iliacus muscles, and, when present, the psoas minor muscle.[20]

The long fusiform psoas major muscle arises from lumbar and T12 transverse processes; the fan-like iliacus muscle arises from the inner iliac fossa. As the 2 muscles merge at the L5-S2 level, a groove is formed at their lateral interface. It is through this fat-filled groove that the femoral nerve and iliolumbar vessels bundle are transmitted.[21] The composite iliopsoas muscle exits the pelvis under the inguinal ligament; its tendon inserts on the lesser trochanter. In addition to its tendinous insertion, the iliacus muscle also inserts directly on the anterior femur and distal lesser trochanter. When fluid distended, the iliopsoas bursa can be seen between the iliacus muscle, the psoas tendon, and the anterior hip joint capsule.[22]

Three things are important about the iliopsoas musculotendinous unit with regards to pathology.

First, the tendons lie in a shallow groove in the pelvic brim as they exit the pelvis. Second, they course immediately adjacent to the anterosuperior aspect of the hip joint on the way to their insertion. Third, the iliacus and psoas tendons may merge together or attach separately on the lesser trochanter, the iliacus tendon more lateral than the psoas, and the identification of 2 separate tendons should not be mistaken for a tear.

Iliopsoas tendinopathy/tendon tear

Iliopsoas tendon pathology in adults is an uncommonly reported cause of anterior hip pain. Whereas lesser trochanteric apophysitis and apophyseal avulsions are common in active children and adolescents, spontaneous lesser tuberosity avulsions in adults are considered pathologic until proved otherwise (**Fig. 9**).[23]

Iliopsoas tendinopathy and tendon rupture in adults are uncommon in radiology. Tendinopathy may present as groin pain exacerbated by hip

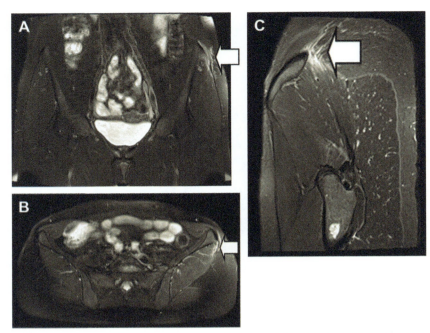

Fig. 8. (A) Coronal, (B) axial, and (C) sagittal fat-suppressed PD-weighted images of the pelvis in a 34-year-old long distance runner who experienced sudden onset pain during marathon run 1 month previously. There is fluid signal around the origin of the ITB at the iliac crest (*white arrows*).

flexion and adduction[24] and has been reported in both kicking sports and in nonathletes.[19] Spontaneous rupture has been reported in elderly individuals who presented with severe groin pain after minor trauma.[25] Bui and colleagues[24] retrospectively studied a small cohort of patients with ruptured iliopsoas tendons and found hip pain the most common presenting symptom and occult fracture the most common clinical diagnosis. Iliopsoas tendon and myotendinous injuries had a prevalence of 0.66% in their series of 4862 pelvic and hip MR images; myotendinous strains and partial tears predominated among those younger than 65 years old, and complete tears made up half of the injuries in those over age 65. Tendon tears are reported to occur close to or at the lesser trochanter insertion and commonly spare the more lateral iliacus muscular component.[26]

MR imaging features seen in tendon rupture include a thickened and discontinuous tendon, a groin mass related to fluid around the torn and retracted psoas tendon and thickened distal iliopsoas muscle, and proximal muscle swelling and edema (**Fig. 10**).[24]

Internal snapping hip syndrome

Snapping hip (coxa saltans) refers to a broad category of dynamic pathology that presents with pain and audible snap. There are 3 categories of snapping hip: external (related to the iliotibial and or gluteus maximus), intra-articular (related to intra-articular processes), and internal (related to the iliopsoas tendon).[27]

Anatomy At the pelvic brim, the iliopsoas tendon lies in a shallow depression between the iliopectineal eminence (medially) and the anterior inferior iliac spine (laterally); it is overlaid by the iliacus and psoas muscles when the hip is flexed.[28]

The tendon undergoes normal medial translation as the hip goes from flexion to extension (**Fig. 11**). Gliding is facilitated by the iliopsoas bursa, which lies between the iliopsoas muscle and the iliopectineal eminence.[29]

In the setting of internal snapping hip syndrome, however, the tendon painfully catches as the hip is brought from a flexed, abducted, and externally rotated position into extension with internal rotation. It may snap over the iliopectineal eminence, the femoral head,[28,30] or over a lesser trochanteric exostosis[31] as it does. The audible or palpable snapping can be voluntarily reproduced and occurs when stair climbing or rising from a seated position.[32] The tendon's proximity to the hip joint may cause one to mistaken its symptoms for intra-articular pathology; furthermore, intra-articular pathology and snapping hip may coexist.[33]

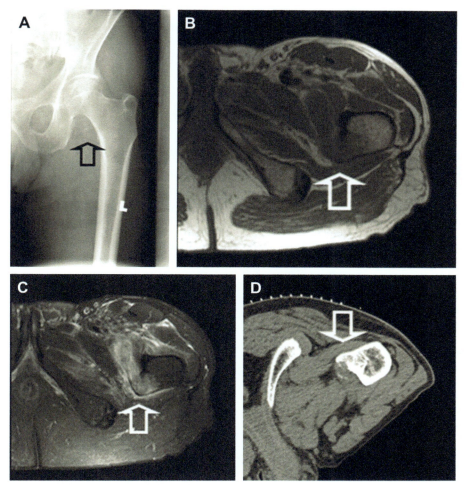

Fig. 9. Frontal radiograph of the left hip (*A*) shows avulsion of the lesser trochanter (*open black arrow*) in this 63-year-old man with history of adenocarcinoma. (*B*) Axial T1 and (*C*) axial fat-suppressed T2-weighted images show a destructive lesion in the lesser trochanter (*open white arrow*) and fluid and debris in the torn tendon gap ([*C*]). (*D*) Prone axial oblique image of the patient obtained at time of CT-guided biopsy shows the lesion in the lesser trochanter (*open white arrow*), histologically proved to be metastasis.

Asymptomatic hip snapping is present in up to 10% of the population and can be differentiated from snapping hip syndrome by the absence of pain.

Imaging There are no MR imaging–specific findings for this entity. Sonography, however, can be diagnostic. Not only can it document tendon dyskinesia and its relationship to the development of pain and symptoms but also it can be used to provide guidance for anesthetic/steroid injections.[34] Sonographic findings (inhomogeneous tendon appearance, hip effusion, and distended iliopsoas bursa),[35] however, are only inconsistently observed in patients with symptomatic snapping hip and have not been corroborated by MR imaging.

Positive response to anesthetic challenge is considered diagnostic. Conservative measures (rest and corticosteroid injections) are the mainstay of treatment. Endoscopic distal tendon release can be considered in recalcitrant cases.[32]

Iliopsoas impingement

Iliopsoas impingement in the setting of total hip arthroplasty Tendon impingement in the setting of total hip arthroplasty (THA) is well known to orthopedic surgeons although it remains a poorly understood reason for postoperative pain. One study reports 4.3% prevalence in patients with pain after THA.[36]

The iliopsoas tendon and the anterosuperior hip joint are closely apposed structures (**Fig. 12**), and mechanical tendon impingement may be caused by presence of a prominent or

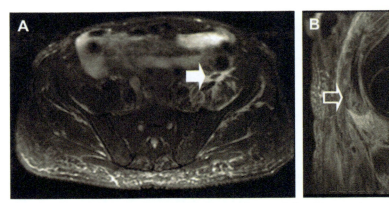

Fig. 10. (*A*) Axial and (*B*) sagittal fat-suppressed intermediate-weighted images in an 80-year-old woman who presented with acute onset left hip pain and numbness. She was clinically suspected of having femoral nerve entrapment. The iliopsoas tendon and muscle are completely torn and retracted ([*B*] *open white arrow*). There is diffuse iliopspoas muscle edema on the left, along with fluid surrounding the femoral nerve in the pelvis ([*A*] *solid white arrow*).

malpositioned acetabular component,[37,38] retained cement,[38] excessively long screws,[38] an acetabular cage, or reinforcement ring.[39] Limb length discrepancy is also another reported cause of impingement.[40]

Metal artifact–reducing MR imaging sequences may increase the role of MR imaging in the future with regards to the work-up of patients with pain after arthroplasty.[41] At present, imaging's role is in guiding diagnostic and therapeutic iliopsoas bursal injections (**Fig. 13**), which are a part of the diagnosis and conservative treatment of affected individuals.[42]

Iliopsoas impingement in the native hip Iliopsoas impingement in the native hip[43] is a subject of debate at society meetings although not widely published in the literature.

The arthroscopic observation of labral tears immediately subjacent to the iliopsoas tendon has led some investigators to postulate a new pathomechanism for labral injury. In small series, these labral tears were observed in patients who underwent arthroscopic iliopsoas tendon release for the treatment of internal snapping hip.[44,45] Heyworth and colleagues[46] observed 7 of 24 patients with a tight psoas tendon overlying and

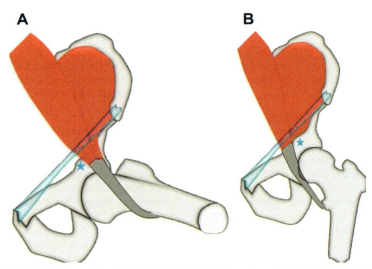

Fig. 11. Internal snapping hip. When the hip is flexed (*A*), the iliopsoas tendon (in grey) is lateral to the iliopectineal eminence (*blue star*). When the hip is extended (*B*), the iliopsoas tendon translates medial to the iliopectineal eminence.

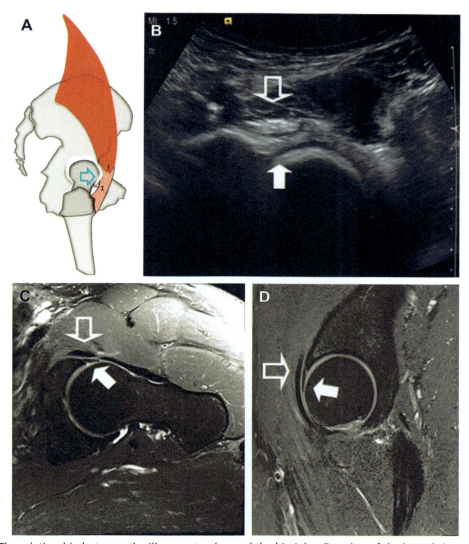

Fig. 12. The relationship between the iliopsoas tendon and the hip joint. Drawing of the lateral view of the hip (*A*) shows that the iliopsoas tendon (I) passes anterior to the anterior aspect of the hip and lies adjacent to the anterosuperior labrum (*open blue arrow*). Long axis view of the femoral neck by ultrasound (*B*), axial oblique (*C*) fat-suppressed PD and sagittal (*D*) fat-suppressed intermediate weighted images show the normally close relationship between the iliopsoas tendon ([*B–D*] *open white arrow*) with the anterior hip joint and the anterosuperior labrum ([*B–D*] *solid white arrow*).

impinging on a torn or inflamed anterior labrum; in these patients, labral impingement was relieved by psoas tendon release. The peculiar location of labral tears in this group (2–3 o'clock as opposed to 11:30–1 o'clock that is characteristic in femoroacetabular impingement) led these investigators to postulate that labral injury was a result of mechanical compression of the capsulolabral complex by the iliopsoas tendon. It remains to be seen if a causal relationship exists, and if so, whether this can be prospectively diagnosed by imaging.

Blankenbaker and colleagues[47] have begun to investigate this entity with MR imaging in patients intraoperatively diagnosed with and arthroscopically treated with tenotomy at the labral level.

Disorders of the Proximal Rectus Femoris Tendon

The long, fusiform muscle of rectus femoris originates from 2 distinct tendons—the direct tendon from the anterior–inferior iliac spine and the

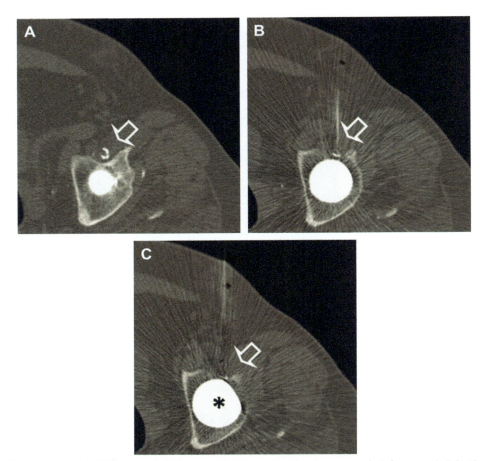

Fig. 13. Contiguous axial CT images (*A–C*) from cranial to caudal after image-guided therapeutic injection of the iliopsoas tendon sheath in a patient with clinically diagnosed iliopsoas impingement. Iodinated hyperdense contrast outlines the iliopsoas tendon in its tendon sheath as it crosses anterior hip joint (*open white arrows*). Proximity to the acetabular cup (*asterisk*) is best seen on the most caudal image (*C*). The patient reported symptomatic relief after the injection.

indirect (also known as reflected) tendon from the superior acetabular ridge and hip joint capsule. The 2 tendons merge shortly after their origins to form a conjoint tendon, with fibers from the direct composing much of the anterior tendon and fibers from the indirect tendon composing much of the posterior.[48]

Rectus femoris extends the knee, flexes the hip, and stabilizes the pelvis on the femur in weight bearing. It is the only component of the powerful quadriceps muscle group that crosses 2 joints and, as such, is the most commonly injured muscle of the 4. Injuries most often occur at the myotendinous junction and most frequently involve the reflected head, where they are also known as central aponeurotic injuries.[48]

Rectus femoris tendon origin injuries, however, are far less common than myotendinous ones. Apophyseal injuries at the origin of rectus femoris

are well known in adolescent athletes, particularly soccer players in whom forceful kicking requires extreme hip hyperextension followed by forceful hip flexion and knee extension.[49] Injuries occur when a player's kick is forcefully blocked or when kicking the air.[50] Avulsion fractures in skeletally mature athletes are also reported; the avulsed fragment is commonly small and can be difficult to detect on plain radiographs.[51] As they heal, the abundant reactive ossification around these injuries can be mistaken for ossified masses (**Fig. 14**).[52]

Pure soft tissue injury of the tendon origin of rectus femoris in adults is less common and there is a paucity of published reports on it. In their retrospective review of more than 3000 pelvic and hip MR studies, Ouellette and colleagues[52] found an overall incidence of 0.5% (17/3160); slightly more than half their patients presented after trauma

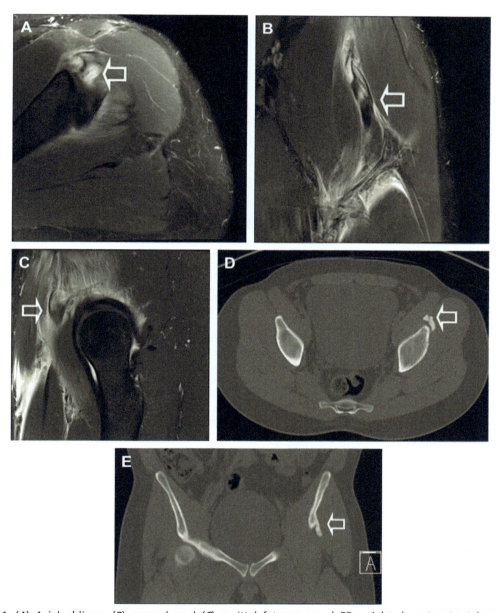

Fig. 14. (A) Axial oblique, (B) coronal, and (C) sagittal fat-suppressed PD-weighted postcontrast images in a 26-year-old man who "fell 10 days ago." There is a high-grade partial tear of the origin of the direct head of rectus femoris (*open arrows*). (D) Axial and (E) coronal reformatted CT images 6 months later when the patient returned for work-up of another condition. Heterotopic ossification has developed at the site of tendon tear ([D,E] *open arrow*).

and indirect head injuries outnumbered direct ones. Rectus femoris origin injuries are also reported to occur an average of once per season in the National Football League, affecting both kicking and nonkicking positions.[49] MR imaging findings include peritendinitis, tendinopathy, and tear (**Figs. 14** and **15**).

LATERAL PAIN AND THE PERITROCHANTERIC SPACE

- Disorders of the hip abductor tendons
- ESHS

Abnormalities of the peritrochanteric space were under-recognized until the widespread use of hip

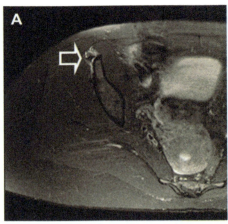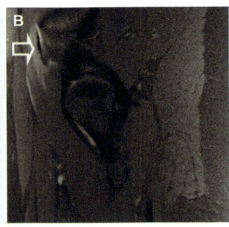

Fig. 15. Axial (*A*) and sagittal (*B*) fat-suppressed intermediate-weighted images in a 42-year-old woman who experienced a pop in her hip during dance class. There is a partial tear or the direct head of rectus femoris from its origin (*open white arrow*).

arthroscopy. They are increasingly implicated as common causes of lateral hip pain. Peritrochanteric pathology falls into 2 major clinical diagnoses: greater trochanteric pain syndrome (GTPS) and ESHS.

Greater Trochanteric Pain Syndrome and Disorders of the Hip Abductor Tendons

Previously known as greater trochanteric bursitis, GTPS is the preferred term for the spectrum of abnormalities of the hip abductor tendons (gluteus medius and minimus) and peritrochanteric bursae. In a study of more than 3000 adults, Sega and colleagues[53] found the prevalence of GTPS 17.6%, with higher prevalence in women and those with coexisting low back pain, osteoarthritis, ITB tenderness, and obesity.[54]

The most common presentation is that of chronic persistent lateral hip and/or buttock pain exacerbated by lying on the affected side, prolonged standing, or transitioning to a standing position. Half of affected individuals complain of lateral thigh pain that radiates to the knee. Patients are tender to palpation over the greater trochanter. Because the hip abductors play an important role in gait and hip joint stability, affected individuals can present with Trendelenburg gait as a result of weak hip abduction.

Anatomy

The peritrochanteric space is an anatomic space between the ITB and the greater trochanteric structures (hip abductor tendons and bursae).

Also known as the rotator cuff of the hip, the gluteus minimus and medius musculotendinous units form a continuous soft tissue envelope over the greater trochanter. Gluteus minimus broadly

arises from the external iliac fossa and inserts on the anterior facet of the greater trochanter (**Fig. 16**B). A second musculotendinous slip attaches to the ventral/superior aspect of the joint capsule. Gluteus minimus is a secondary hip abductor and helps stabilize the femoral head in the acetabulum.[55] Gluteus medius has 2 distinct insertion sites (see **Fig. 16**C). The posterior muscle fibers coalesce into a stout posterior tendon that inserts on the posterior facet; the central and anterior fibers form a rectangular muscular insertion on the lateral facet. This tendon arrangement can be seen on far lateral sagittal MR images (see **Fig. 16**C).

Imaging

Axial/axial oblique images show the tendons to best advantage. On contiguous images, broad posterior gluteus medius tendon fibers coalesce into a stout tendon that inserts on the posterior facet. At the same level, central and anterior fibers form the predominantly muscular lateral facet insertion. The greater trochanter has a smoothly curved posterolateral surface on straight axial images at the insertion of gluteus medius (see **Fig. 16**A).

The gluteus minimus insertion is more distal and is located on the anteriorly-facing surface of the anterior facet, identified by the angular lateral contour of the greater trochanter (see **Fig. 3**B). Because of the anterior facet's orientation, the trochanteric insertion of the gluteus minimus is rarely seen to advantage on the coronal images.

Gluteus medius and minimus tendinopathy/ tear

The abductor tendons can be affected by peritenditinitis (see **Fig. 3**), tendinopathy (see **Fig. 3**), and tendon tears (**Fig. 17**). Tendon pathology may or may not be accompanied by distension of

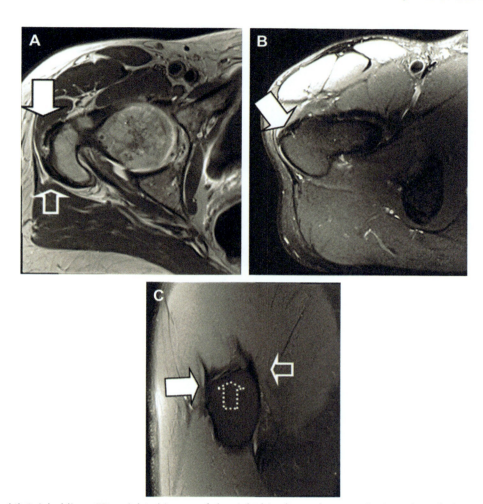

Fig. 16. (*A*) Axial oblique PD-weighted image of the right hip shows the posterior insertion of gluteus medius (*open white arrow*) and the tendon of gluteus minimus (*white arrow*) proximal to its insertion. (*B*) Axial oblique fat-suppressed PD-weighted image caudal to A at the insertion of gluteus minimus (*white arrow*). (*C*) Sagittal fat-suppressed PD-weighted image shows the insertions of gluteus minimus (*white arrow*) and both the lateral (*dotted arrow*) and posterior (*open white arrow*) insertions of gluteus medius.

anatomic bursae located deep to and named for their corresponding tendon.

In a sonographic study of 75 patients with GTPS, gluteus medius tendinosis manifested as tendon enlargement and diffuse echogenicity.[56] Tears most commonly affected the deep anterior fibers of the lateral muscular insertion of gluteus medius. Tendon gaps were frequently filled with fluid.[56]

Tendon discontinuity on MR imaging can be detected and corroborated in multiple planes. As is true in the shoulder, deep undersurface tears are not apparent during arthroscopy of the peritrochanteric space, and a comment about tear location is helpful to arthroscopists; similarly the presence of muscle atrophy have implications in management (see **Fig. 5**C).

MR imaging had sensitivity of 33% to 100%, specificity of 92% to 100%, positive predictive value of 71% to 100%, and negative predictive value of 50% for the detection of hip abductor pathology in a recent meta-analysis. Sonography had a sensitivity of 79% to 100% and positive predictive value of 95% to 100%.[20]

This level of detail, however, is not always possible on large FOV sequences of the pelvis and examinations done at lower field strengths, where even tendon discontinuity can be undetectable in the absence of significant tendon retraction. Secondary signs of tendon pathology become more important in this circumstance. Cvitanic and colleagues[57] found high T2 signal above the greater trochanter larger than 1 cm or thin high T2 signal lateral and superior to the greater trochanter

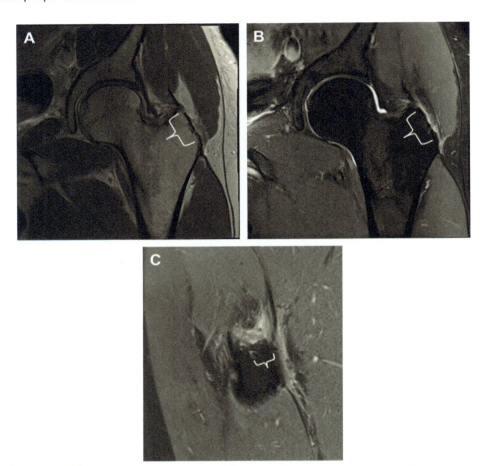

Fig. 17. (*A*) Coronal PD, (*B*) coronal fat-suppressed PD, and (*C*) sagittal fat-suppressed PD-weighted images in a 46-year-old who woman who presented with atraumatic hip pain. The lateral trochanteric facet is bare (*brackets*) due to a completely retracted tear of the lateral portion of gluteus medius.

to be the most specific secondary signs. High T2 signal had the greatest positive and negative predictive value for abductor tendon tears. Elongation of the gluteus medius tendon greater than 2 cm in the coronal plane also proved helpful in the detection of tendon pathology.

GTPS is treated by rest, physical therapy, anti-inflammatory medications, and corticosteroid injections, which are successful in the vast majority of patients. Open repair, particularly for full thickness tears, is an option in cases recalcitrant to conservative measures.[58] Endoscopic repair has emerged as a less-invasive treatment option requiring less rehabilitation and has been associated with relief of pain and return of hip abductor strength in small series.[59]

External Snapping Hip Syndrome

The ITB is not a static structure. Its tension can be increased by contraction of gluteus maximus and tensor fascia lata.[16] The ITB also translates anterior-posterior during hip and knee flexion and extension (**Fig. 18**) and is subject to biomechanical forces as it traverses lateral to the greater trochanter at the hip and lateral to the lateral femoral condyle as it crosses the knee.

Coxa saltans externa, or external snapping hip, is the most common of the 3 types of hip snapping. ESHS refers to painful catching of a pathologically thickened posterior third of the ITB or anterior edge of gluteus maximus as it translates anterior and posterior to the greater trochanter during hip flexion and extension. Patients may report a subjective sensation of subluxation and dislocation, leading some investigators to refer to this entity as *pseudosubluxation*.

The cause of ITB thickening is likely multifactorial but not completely understood. Although symptoms may manifest after trauma, most are associated with repetitive motions related to work or sport and have been reported in ballet dancers, cyclists, runners, and soccer players.[60] ESHS is also reported after surgery where the

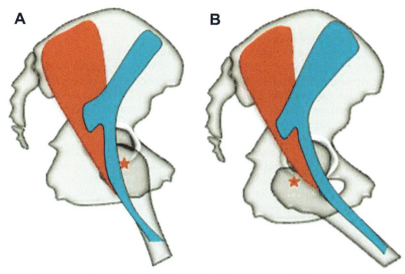

Fig. 18. Anteroposterior translation of the ITB. When the hip is extended (A), the ITB (*blue*) and the margin of gluteus maximus (*red*) are posterior to the greater trochanter (*red star*). As the hip is flexed (B), the ITB and gluteus maximus translate anterior to the greater trochanter.

ITB was the source of graft, or when surgery results in an overly prominent greater trochanter. Coxa valga and reduced bi-iliac width are also cited as potential predisposing conditions.[61,62]

Little has been written on the imaging findings of this entity. Pelsser and colleagues[35] studied a small group of patients with sonography in whom half the snapping hips were painful. Although they demonstrated the dynamic aspects of this entity and their association with pain under direct sonography, they could not establish an association with increased ITB thickness and trochanteric bursitis.

Treatment is conservative. Surgery is reserved for recalcitrant cases and includes arthroscopic release of the thickened tissue.

POSTERIOR PAIN

- Disorders of the proximal hamstring tendons
  - Hamstring tendinopathy
  - Hamstring tendon tear

Posterior pain is less common than anterior, lateral, and medial pain[63] and is most frequently secondary to lumbar spine disease or sacroiliac joint dysfunction. Proximal hamstring pathology, including tendinopathy and tendon rupture, is less commonly encountered. Gluteal/posterior thigh pain can present a diagnostic challenge to clinicians, and MR imaging is often enlisted for its work-up.[64]

Disorders of the Hamstring Tendons

Injuries to the hamstring myotendinous unit are common, particularly in athletes. Eccentric muscle contraction plays an important role in these injuries.

Whereas concentric muscle contraction results in an increase in muscle tension coincident with muscle shortening (as occurs during the flexion portion of a biceps curl), eccentric muscle contraction results in an increase in muscle tension coincident with muscle lengthening (as occurs during the extension portion of a biceps curl). This serves to dissipate/store energy and absorb shock, which are crucial in decelerating a limb or body segment. Generally, eccentric contractions generate greater loads than concentric ones; correspondingly tendons of muscles, which participate in eccentric contractions are subject to greater tensile loads. In the case of the hamstring muscle group, eccentric contraction occurs during walking and running; it decelerates the extended knee before foot strike, assists with hip extension after foot strike, then extends the knee during the takeoff phase. If the forces needed to decelerate exceed the strength of the myotendinous unit, the muscle, the myotendinous unit or the tendon can fail.

The hamstring muscle group is most commonly injured at its weak myotendinous junction; this most often affects the long head of biceps femoris.[65] Myotendinous junction injuries are clinically evaluated, treated conservatively, and generally do well.

Proximal hamstring tendinopathy is the result of chronic repetitive eccentric overload.[66] Also known as hamstring syndrome, ischiatic intersection syndrome, hamstring enthesopathy, high hamstring tendinopathy, and hamstring origin tendinopathy,[67] this is commonly seen in running athletes and in soccer and football players.

The most serious hamstring injuries are tendon ruptures.[68] They affect both the athletic and middle-aged nonathletic populations and are the result of voluntary or involuntary forceful eccentric muscle contraction, as can occur when there is sudden and simultaneous forced hip flexion and knee extension. Excessive passive lengthening, seen in ballet dancers, is a less common cause.

Surprisingly, distinguishing between myotendinous strain (treated conservatively) and tendon rupture (potentially treated surgically) can be difficult. Approximately 25% of hamstring strength comes from the short head biceps femoris; therefore, some hamstring strength may remain despite complete proximal tendon rupture. The presence of blood products may make palpation of a tendon gap difficult on physical examination. MR imaging is often necessary to make the diagnosis and define the extent of injury.

Anatomy

The hamstring muscle group consists of semimembranosus, semitendinosus and the long head of biceps femoris; together they play a role in knee flexion and hip extension and affect pelvic tilt and rotation, sacral rotation and extension, and hip rotation.[69]

The hamstring muscles arise from the ischial tuberosity, with the exception of the short head of the biceps femoris, which takes its origin from the lower lateral linea aspera at the midfemoral shaft and lateral supracondylar line of the femur.

Semitendinosus and long head of the biceps femoris have a conjoint origin from the posteromedial aspect of the ischial tuberosity. Semimembranosus arises from a long flat tendon at the

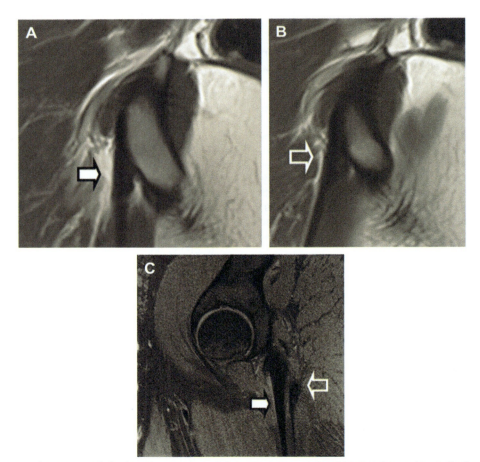

Fig. 19. Normal anatomy of the hamstring origin. (*A*) Coronal PD-weighted image shows the vertically oriented origin of semimembranosus (*white arrow*). (*B*) Coronal PD-weighted image shows the oblique origin of the conjoint biceps femoris and semitendinosus tendon, which points laterally (*open white arrow*). (*C*) Sagittal fat-suppressed T2-weighted image shows semimembranosus tendon (*white arrow*) anterior to the conjoint tendon (*open white arrow*).

posterolateral aspect of the ischial tuberosity, lateral to the conjoint tendon of the biceps femoris and semitendinosus.

Imaging

Although the hamstring origin consists of 3 structures, on MR imaging, the origin of the hamstring muscle complex is dominated by the appearance of 2 tendons—those of semimembranosus and biceps femoris.

The 2 can be distinguished in the coronal plane; whereas the semimembranosus tendon is vertically oriented at its origin (**Fig. 19**A), the biceps femoris tendon points lateral toward its ultimate distal insertion at the fibula (see **Fig. 19**B). In the sagittal plane, the semimembranosus tendon is located anterior and lateral to the conjoint (see **Fig. 19**C).

In contrast, the semitendinosus origin is predominantly muscular; its small tendon seen may not be appreciated on MR imaging. Semitendinosus arises from the medial surface of the long head biceps femoris tendon and from the ischial tuberosity.[70]

Hamstring Tendinopathy

High hamstring tendinopathy (see **Fig. 4**) is an uncommon overuse injury seen in young athletes involved in sports that require bursts of speed and repetitive hip stretch, such as football, soccer, basketball, sprinting, rowing, and kickboxing. Patients typically report deep buttock or thigh pain when running and when seated.[71] Pain radiating

into the popliteal fossa often suggests sciatic nerve involvement,[72] which can result in chronic pain if scar forms around the secondarily involved nerve.

There is little information on the imaging of this entity in the published literature. Zissen and colleagues' retrospective review of 65 patients treated by sonographic guided tendon injection[73] revealed peritendinitis (63%) as the most common preinjection MR imaging finding. Tendinopathy was seen in 25%, and no tendon abnormalities were seen in 22%. Of the 3 tendons, semimembranosus is the most commonly affected.[64] De Smet and colleagues[13] found that symptomatic patients were more likely to have a thickened tendon, peritendinous increased T2 signal, and reactive edema of the ischial tuberosity, although there was considerable overlap between symptomatic and asymptomatic patients with regards to the presence of signal abnormality.

Anti-inflammatory medications and physical therapy are successful in the majority of patients. Semimembranosus tenotomy is considered when conservative management fails.[64]

Hamstring Tendon Tear

Proximal hamstring tendon avulsions are common in adult football players, runners, water skiers, cheerleaders, gymnasts, and dancers. These most commonly occur at their origin, and most frequently affect the conjoint tendon with variable involvement of semimembranosus. In contrast to

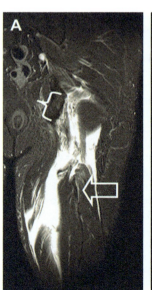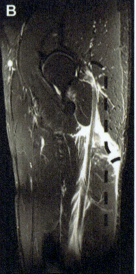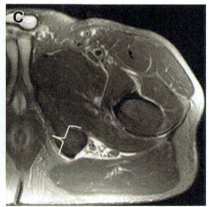

Fig. 20. (A) Coronal and (B) sagittal STIR and (C) axial fat-suppressed T2-weighted images in a 50-year-old man who presented after water-skiing injury. The ischial tuberosity is bare ([A and C] *white bracket*) where the tendons were avulsed and retracted ([A] *open white arrow*). Note the extensive edema along the length of the sciatic nerve (*black bracket*).

children, in whom osseous avulsions are common, adult injuries are often soft tissue (**Fig. 20**). Patients report a pop or snap; this is followed by posterior thigh pain, weakness, and sensation of giving away and avoid sitting on the affected side because of pain.

The role of imaging is to confirm the diagnosis and evaluate the extent of the disease. Although there is some variation among practitioners, most agree that single tendon ruptures and multitendon ruptures retracted less than 2 cm may be treated conservatively[74] because torn tendons tend to scar to intact tendons, allowing for return to full strength.

SUMMARY

Tendon pathology is a common cause of hip pain but can be difficult to diagnose by physical examination. Imaging, in particular MR imaging, is integral in the work-up because of its ability to evaluate both the hip joint and its surrounding tendons. An anatomy-based search process can facilitate MR imaging interpretation and ensure that tendon abnormalities are considered in the differential diagnosis of nonarthritic hip pain.

REFERENCES

1. Anon. National ambulatory medical care survey. Hyattsville (MD): National Center for Health Statistics; 1995. CHS CD-ROM series 13, no. 11. Issued July 1997.

2. Martin RL, Irrgang JJ, Sekiya JK. The diagnostic accuracy of a clinical examination in determining intra-articular hip pain for potential hip arthroscopy candidates. Arthroscopy 2008;24(9):1013–8.

3. Maffulli N, Wong J, Almekinders LC. Types and epidemiology of tendinopathy. Clin Sports Med 2003;22(4):675–92.

4. Anon. American College of Radiology. ACR Appropriateness Criteria®: Chronic Hip Pain. Available at: http://www.acr.org/~/media/ACR/Documents/AppCriteria/Diagnostic/ChronicHipPain.pdf. Accessed July 12, 2012.

5. Kong A, Van der Vliet A, Zadow S. MRI and US of gluteal tendinopathy in greater trochanteric pain syndrome. Eur Radiol 2007;17(7):1772–83.

6. Li T, Mirowitz SA. Manifestation of magic angle phenomenon: comparative study on effects of varying echo time and tendon orientation among various MR sequences. Magn Reson Imaging 2003;21(7):741–4.

7. Kraemer EJ, El-Khoury GY. Atypical calcific tendinitis with cortical erosions. Skeletal Radiol 2000; 29(12):690–6.

8. Bui-Mansfield LT, Moak M. Magnetic resonance appearance of bone marrow edema associated with hydroxyapatite deposition disease without cortical erosion. J Comput Assist Tomogr 2005;29(1):103–7.

9. Yang I, Hayes CW, Biermann JS. Calcific tendinitis of the gluteus medius tendon with bone marrow edema mimicking metastatic disease. Skeletal Radiol 2002; 31(6):359–61.

10. Flemming DJ, Murphey MD, Shekitka KM, et al. Osseous involvement in calcific tendinitis: a retrospective review of 50 cases. AJR Am J Roentgenol 2003;181(4):965–72.

11. Hottat N, Fumière E, Delcour C. Calcific tendinitis of the gluteus maximus tendon: CT findings. Eur Radiol 1999;9(6):1104–6.

12. Blankenbaker DG, Ullrick SR, Davis KW, et al. Correlation of MRI findings with clinical findings of trochanteric pain syndrome. Skeletal Radiol 2008; 37(10):903–9.

13. De Smet AA, Blankenbaker DG, Alsheik NH, et al. MRI appearance of the proximal hamstring tendons in patients with and without symptomatic proximal hamstring tendinopathy. AJR Am J Roentgenol 2012;198(2):418–22.

14. Micheli LJ, Fehlandt AF Jr. Overuse injuries to tendons and apophyses in children and adolescents. Clin Sports Med 1992;11(4):713–26.

15. Sher I, Umans H, Downie SA, et al. Proximal iliotibial band syndrome: what is it and where is it? Skeletal Radiol 2011;40(12):1553–6.

16. Birnbaum K, Siebert CH, Pandorf T, et al. Anatomical and biomechanical investigations of the iliotibial tract. Surg Radiol Anat 2004;26(6):433–46.

17. Kaplan EB. The iliotibial tract; clinical and morphological significance. J Bone Joint Surg Am 1958; 40(4):817–32.

18. Hébert KJ, Laor T, Divine JG, et al. MRI appearance of chronic stress injury of the iliac crest apophysis in adolescent athletes. AJR Am J Roentgenol 2008; 190(6):1487–91.

19. Shabshin N, Rosenberg ZS, Cavalcanti CF. MR imaging of iliopsoas musculotendinous injuries. Magn Reson Imaging Clin N Am 2005;13(4):705–16.

20. Torres GM, Cernigliaro JG, Abbitt PL, et al. Iliopsoas compartment: normal anatomy and pathologic processes. Radiographics 1995;15(6):1285–97.

21. Ishigami K, Yoshimitsu K, Irie H, et al. Lesions arising in or involving the iliopsoas groove. J Comput Assist Tomogr 2008;32(6):975–81.

22. Aliabadi P, Baker ND, Jaramillo D. Hip arthrography, aspiration, block, and bursography. Radiol Clin North Am 1998;36(4):673–90.

23. Phillips CD, Pope TL Jr, Jones JE, et al. Nontraumatic avulsion of the lesser trochanter: a pathognomonic sign of metastatic disease? Skeletal Radiol 1988;17(2):106–10.

24. Bui KL, Ilaslan H, Recht M, et al. Iliopsoas injury: an MRI study of patterns and prevalence correlated with clinical findings. Skeletal Radiol 2008;37(3):245–9.

25. Lecouvet FE, Demondion X, Leemrijse T, et al. Spontaneous rupture of the distal iliopsoas tendon: clinical

and imaging findings, with anatomic correlations. Eur Radiol 2005;15(11):2341–6.

26. Blankenbaker D, Tuite M. Iliopsoas musculotendinous unit. Semin Musculoskelet Radiol 2008;12(1):013–27.

27. Blankenbaker DG, De Smet AA. Hip injuries in athletes. Radiol Clin North Am 2010;48(6):1155–78.

28. Jacobson T, Allen WC. Surgical correction of the snapping iliopsoas tendon. Am J Sports Med 1990;18(5):470–4.

29. Tatu L, Parratte B, Vuillier F, et al. Descriptive anatomy of the femoral portion of the iliopsoas muscle. Anatomical basis of anterior snapping of the hip. Surg Radiol Anat 2001;23(6):371–4.

30. Byrd JW. Hip arthroscopy: patient assessment and indications. Instr Course Lect 2003;52:711–9.

31. Schaberg JE, Harper MC, Allen WC. The snapping hip syndrome. Am J Sports Med 1984;12(5):361–5.

32. Ilizaliturri VM Jr, Camacho-Galindo J. Endoscopic treatment of snapping hips, iliotibial band, and iliopsoas tendon. Sports Med Arthrosc 2010;18(2):120–7.

33. Byrd JW. Snapping hip. Operat Tech Sports Med 2005;13(1):46–54.

34. Adler RS, Buly R, Ambrose R, et al. Diagnostic and therapeutic use of sonography-guided iliopsoas peritendinous injections. AJR Am J Roentgenol 2005;185(4):940–3.

35. Pelsser V, Cardinal E, Hobden R, et al. Extraarticular snapping hip: sonographic findings. AJR Am J Roentgenol 2001;176(1):67–73.

36. Bricteux S, Beguin L, Fessy MH. Iliopsoas impingement in 12 patients with a total hip arthroplasty. Rev Chir Orthop Reparatrice Appar Mot 2001;87(8):820–5 [in French].

37. Trousdale RT, Cabanela ME, Berry DJ. Anterior iliopsoas impingement after total hip arthroplasty. J Arthroplasty 1995;10(4):546–9.

38. Dora C, Houweling M, Koch P, et al. Iliopsoas impingement after total hip replacement: the results of non-operative management, tenotomy or acetabular revision. J Bone Joint Surg Br 2007;89(8):1031–5.

39. Bader R, Mittelmeier W, Zeiler G, et al. Pitfalls in the use of acetabular reinforcement rings in total hip revision. Arch Orthop Trauma Surg 2005;125(8):558–63.

40. Heaton K, Dorr LD. Surgical release of iliopsoas tendon for groin pain after total hip arthroplasty. J Arthroplasty 2002;17(6):779–81.

41. Hayter CL, Koff MF, Potter HG. Magnetic resonance imaging of the postoperative hip. J Magn Reson Imaging 2012;35(5):1013–25.

42. Nunley RM, Wilson JM, Gilula L, et al. Iliopsoas bursa injections can be beneficial for pain after total hip arthroplasty. Clin Orthop Relat Res 2010;468(2):519–26.

43. Domb BG, Shindle MK, McArthur B, et al. Iliopsoas impingement: a newly identified cause of labral pathology in the hip. HSS J 2011;7(2):145–50.

44. Ilizaliturri VM Jr, Villalobos FE Jr, Chaidez PA, et al. Internal snapping hip syndrome: treatment by endoscopic release of the iliopsoas tendon. Arthroscopy 2005;21(11):1375–80.

45. Flanum ME, Keene JS, Blankenbaker DG, et al. Arthroscopic treatment of the painful "internal" snapping hip: results of a new endoscopic technique and imaging protocol. Am J Sports Med 2007;35(5):770–9.

46. Heyworth BE, Shindle MK, Voos JE, et al. Radiologic and intraoperative findings in revision hip arthroscopy. Arthroscopy 2007;23(12):1295–302.

47. Blankenbaker DG, Tuite MJ, Keene JS, et al. Labral Injuries Due to Iliopsoas Impingement: Can They Be Diagnosed on MR Arthrography? AJR Am J Roentgenol 2012;199(4):894–900.

48. Hasselman CT, Best TM, Hughes C, et al. An explanation for various rectus femoris strain injuries using previously undescribed muscle architecture. Am J Sports Med 1995;23(4):493–9.

49. Hsu JC. Proximal rectus femoris avulsions in national football league kickers: a report of 2 cases. Am J Sports Med 2005;33(7):1085–7.

50. Gamradt SC, Brophy RH, Barnes R, et al. Nonoperative treatment for proximal avulsion of the rectus femoris in professional American football. Am J Sports Med 2009;37(7):1370–4.

51. Sanders T, Zlatkin M. Avulsion injuries of the pelvis. Semin Musculoskelet Radiol 2008;12(1):042–53.

52. Resnick JM, Carrasco CH, Edeiken J, et al. Avulsion fracture of the anterior inferior iliac spine with abundant reactive ossification in the soft tissue. Skeletal Radiol 1996;25(6):580–4.

53. Ouellette H, Thomas BJ, Nelson E, et al. MR imaging of rectus femoris origin injuries. Skeletal Radiol 2006;35(9):665–72.

54. Segal NA, Felson DT, Torner JC, et al. Greater trochanteric pain syndrome: epidemiology and associated factors. Arch Phys Med Rehabil 2007;88(8):988–92.

55. Beck M, Sledge JB, Gautier E, et al. The anatomy and function of the gluteus minimus muscle. J Bone Joint Surg Br 2000;82(3):358–63.

56. Labrosse JM, Cardinal E, Leduc BE, et al. Effectiveness of ultrasound-guided corticosteroid injection for the treatment of gluteus medius tendinopathy. AJR Am J Roentgenol 2010;194(1):202–6.

57. Cvitanic O, Henzie G, Skezas N, et al. MRI diagnosis of tears of the hip abductor tendons (gluteus medius and gluteus minimus). AJR Am J Roentgenol 2004;182(1):137–43.

58. Voos JE, Maak T, Kelly BT. Arthroscopic hip "rotator cuff repair" of gluteus medius tendon avulsions. In: Techniques in hip arthroscopy and joint preservation surgery. Elsevier; 2011. p. 144–51. Available at: http://linkinghub.elsevier.com/retrieve/pii/B9781416056423000177; 2011. Accessed July 7, 2012.

59. Voos JE, Shindle MK, Pruett A, et al. Endoscopic repair of gluteus medius tendon tears of the hip. Am J Sports Med 2009;37(4):743–7.

60. Wahl CJ. Internal coxa saltans (snapping hip) as a result of overtraining: a report of 3 cases in professional athletes with a review of causes and the role of ultrasound in early diagnosis and management. Am J Sports Med 2004;32(5):1302–9.

61. Reid DC. Prevention of hip and knee injuries in ballet dancers. Sports Med 1988;6(5):295–307.

62. Larsen E, Johansen J. Snapping hip. Acta Orthop Scand 1986;57(2):168–70.

63. Frank RM, Slabaugh MA, Grumet RC, et al. Posterior hip pain in an athletic population: differential diagnosis and treatment options. Sports Health 2010; 2(3):237–46.

64. Lempainen L, Sarimo J, Mattila K, et al. Proximal hamstring tendinopathy: results of surgical management and histopathologic findings. Am J Sports Med 2009;37(4):727–34.

65. Koulouris G, Connell D. Evaluation of the hamstring muscle complex following acute injury. Skeletal Radiol 2003;32(10):582–9.

66. LaStayo PC, Woolf JM, Lewek MD, et al. Eccentric muscle contractions: their contribution to injury, prevention, rehabilitation, and sport. J Orthop Sports Phys Ther 2003;33(10):557–71.

67. Cacchio A, Borra F, Severini G, et al. Reliability and validity of three pain provocation tests used for the diagnosis of chronic proximal hamstring tendinopathy. Br J Sports Med 2012. Available at: http://www.ncbi.nlm.nih.gov/pubmed/22219215. Accessed July 16, 2012.

68. Koulouris G, Connell D. Hamstring muscle complex: an imaging review. Radiographics 2005;25(3): 571–86.

69. Carlson C. The natural history and management of hamstring injuries. Curr Rev Musculoskelet Med 2008;1(2):120–3.

70. Sato K, Nimura A, Yamaguchi K, et al. Anatomical study of the proximal origin of hamstring muscles. J Orthop Sci 2012. Available at: http://www.ncbi.nlm.nih.gov/pubmed/22669443. Accessed July 25, 2012.

71. Fredericson M, Moore W, Guillet M, et al. High hamstring tendinopathy in runners: meeting the challenges of diagnosis, treatment, and rehabilitation. Phys Sportsmed 2005;33(5):32–43.

72. Young IJ, van Riet RP, Bell SN. Surgical release for proximal hamstring syndrome. Am J Sports Med 2008;36(12):2372–8.

73. Zissen MH, Wallace G, Stevens KJ, et al. High hamstring tendinopathy: MRI and ultrasound imaging and therapeutic efficacy of percutaneous corticosteroid injection. AJR Am J Roentgenol 2010;195(4): 993–8.

74. Cohen S, Bradley J. Acute proximal hamstring rupture. J Am Acad Orthop Surg 2007;15(6):350–5.

Magnetic Resonance Imaging of Athletic Pubalgia and the Sports Hernia
Current Understanding and Practice

Waseem Khan, MD[a], Adam C. Zoga, MD[b],*,
William C. Meyers, MD, MBA[c,d,e]

KEYWORDS

- Magnetic resonance imaging • Sports hernia • Athletic pubalgia • Musculoskeletal groin pain

KEY POINTS

- Magnetic resonance imaging (MRI) is an essential tool for accurately identifying the various lesions seen with athletic pubalgia and core injuries.
- A dedicated athletic pubalgia MRI protocol is a useful adjunct in delineation of injury extent and can help with appropriate subspecialist referral.

INTRODUCTION

Groin pain in athletes has long been a diagnostic and therapeutic conundrum for orthopedic surgeons, sports medicine physicians, and the entire training staff for athletic teams and departments. The groin region is commonly injured during activities involving rapid acceleration, twisting and lateral motion, and abrupt changes in direction at the body's musculoskeletal core. Sports including soccer, American rules football, hockey, and baseball have been associated with particularly high rates of activity-induced groin pain, or athletic pubalgia. Up to 13% of soccer injuries involve the groin.[1,2] In 1 series, 58% of soccer players had experienced a groin injury.[3] But as the understanding of the specific musculoskeletal lesions associated with athletic pubalgia has grown, so has the incidence of its diagnosis across a diverse population with wide variations in age, activity level, and favored athletic endeavor.

The clinical assessment of athletic pubalgia remains challenging, as multiple possible pathologies may yield similar presentations and findings on physical examination. Patients often present with inguinal pain, which may radiate into the perineum or medial thigh. Patients can experience an insidious onset of symptoms or an acute injury, but an acute on chronic presentation seems most prevalent. Symptoms may persist for unnecessarily long periods before the correct diagnosis is made, hindering participation and causing delays in return to activity. Such sports-related injuries of the groin were often labeled sports hernias early on. This term may have developed as a consequence of the anatomic proximity of the superficial inguinal ring to the true location of injury, causing confounding symptoms not unlike those produced by true hernias. This term is a misnomer, however, as magentic resonance imaging (MRI) has shown that there is very infrequently a true hernia in this patient

[a] Thomas Jefferson University Hospital, 132 South 10th Street, Philadelphia, PA 19107, USA; [b] Musculoskeletal MRI and Ambulatory Imaging Centers, Thomas Jefferson University Hospital, 132 South 10th Street, 1083A, Philadelphia, PA 19107, USA; [c] Vincera Core Physicians, Philadelphia, PA, USA; [d] Drexel University College of Medicine, Philadelphia, PA, USA; [e] Thomas Jefferson University Hospital, 4623 South Broad Street, Philadelphia, PA 19112, USA
* Corresponding author.
E-mail address: adam.zoga@jefferson.edu

Magn Reson Imaging Clin N Am 21 (2013) 97–110
http://dx.doi.org/10.1016/j.mric.2012.09.008
1064-9689/13/$ – see front matter © 2013 Elsevier Inc. All rights reserved.

population. Athletic pubalgia is better, as it implies a more clinical diagnosis, but it still falls short in identifying a true musculoskeletal lesion, of which there are many. More recently, the term core injury has been used to broaden the spectrum of musculoskeletal lesions that should be considered. In a general sense, these terms imply a clinical syndrome in which groin pain does not originate from intrinsic pathology of the hip (**Fig. 1**).[4]

Over the past 5 years, MRI has taken a central role in the diagnosis of athletic pubalgia or core injury, and in many cases, referral to the most appropriate subspecialist. There has been a great focus on lesions involving the aponeurosis of the rectus abdominis and adductor longus anterior to the pubic bone and pubic symphysis, but many other sites of injury can be encountered at MRI. This article reviews the basic anatomy of the musculoskeletal pubic region as well as specific lesions leading to clinical athletic pubalgia or core injury. A dedicated MRI protocol will be detailed, as well as patterns of MRI findings reproducibly seen at MRI in these patients. Common confounding and concomitant inuries will be briefly discussed, and the expected post-operative MRI appearance as well as commonly observed complications will be described.

ANATOMY

The pubic symphysis includes 2 pubic bones with an articular disc interposed between the medial articular surfaces, resulting in an amphiarthrodial joint. The pubic bone forms the anterior aspect of the overall innominate bone, and is composed of superior and inferior pubic rami and the pubic

body, which is situated medially. The medial aspect of the pubic body is ovoid, and covered by a thin layer of hyaline cartilage. The intervening disc is composed of fibrocartilage, and along with transversely oriented subarticular osseous ridges and grooves, helps stabilize the joint by dispersing shear forces. The pubic crest forms the superior and anterior margin of the pubic body. The pubic tubercle, which is the attachment site for the caudal rectus abdominis and the inguinal ligament, is a bony excrescence at the inferolateral margin of the pubic crest.[4–6]

Beyond the articular disc, the joint is stabilized by 4 ligaments and multiple tendon attachments. The arcuate and the superior, anterior, and posterior pubic ligaments encase the pubis, although the former 2 ligaments are more functionally important, particularly for resisting shear forces. The arcuate ligament lines the inferior margin of the pubic symphysis, intimate to the articular disc and the rectus abdominis/adductor longus aponeurosis. The superior pubic ligament courses between the pubic tubercles. The anterior pubic ligament is comprised of a deep bundle that blends with the articular disc, and a superficial bundle that merges with the aponeuroses of the rectus abdominis and external oblique muscles. The posterior pubic ligament is thin, and least clinically important.[5–7] These ligaments are generally not easily identifiable with MRI, but the arcuate ligament in particular is often injured and likely plays a central role in athletic pubalgia lesions.[4]

The pubic symphysis stabilizes the anterior pelvis, while still allowing a small degree of craniocaudal movement at the joint.[8–10] The large ovoid surface of the joint distributes craniocaudal shear forces produced while ambulating.[6] While primarily a stabilizer of the anterior pelvis, anatomy at the symphysis allows for laxity and diastasis during pregnancy and childbirth (**Fig. 2**).[8]

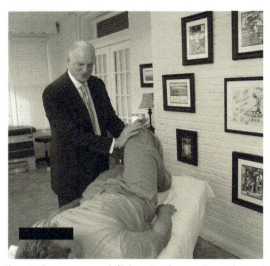

Fig. 1. Surgeon specializing in diagnosis and treatment of athletic pubalgia performs a physical examination maneuver directed to musculoskeletal core injury.

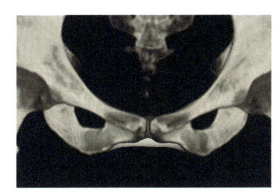

Fig. 2. Diagram of pubic symphysis demonstrates the midline pubic disc in red and the anteroinferior arcuate ligament in green.

The pubic symphysis is also a focal point for multiple musculotendinous attachments, contributing to overall pelvic stabilization. Abdominal wall muscles attaching to this location include the rectus abdominis, internal and external obliques, and the transversus abdominis. The adductor compartment muscles in the medial thigh attaching to the pubis include the pectineus, adductor longus, adductor brevis, adductor magnus, and gracilis. These extensive muscular, tendinous and ligamentous attachments, and the biomechanical forces distributed in the region are the impetus for labeling the region as the musculoskeletal core.

Functionally, the rectus abdominis and adductor longus are critical for stability at the anterior pelvis.[8] These paired muscles attach on a broad aponeurotic plate spanning the midline from the pubic tubercles to the anteroinferior pubic bodies. Medially, the rectus abdominis tendons merge with the anterior pubic ligament. Laterally, the caudal rectus abdominis lies just posteromedial to the superficial inguinal ring, and likely plays a role in reinforcing the wall of the posteromedial superficial inguinal canal.[4] At the lateral margin of the pubis, the adductor longus, the most anterior muscle among the adductors, blends with the caudal rectus abdominis attachment. At the midline, the caudal rectus abdominis, adductor fibers, arcuate ligament, and anterior pubic periosteum form the previously mentioned aponeurotic plate, which represents a merging of the right and left aponeuroses already described (**Fig. 3**).[4,6,11]

During core rotation and extension, the rectus abdominis and adductor longus are relative antagonists. While the rectus elevates the anterior pelvis, the adductor longus depresses it. Injury of 1 of the components tends to cause abnormal biomechanical forces on the opposing muscles

and tendons, leading to further injury at the aponeurosis and its tenoperiosteal attachments.[12] This can lead to pelvic instability, and ultimately osteitis pubis, any of which can contribute to chronic pelvic pain in athletes.[4] Continued activity in the setting of pelvic instability establishes a cycle of additional injury reflecting the altered biomechanics, which often leads to further and more extensive core injury.

IMAGING PROTOCOL

A dedicated athletic pubalgia MRI protocol is the study of choice for a specific subset of young athletic patients with groin pain, particularly if the pathology is felt to be extrinsic to the hip. Imaging is generally performed in a supine position for patient comfort, and the bladder should be emptied just before image acquisition. Either 1.5 T or 3 T systems should provide high-quality imaging of the pubic region. Coil selection and positioning are generally more important imaging considerationa than field strength with late model MRI systems. A receiver coil should be positioned over midline, centered on the pubic symphysis. Ideally, the coil will allow for imaging over a large field of view from hip to hip and midthigh to midthigh. The authors have found that phased array torso coils generally allow for at least survey imaging of the hips and thighs as well as high-resolution imaging of the pubic symphysis region of the smaller field-of-view sequences.

Three large field-of-view sequences of the pelvis are first obtained using a body coil. A coronal T1-weighted sequence is useful for assessment of marrow abnormalities, including fracture, neoplasm, or infection. A coronal short tau inversion recovery (STIR) sequence is useful for both

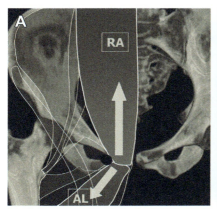
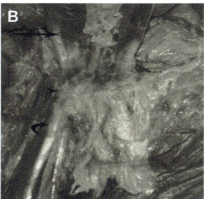

Fig. 3. (*A*) Diagram shows apposing functions of rectus abdominis (RA) and adductor longus (AL) muscles at the pubic tubercle. Black oval denotes superficial inguinal ring. (*B*) Gross specimen demonstrating the rectus abdominis (*straight arrow*), pubic attachment site (*arrowhead*), and adductor longus tendon (*curved arrow*).

osseous and soft tissue pathology, as well as abnormal fluid, and allows for homogenous suppression of fat, despite relatively poor signal-to-noise ratio. An axial large field-of-view fast spin echo (FSE) T2-weighted fat-saturated sequence allows for adequate contrast and coverage to identify marrow edema, bursitis, hip flexor injury, and even visceral pelvic lesions, as well as high enough resolution to delineate rectus abdominis injury.

Following large field-of-view sequences, higher-resolution sequences dedicated to the pubic symphysis region are acquired. Coronal oblique (axial oblique) images, including proton density (PD) and axial fat-saturated FSE T2-weighted images, are obtained by paralleling the arcuate line of the pelvis or the anterior iliac crest, as defined from a sagittal localizer sequence. The primary benefit of these oblique sequences is that they allow a better angle for evaluation of the adductor longus tendons and rectus abdominis/adductor aponeurosis. These sequences are also useful to assess for true inguinal hernias. Sagittal PD and FSE fat-saturated T2-weighted sequences using the small field of view are also obtained, allowing for excellent evaluation of the aponeurosis and its periosteal attachment to the anterior and anteroinferior pubic ramus.[4] The nonfat-suppressed PD FSE sequences in particular are useful in assessing prior inguinal or core surgeries and potential reinjury. The imaging protocol is summarized in **Table 1**.[4,8]

MRI FINDINGS

Systematic assessment of images allows diagnosis of not only rectus abdominis/adductor longus aponeurosis injuries, but other possible etiologies of groin pain, including pelvic muscle strains and tears, osteitis pubis, fracture, sacroiliitis, visceral pathology, and intrinsic hip disorders. This, in turn, can dictate referral to the appropriate clinical subspecialist.[4,13]

Rectus Abdominis/Adductor Aponeurosis Injury

In the clinical setting of athletic pubalgia, rectus abdominis/adductor aponeurosis injuries are the most frequently encountered lesions at MRI.[4] These injuries involve the caudal rectus abdominis, adductor longus origin, and pubic tubercle periosteum. Frequently, interstitial tearing or detachment of the lateral edge of the caudal rectus abdominis is noted, with confluent involvement of the adductor longus tendon.[4,12–16] Morphologic symmetry is key in diagnosing this lesion, and its identification shows a high correlation with the

situs of unilateral symptomatology. On axial images, the lesion can manifest as a visible deficiency of the rectus abdominis on cross section just anterior to the pubic tubercle. This deficiency is often positioned immediately posteromedial to the superficial ring, where the injured rectus abdominis shows an acutely angled contour in contrast to the normal, curvilinear morphology on the noninjured side. These patients often present with insidious groin pain and focal tenderness at the pubic tubercle. This lesion, in particular, is commonly treated with surgical pelvic floor repair.[13]

In the setting of a unilateral rectus abdominis/adductor aponeurosis lesion, MRI often demonstrates subenthesial marrow edema at the pubic tubercle, the site of the caudal rectus abdominis insertion. This edema is confined to the anteroinferior aspect of the pubic body at the site of the attachment of the aponeurosis, unlike osteitis pubis, which spans the full anteroposterior course of the pubic body.[17] The adductor longus tendon may be enlarged, demonstrate interstitial tearing, or be completely detached from the pubis. Interstitial tearing is manifested by fluid signal interspersed within the tendon. Detachment is often accompanied by a hematoma interposed between the tendon and the underlying pubis (**Fig. 4**).

An aponeurosis lesion also often presents with a secondary cleft sign on MRI, which has a high correlation with the side of pain. This sign was initially described in reference to arthrography of the pubic symphysis, but is visible by MRI, and is thought to reflect a tear at the origin of the adductor longus and gracilis tendons.[18–20] While the primary cleft is developmental and vertical in configuration at the posterosuperior aspect of the pubic symphyseal disc, the secondary cleft has the appearance of an inferior extension of the primary cleft, coursing around the anteroinferior periphery of the pubic body, and is hyperintense on T2-weighted images.[8] The cleft may be positioned between the rectus abdominis/adductor aponeurosis and the underlying pubic bone, or less often, it may be subapophyseal (**Fig. 5**).[4]

Midline Rectus Abdominis/Adductor Aponeurotic Plate Injury (Pubic Plate Injury)

More recently, it has been noted that some patients with athletic pubalgia show a midline lesion at MRI extending into both rectus abdominis/adductor aponeuroses. Patients often present with bilateral groin pain, although symptomatology is frequently more acute or severe on 1 side. At MRI, there is often a confluent bilateral secondary

Table 1
Imaging protocol of the pubic symphysis region

Sequence	Field of View	Matrix	NEX	Slice Thickness/Skip	TR	TE	TI	Echo Train Length	Bandwidth
Coronal STIR	28–36 (both hips)	256 × 192	2–3	4 mm/1 mm	>2000	20–40	150	8	16
Coronal T1 SE	28 (both hips)	256 × 256	1–2	4 mm/1 mm	400–800	Minimum	N/A	N/A	16
Axial T2 FSE fat-saturated	28 (both hips)	256 × 256	2–3	5 mm/1 mm	>2000	50–60	N/A	8	16
Axial oblique PD FSE fat-saturated	20	256 × 192	1–2	4 mm/0.5 mm	3000 (maximum)	25–30	N/A	4	16
Axial oblique T2 FSE fat-saturated	20	256 × 192	2–3	4 mm/0.5 mm	>2000	50–60	N/A	8	16
Sagittal T2 FSE fat-saturated	20–22	256 × 192	2–3	4 mm/0.5 mm	>2000	50–60	N/A	8	16
Sagittal PD FSE fat-saturated	20–22	256 × 256	2–3	4 mm/0.5 mm	>2000	20–30	N/A	8	16

Abbreviations: NEX, Number of excitations; TE, Time to echo; TI, Time to inversion; TR, Repetition time.

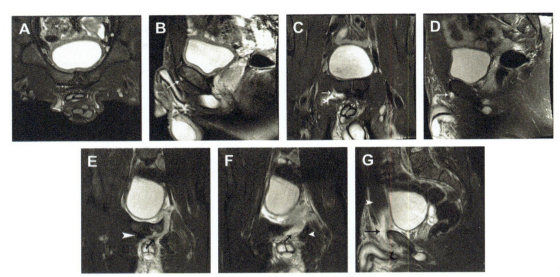

Fig. 4. (*A*) Coronal oblique FSE fat-saturated T2-weighted image from a dedicated athletic pubalgia MRI protocol shows a small tear at the lateral edge of the right rectus abdominis–adductor aponeurosis in a football player (*arrow*). (*B*) Sagittal FSE fat-saturated T2-weighted image from the same examination as Fig. 4A again shows the lateral edge aponeurosis tear (*arrow*). (*C*) Coronal oblique FSE fat-saturated T2-weighted image demonstrates a large tear at the lateral edge of the right aponeurosis (*arrow*), with retraction of the adductor longus tendon (*arrowhead*), and an interposed hematoma in a professional basketball player with an acute-on-chronic injury. (*D*) Sagittal FSE fat-saturated T2-weighted image from the same examination as Fig. 4C shows the elongated tenoperiosteal detachment of the rectus abdominis (*arrow*). (*E*) Coronal oblique FSE fat-saturated T2-weighted image in a football player shows a very large aponeurotic lesion with an adductor avulsion on the left (*black arrow*). Normal right aponeurosis is seen on the right (*white arrowhead*). (*F*) More anterior image from the same examination and sequence as Fig. 4E confirms an avulsed osseous fragment (*white arrowhead*) arising from the pubic attachment site of the aponeurosis, while the black arrow shows hematoma. (*G*) Sagittal fat-saturated T2-weighted FSE image from same patient reveals torn (*black arrow*) and partially retracted rectus abdominis (*white arrowhead*). There is complete avulsion at the level of the aponeurosis (*curved arrow*).

cleft anteroinferior to the pubic symphysis. Abnormal T2 hyperintense signal undercuts the medial edge of both rectus abdominis attachments, extending into both aponeurosis, and sometimes even the lateral edge of the caudal rectus abdominis either unilaterally or bilaterally. The injury seems to manifest as a disruption or lifting of the entire apparatus at the pubic symphysis

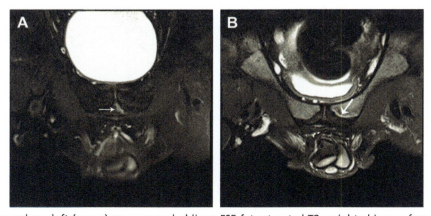

Fig. 5. (*A*) Secondary cleft (*arrow*) on a coronal oblique FSE fat saturated T2-weighted image from a dedicated athletic pubalgia protocol. (*B*) Coronal oblique fat saturated T2-weighted FSE image identifies a subapophyseal athletic pubalgia lesion (*arrow*) in a teenaged soccer player.

region, and thus it has been termed a pubic plate disruption. Osteitis pubis is common, but can be asymmetric, and often aponeurotic plate lesions extend as interstitial tearing into 1 adductor longus tendon origin.[14–16] Anecdotally, there is a trend for this injury to occur in women, which may be related to anatomic differences in the pubic symphysis between men and women.[4]

When a midline pubic plate lesion is identified, extent, lateral edge rectus abdominis involvement, adductor longus involvement, and asymmetric osteitis pubis should all be meticulously delineated at MRI. It is the authors' experience that unilateral treatment in the setting of these midline lesions can lead to contralateral injury and subsequent recurrent athletic pubalgia months or years later (**Fig. 6**).

Osteitis Pubis

Osteitis pubis is an osseous response to instability at the pubic symphysis. Most often, repetitive chronic shear forces and tensile forces from injured muscle attachments lead to deranged biomechanics, which sets up an inflammatory response leading to osteitis and periostitis.[8] The resultant instability may further exacerbate soft tissue injuries, including adductor and rectus abdominis tears. While primary soft tissue core lesions in athletes may lead to altered biomechanics and ultimately to osteitis pubis, ligamentous injury related to single trauma or childbirth can also lead to instability at the symphysis and a similar pattern of osteitis pubis.[20] In fact, in the authors' experience, severe osteitis pubis is not an infrequent diagnosis in postpartum athletes soon after their return to activity after childbirth.[4]

On imaging, marrow edema spanning essentially the full anteroposterior course of the subchondral bone in the pubic body is noted. Marrow edema is generally bilateral, but may asymmetrically predominate on the side of symptoms. This should be differentiated from the focal marrow edema at the pubic tubercles often seen with avulsive injuries of the rectus abdominis–adductor aponeurosis. Osteitis pubis can manifest with several different patterns on MRI. Sometimes, there is intense subchondral bone marrow edema without osseous productive change or erosion. This is considered acute osteitis pubis, likely with an inflammatory component, and superimposed stresses or insufficiency fractures are not infrequent in the parasymphyseal region with this scenario. In other cases, there is very little bone marrow edema but more osseous productive change and subchondral cyst formation. This is considered chronic osteitis pubis and likely reflects chronic instability at the symphysis. Another pattern shows subchondral bone marrow edema with articular erosion somewhat analogous to distal clavicular osteolysis at the acromioclavicular joint. With these more severe lesions, potential for healing at the symphysis is unclear (**Fig. 7**).[21–23]

Rectus Abdominis Strain

Although the rectus abdominis may be strained anywhere in its course, at its caudal end, a strain is generally seen in conjunction with a rectus abdominis/adductor aponeurosis injury. As in any other muscle, a strain is identified by T2 hyperintensity in the muscle belly. The contralateral rectus abdominis may serve as an internal control.[16] The key observation is whether there is involvement of the aponeurosis, which may require surgery, or whether the strain is isolated, in which case it may heal with conservative measures. Chronically, asymmetric atrophy of the rectus abdominis may be seen (**Fig. 8**).

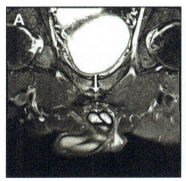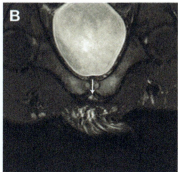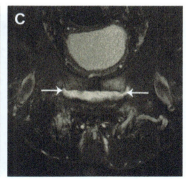

Fig. 6. (*A*) Coronal oblique FSE fat-saturated T2-weighted image shows a midline rectus abdominis–adductor aponeurotic plate lesion (*arrow*) in a professional female distance runner. (*B*) Another midline aponeurotic plate defect (*arrow*) in a 17-year-old male basketball player. (*C*) A large midline aponeurotic plate defect extending to the lateral edges of both aponeurosis (*arrows*) in a middle-aged recreational athlete.

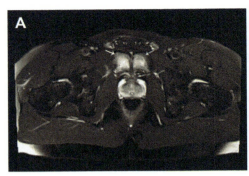
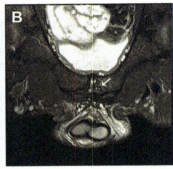

Fig. 7. (*A*) Bone marrow edema spanning the subchondral region of the pubic symphysis anterior to posterior on an axial FSE fat-saturated T2-weighted image (*arrows*) typical for severe osteitis pubis. (*B*) Coronal oblique FSE fat-saturated T2-weighted image shows chronic osteitis pubis with osseous productive change and subchondral cyst formation (*arrow*).

Adductor Injury

Adductor injury is a frequent cause of groin pain among athletes, and it may occur proximally concurrent with rectus abdominis injury, but also more distally within the tendon or muscle itself. These latter injuries more often respond to conservative measures, while proximal aponeurosis injuries are best treated surgically.[8] Chronic repetitive overuse is most frequently implicated as the source of adductor injury, although acute injuries may also occur.[17,24–26]

On MRI, acute strains present with edema in the adductor compartment muscle bellies or myotendinous junctions, especially the adductor longus, and less so the adductor brevis and pectineus. Avulsion and retraction of the adductor longus should prompt assessment of the caudal rectus abdominis, as these injuries are often concurrently seen.[4,8,17,27]

Chronic tendinopathy may be manifested by enlargement and hypointense signal of the tendon in the setting of hypoxic degeneration. Focal rounded hypointensity also may be seen, and represents hydroxyapatite deposition, or calcific tendinosis.[8]

Occasionally, injury of the adductor compartment at the level of the myotendinous junction may lead to disruption of the muscle sheath with subsequent herniation of muscle fibers through the defect.[28] This has been termed baseball pitcher/hockey goalie syndrome, and it responds poorly to conservative management. It may result from chronic repetitive stress at sites of relative weakness, such as entry points of neurovascular structures.[29] MRI findings are not well described, although one may see focal edema in the adductor longus muscle belly, and a focal bulge at the site of herniation.[30] Distal myotendinous adductor injury is sometimes seen in the setting of recurrent pain after pelvic floor repair or adductor tendon release for a proximal lesion (**Fig. 9**).[4,31]

CONFOUNDING PATHOLOGIES

Groin pain is an elusive clinical presentation, and numerous other pathologies may lead to symptoms akin to athletic pubalgia lesions. Many of these entities may be imaged during the MRI athletic pubalgia protocol, particularly on the large field-of-view sequences. One should also remember to assess pelvic visceral structures, as incidental masses or other pathologies may be identified. Sometimes, the groin pain may be attributed to visceral pathology, such as endometriosis, adenomyosis, or inflammatory bowel disease. Some of the more common musculoskeletal pathologies presenting with groin pain similar to athletic pubalgia lesions are briefly discussed in this section.

Fig. 8. Right rectus abdominis atrophy (*arrow*) on an axial fat-saturated FSE T2-weighted image in a patient with chronic right-sided groin pain.

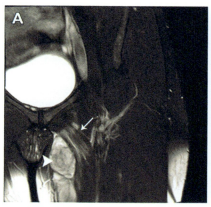
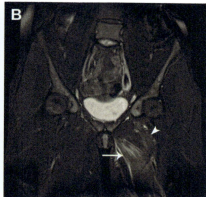

Fig. 9. (*A*) Grade 2 strain of the left adductor longus (*arrow*) with an associated hematoma (*arrowhead*) on coronal STIR image from an athletic pubalgia protocol. (*B*) Coronal oblique FSE fat-saturated T2-weighted image reveals left adductor longus (*arrow*) and pectineus (*arrowhead*) strains in a football player with an acute groin strain.

Inguinal Hernia

Athletic pubalgia symptoms may mimic those of inguinal hernia, which may account for the misnomer of sports hernia. The anatomic proximity of the superficial inguinal ring to the rectus attachment at the pubic tubercle may account for similarities in clinical presentation. In athletes, direct inguinal and femoral hernias are more common than indirect inguinal hernias.[32] Inguinal hernias are best evaluated on the coronal oblique PD sequence. One should look for symmetry in the inguinal canal, which should contain a small amount of fat, and in males, the spermatic cord, and females, the round ligament. There should be no fluid, mass effect, or enteric contents. Susceptibility artifact in this region may indicate a mesh from prior herniorrhaphy.[33] In some cases, inappropriate herniorrhaphy may have been performed to treat an athletic pubalgia lesion. Although this may transiently improve symptoms, they inevitably return after the patient resumes athletic activity (**Fig. 10**).[8]

Hip Pathology

In the authors' experience, among the most common etiologies of pain in athletes who do not have athletic pubalgia lesions on dedicated MRI are lesions of the hip, particularly acetabular labral tears. Although noncontrast MRI has limited sensitivity for detection of labral tears, coronal large field-of-view STIR and the limited views of the hips on sagittal small field-of-view fat-saturated FSE T2 images should be assessed for tears, particularly detached tears, which may be easier to detect than more subtle undersurface tears. Tears are most often located at the anterosuperior

aspect of the acetabular labrum.[34] Other secondary signs should be sought, including paralabral cysts, evidence for cartilage loss such as subchondral marrow edema and cysts, and findings of femoroacetabular impingement. Sometimes, follow-up dedicated imaging of the hip after intra-articular administration of a gadolinium-based contrast is necessary for more thorough evaluation (**Fig. 11**).

Other pathology in the hip is less often seen in this relatively young and athletic population. However, osteoarthritis, effusion and synovitis, and intra-articular bodies may be recognized.

Stress Fracture

In the active population, overuse may lead to stress response, and eventually stress fracture. It

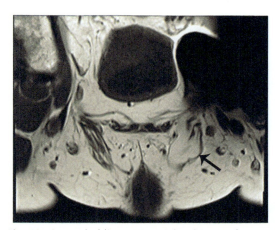

Fig. 10. Coronal oblique PD-weighted image from an athletic pubalgia MRI protocol identifies a left inguinal hernia (*arrow*).

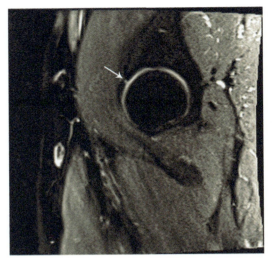

Fig. 11. Anterior acetabular labrum tear (*arrow*) identified on sagittal FSE fat-saturated T2-weighted image at the most lateral aspect of the field of view in an athletic pubalgia protocol.

is important to recognize these findings, as continued activity may lead to completion of the fracture. Typical locations include the medial femoral neck, inferior pubic ramus, and parasymphyseal region. MRI may reveal periosteal edema, marrow edema (increased signal on STIR or fat-saturated T2-weighted images within the marrow space), and a low signal line on T1- and T2-weighted images, which is generally oriented perpendicular to trabeculae (**Fig. 12**).[35]

Lumbar Spine and Sacroiliac Joints

Lumbar spine and sacroiliac joint pathology may sometimes present with groin pain. Therefore, images should be scrutinized for disc herniations and other pathology (**Fig. 13**). The sacroiliac joints are well visualized on the pubalgia protocol, and must be evaluated for subchondral marrow edema, erosion, and adjacent fluid collections. Inflammatory, infectious, and degenerative conditions may produce pathology at this site. Unilateral sacroiliitis must be considered infectious until proven otherwise.[16]

Bursitis

Iliopsoas bursitis may present with groin pain, and it is exacerbated by hip flexion.[36] MRI will demonstrate a T2 hyperintense fluid collection located between the anterior hip capsule and the distal iliopsoas tendon, lateral to the femoral vessels.[37] At least 10% 15% of these collections communicate with the hip joint. Obturator externus bursitis may also present with groin pain. MRI reveals fluid between the obturator externus muscle and the subjacent ischium (**Fig. 14**).

Apophysitis

In the skeletally immature patient, apophysitis may present with groin pain. These apophyses abound in and around the pelvis. Overuse may lead to injury to the anterior inferior iliac spine, where the rectus femoris originates, and the anterior superior iliac spine, the site of origin of the sartorius and tensor

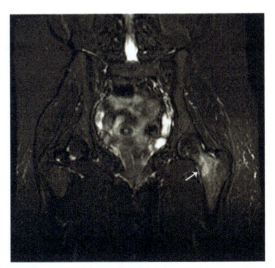

Fig. 12. Coronal, large field-of-view STIR image shows a left femoral neck stress fracture in a runner with acute-on-chronic left-sided groin pain. There is extensive bone marrow edema and a faint low signal fracture line (*arrow*).

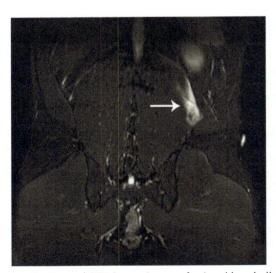

Fig. 13. Coronal STIR image in a professional baseball outfielder with deep, posterior groin pain reveals a left quadratus lumborum strain (*arrow*), a more posterior musculoskeletal core injury.

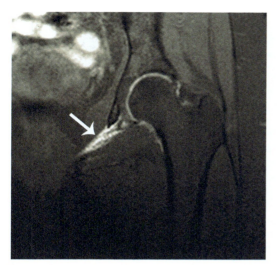

Fig. 14. Coronal, large field-of-view STIR image from an athletic pubalgia protocol shows left obturator externus bursitis (*arrow*).

fascia lata. Athletes involved in kicking are particularly susceptible.[8,38] On MRI, fluid-sensitive sequences demonstrate increased signal within the apophysis, as well as adjacent cartilage and tendinous attachments. T1-weighted images may reveal fragmentation of the apophysis.[4] The pubic apophyses may also undergo such changes, and persistent activity may lead to delay in fusion, fragmentation, or even osteonecrosis (**Fig. 15**).

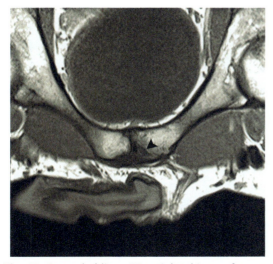

Fig. 15. Coronal oblique PD-weighted image from an athletic pubalgia MRI protocol in a 17 year-old soccer player with chronic left-sided groin pain shows diffusely low signal in an un-united pubic apophysis (*arrowhead*). The apophysis showed low signal on all sequences, compatible with osteonecrosis.

TREATMENT AND POSTOPERATIVE IMAGING EVALUATION

The rectus abdominis–adductor aponeurosis and aponeurotic plate injuries described previously are often treated surgically. However, a poor understanding of the underlying pathology behind athletic pubalgia has led to misguided surgical attempts, including placement of mesh either cranial to the aponeurosis, or even at the inguinal canal.[13] These approaches may reflect the misguided belief that there is in fact a hernia leading to the symptoms of athletic pubalgia. Although symptoms may abate for the short term after such procedures, they inevitably return some time after resumption of athletic activity. Imaging of such types of repairs should be investigated for susceptibility at the site of the mesh and its relation to the aponeurosis. Scarring and fibrosis, seen as low T1 signal, and fat necrosis, as denoted by lobulated areas of hypointense fat on all sequences, are important to identify.[39–42] Although true hernias through or adjacent to a mesh repair are uncommon, there may be associated ipsilateral muscle atrophy, particularly at the lateral margin of the caudal rectus abdominis.[39]

There is limited literature describing imaging findings after recurrent groin pain following mesh repair or herniorrhaphy, especially if the repair is directed toward an athletic pubalgia lesion. The authors possess the most experience with postoperative imaging after open pelvic floor repair, which directly reinforces the rectus abdominis–adductor aponeurosis.[43] After such repair, patients occasionally return with recurrent or new groin pain, sometimes on the contralateral side. The incidence of reinjury at the site of previous unilateral pelvic floor repair, or after bilateral repair, is less than 1%. However, in patients with a unilateral pelvic floor repair, a contralateral injury leading to recurrent athletic pubalgia is reported with an incidence of approximately 4%.[13] This incidence of contralateral injury may reflect an initial midline pubic plate lesion treated unilaterally in accordance with symptoms, but ultimately progressing away from the repair toward the other aponeurosis (**Fig. 16**).

Postoperative imaging generally implements the same MRI protocol as described previously. There are some caveats, however. If there is clinical concern for postoperative infection, the use of a gadolinium-based contrast agent can be helpful and should be considered. If there is concern for repair failure or retear, imaging on a 3 T system may be beneficial in the effort to distinguish fluid signal from T2 hyperintense granulation tissue at sites of repair, although this is only theoretical.[39]

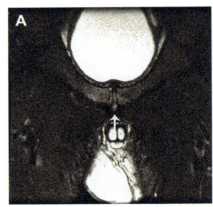
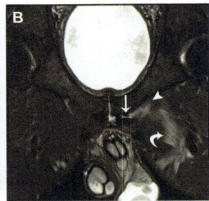

Fig. 16. (*A*) Initial coronal oblique FSE fat-saturated T2-weighted image in National Football League safety shows a small midline aponeurotic plate disruption (*arrow*). The patient went on to have unilateral right-sided pelvic floor repair due to predominant right-sided symptoms. (*B*) Follow-up MRI 9 months later after developing left-sided groin pain in the same patient reveals new aponeurotic lesion (*straight arrow*) and strains of the obturator externus (*arrowhead*) and adductor brevis (*curved arrow*).

First, one should attempt to identify the site of surgery or the suture rows from pelvic floor repair, most often seen as a hypointense region at the caudal aspect of the lateral edge of the rectus abdominis. T2 hyperintense signal at this location is expected, but there should be no gap or fluid signal. Osteitis pubis should improve or completely resolve when compared with preoperative imaging, as surgical repair should stabilize the symphysis pubis, thereby improving findings of osteitis pubis.[23,39] If there is increasing marrow edema in the pubic body after surgery, this may indicate either failure of the repair, persistent instability, premature return to athletic activity, or an overly ambitious rehabilitation program.[39]

A secondary cleft will generally persist on postoperative imaging, if it was present before the procedure.[4,17,40] However, if the cleft is smaller and less intense on T2-weighted images, this is a promising finding. This is felt to represent hyperintense granulation tissue rather than fluid or hematoma. If the secondary cleft becomes larger, or there is a new fluid signal gap at the cleft, this may indicate surgical failure with a new or recurrent tear (**Fig. 17**).[14]

Another finding for which to look is ipsilateral rectus abdominis atrophy. Although atrophy present on preoperative imaging will persist, it should not exacerbate. This finding is associated with ipsilateral recurrent groin pain. Some surgeons will concurrently perform debridement of the adductor longus tendon to promote healing. On MRI, this appears as an enlarged tendon with peritendinous hyperintense signal reflecting granulation tissue.[17,21,39]

One of the most commonly identified findings in the setting of new postoperative groin pain is a strain of the proximal myotendinous junction of the adductor longus. However, this injury occurs more distally, approximately 8 to 12 cm caudal to the origin (**Fig. 18**). The cause for this injury remains unclear, but may be related to a combination of postoperative physical therapy and tautening of the muscle after surgery.[39] Finally, one should not

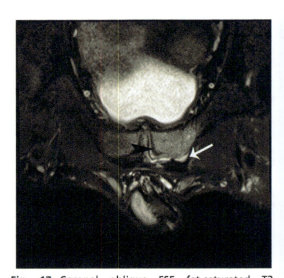

Fig. 17. Coronal oblique FSE fat-saturated T2-weighted image shows recurrent tear of left rectus abdominis–adductor aponeurosis after prior left-sided repair. The tear extends to the lateral edge (*white arrow*). Associated marrow edema from osteitis pubis is noted (*black arrowhead*).

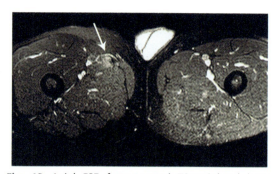

Fig. 18. Axial FSE fat-saturated T2-weighted large field-of-view image in a runner with prior athletic pubalgia lesion presented 9 months after pelvic floor repair with new pain. Arrow denotes strain of myotendinous junction of right adductor longus, 11 cm distal to origin.

forget to assess for the confounding lesions described previously, which may present as a new cause for groin pain after surgery.

SUMMARY

Groin pain is a challenging scenario for even the most experienced clinician. A better understanding of the anatomy of the rectus abdominis–adductor aponeurosis has allowed for more definitive diagnosis of pathology in this region. MRI is an essential tool for accurately identifying the various lesions seen with athletic pubalgia and core injuries as well as delineating injury extent. A dedicated athletic pubalgia MRI protocol is a useful adjunct for assessment, where patients may be referred to the appropriate subspecialist depending on their respective pathology. For example, rectus abdominis–adductor aponeurosis lesions may be referred to a surgeon experienced in pelvic floor repair, while patients with hip flexor injuries can be treated with physical therapy, and those with acetabular labral tears can be directed to a hip arthroscopy specialist.

REFERENCES

1. Ekstrand J, Gillquist J. The avoidability of soccer injuries. Int J Sports Med 1983;4(2):124–8.
2. Ekstrand J, Hilding J. The incidence and differential diagnosis of acute groin injuries in male soccer players. Scand J Med Sci Sports 1999;9:98–103.
3. Harris NH, Murray RO. Lesions of the symphysis in athletes. Br Med J 1974;4(5938):211–4.
4. Zoga A, Mullens F, Meyers W. The spectrum of MR imaging in athletic pubalgia. Radiol Clin North Am 2000;48:1179–97.
5. Williams A. Thigh. In: Stranding S, editor. Gray's anatomy: the anatomical basis of clinical practice.
39th edition. Edinburgh (Scotland): Elsevier; 2008. p. 1349–87.
6. Gamble JG, Simmons SC, Freedman M. The symphysis pubis: anatomic and pathologic considerations. Clin Orthop Relat Res 1986;203:261–72.
7. Putschar WG. The structure of the human symphysis pubis with special consideration of parturition and its sequelae. Am J Phys Anthropol 1976;45(3 pt 2): 589–94.
8. Omar IM, Zoga AC, Kavanagh EC, et al. Athletic pubalgia and "sports hernia": optimal MR imaging technique and findings. Radiographics 2008;28: 1415–38.
9. Walheim GG, Selvik G. Mobility of the pubic symphysis: in vivo measurements with an electromechanic method and a roentgen stereophotogrammetric method. Clin Orthop Relat Res 1984;191: 129–35.
10. Walheim G, Olerud S, Ribbe T. Mobility of the pubic symphysis: measurements by an electromechanical method. Acta Orthop Scand 1984;55(2):203–8.
11. Vix VA, Ryu CY. The adult symphysis pubis: normal and abnormal. Am J Roentgenol Radium Ther Nucl Med 1971;112:517–25.
12. Zoga AC, Kavanaugh EC, Omar IM, et al. Athletic pubalgia and the "sports hernia": MR imaging findings. Radiology 2008;247(3):797–807.
13. Meyers WC, McKechnie A, Philippon MJ, et al. Experience with "sports hernia" spanning two decades. Ann Surg 2008;248(4):656–65.
14. Shortt CP, Zoga AC, Kavanagh EC, et al. Anatomy, pathology, and MRI findings in the sports hernia. Semin Musculoskelet Radiol 2008;12(1):54–61.
15. Kavanagh EC, Zoga AC, Omar I, et al. MR imaging of the rectus abdominis/adductor aponeurosis: findings in the 'sports hernia'. Proceedings of the American Roentgen Ray Society. AJR Am J Roentgenol 2007;188:A13–6.
16. Mullens FE, Zoga AC, Meyers WC. Review of MRI technique and imaging findings in athletic pubalgia and the "sports hernia". Eur J Radiol 2011 Sep 3. [Epub ahead of print].
17. Robinson P, Barron DA, Parsons W, et al. Adductor-related groin pain in athletes: correlation of MR imaging with clinical findings. Skeletal Radiol 2004; 33:451–7.
18. O'Connell MJ, Powell T, McCaffrey NM, et al. Symphyseal cleft injection in the diagnosis treatment of osteitis pubis in athletes. AJR Am J Roentgenol 2002;179:955–9.
19. Brennan D, O'Connell MJ, Ryan M, et al. Secondary cleft sign as a marker of injury in athletes with groin pain. MR image appearance and interpretation. Radiology 2005;235:162–7.
20. Gibbon WW, Hession PR. Diseases of the pubis and pubic symphysis: MR imaging appearances. AJR Am J Roentgenol 1997;169:849–53.

21. Cunningham PM, Brennan D, O'Connell M, et al. Patterns of bone and soft-tissue injury at the symphysis pubis in soccer players: observations at MRI. AJR Am J Roentgenol 2007;188:W291–6.

22. Verrall GM, Slavotinek JP, Fon GT. Incidence of pubic bone marrow oedema in Australian rules football players: relation to groin pain. Br J Sports Med 2001;35:28–33.

23. Kunduracioglu B, Yilmaz C, Yorubulut M, et al. Magnetic resonance findings of osteitis pubis. J Magn Reson Imaging 2007;25(3):535–9.

24. Akermark C, Johansson C. Tenotomy of the adductor longus tendon in the treatment of chronic groin pain in athletes. Am J Sports Med 1992;20:640–3.

25. Anderson K, Strickland SM, Warren R. Hip and groin injuries in athletes. Am J Sports Med 2001;29:521–33.

26. Garrett WE Jr. Muscle strain injuries. Am J Sports Med 1996;24(Suppl 6):S2–8.

27. Nicholas SJ, Tyler TF. Adductor muscle strains in sports. Sports Med 2002;32:339–44.

28. Meyers WC, Lanfranco A, Castellanos A. Surgical management of chronic lower abdominal and groin pain in high-performance athletes. Curr Sports Med Rep 2002;1:301–5.

29. Gokhale S. Three-dimensional sonography of muscle hernias. J Ultrasound Med 2007;26:239–42.

30. Mellado JM, Perez del Palomar L. Muscle hernias of the lower leg: MRI findings. Skeletal Radiol 1999;28: 465–9.

31. Zoga AC, Morrison WB, Roth CG, et al. MR findings in athletic pubalgia: normal postoperative appearance and reinjury patterns after pelvic repairs and releases for 'sports hernia'. In: Proceedings of the Radiologic Society of North America. Chicago: Radiologic Society of North America; 2009.

32. Gullmo A. Herniography: the diagnosis of hernia in the groin and incompetence of the pouch of Douglas and pelvic floor. Acta Radiol Suppl 1980;361:1–76.

33. Van den Berg JC, de Valois JC, Go PM, et al. Detection of groin hernia with physical examination, ultrasound, and MRI compared with laparoscopic findings. Invest Radiol 1999;34:739–43.

34. Overdeck KH, Palmer WE. Imaging of hip and groin injuries in athletes. Semin Musculoskelet Radiol 2004;8:41–55.

35. Hwang B, Fredericson M, Chung C, et al. MRI Findings of Femoral Diaphyseal Stress Injuries in Athletes. AJR Am J Roentgenol 2005;185(1): 166–73.

36. Parziale JR, O'Donnell CJ, Sandman DN. Iliopsoas bursitis. Am J Phys Med Rehabil 2009; 88(8):690–1.

37. Varma D, Richli W, Charnsangavej C. MR appearance of the distended iliopsoas bursa. AJR Am J Roentgenol 1991;156:1025–8.

38. Peck DM. Apophyseal injuries in the young athlete. Am Fam Physician 1995;51:1891–5, 1897–8.

39. Zoga AC, Meyers WC. Magnetic resonance imaging for pain after surgical treatment for athletic pubalgia and the "sports hernia". Semin Musculoskelet Radiol 2011;15:372–82.

40. Meyers WC, Foley DP, Garrett WE, et al. PAIN (Performing Athletes with Abdominal or Inguinal Neuromuscular Pain Study Group). Management of severe lower abdominal or inguinal pain in high-performance athletes. Am J Sports Med 2000; 28(1):2–8.

41. Garvey JF, Read JW, Turner A. Sportsman hernia: what can we do? Hernia 2010;14(1):17–25.

42. Ziprin P, Prabhudesai SG, Abrahams S, et al. Transabdominal preperitoneal laparoscopic approach for the treatment of sportsman's hernia. J Laparoendosc Adv Surg Tech A 2008;18(5):669–72.

43. Caudill P, Nyland J, Smith C, et al. Sports hernias: a systematic literature review. Br J Sports Med 2008;42(12):954–64.

MR Imaging of Osseous Lesions of the Hip

Adnan Sheikh, MD[a],*, Khaldoun Koujok, MD[b],
Marcos Loreto Sampaio, MD[a], Mark E. Schweitzer, MD[a]

KEYWORDS

- MR imaging • Hip • Developmental dysplasia of the hip • Proximal femoral fractures
- Legg-Calvé-Perthes disease • Slipped capital femoral epiphysis • Avascular necrosis

KEY POINTS

- MR imaging, because of its superior contrast, plays a vital role in the workup of osseous abnormalities of the hip.
- MR imaging is an excellent modality to diagnose early Legg-Calvé-Perthes disease and slipped capital femoral epiphysis when radiographs are negative.
- MR imaging is essential to differentiate transient synovitis from other serious abnormalities, such as septic arthritis and osteomyelitis.
- Avascular necrosis is characterized by the "double line" sign on MR imaging.
- MR imaging plays an important role in the assessment of occult fractures, particularly in patients with osteoporosis.

INTRODUCTION

Painful conditions of the hip are often difficult to assess clinically, which leads to a reliance on imaging for diagnosis. Although radiography remains the cornerstone of investigation, MR imaging, because of its superior soft tissue resolution, has emerged as the preferred modality for evaluating osseous and soft tissue abnormalities around the hip. This article summarizes the clinical presentation, underlying disease processes, and essential radiologic features of common conditions affecting the osseous structures in the pediatric and adult hip. The first part reviews the pediatric hip conditions of Legg-Calvé-Perthes (LCP) disease, slipped capital femoral epiphysis (SFCE), and developmental dysplasia of the hip (DDH). The second part of the article discusses the clinical features and MR imaging findings of avascular necrosis (AVN) and proximal femoral fractures.

LCP DISEASE

LCP disease is an idiopathic ischemic necrosis of the proximal femoral epiphysis. It usually affects children between 3 and 12 years of age, most commonly between 5 and 7 years.[1] The disease occurs bilaterally in 8% to 20% and is 4 to 5 times more common in boys than girls.[1,2] Caucasians are more commonly affected with this disease, with a reported annual incidence ranging between 5.1 and 15.6 per 100,000.[3] Most patients with LCP disease have delayed skeletal maturation.[4]

Although the causes of LCP disease is unknown, impairment of the blood supply to the femoral head by extrinsic compression of vessels or intravascular occlusion is believed to be the cause.[5] In some cases, more than one episode of infarction occurs.

Most affected children present with limping caused by groin, thigh, or referred knee pain. The

Disclosures: No disclosures.
[a] The Ottawa Hospital, University of Ottawa, General Campus, 501 Smyth Road, Ottawa, Ontario K1H 8L6, Canada; [b] Department of Diagnostic Imaging, Children's Hospital of Eastern Ontario, University of Ottawa, 401 Smyth Road, Ottawa, Ontario K1H 8L1, Canada
* Corresponding author.
E-mail address: asheikh@ottawahospital.on.ca

Magn Reson Imaging Clin N Am 21 (2013) 111–125
http://dx.doi.org/10.1016/j.mric.2012.09.001

symptoms may sometimes be intermittent. The clinical examination may show restricted internal rotation and muscle atrophy around the hip. The standard radiologic evaluation should include supine anteroposterior neutral (AP) and external rotation-abduction (frog-leg) positions. These views should be obtained at the initial evaluation and follow-up studies.

Radiographic Findings

Radiographic findings of LCP disease are the result of osteonecrosis and subsequent repair. In the early stages of LCP disease, all or some of the following signs may be seen on radiographs: small and sclerotic proximal femoral epiphysis (compared with the contralateral side), ossification center lateralization, and subchondral fissure (crescent sign). Ossification center lateralization is caused by overgrowth of the acetabular cartilage and femoral head cartilage.[6] Subchondral lucency or fissure is commonly seen in the frog-leg position (Fig. 1A, B). This fissure appears as a thin line paralleling the outer contour of the anterolateral aspect of the epiphysis.[6] As the disease progresses, resorption and reossification continue simultaneously, giving the fragmented appearance of the femoral head. In advanced stages, flattening and

fragmentation associated with deformity, broadening, and lateral subluxation of the femoral epiphysis are seen. These changes are accompanied by broadening and shortening of the femoral neck, with cystic changes along the physis (Fig. 2A).

MR Imaging Findings

MR imaging has proved to be sensitive even in the early phase of LCP disease when radiographs are normal or equivocal. MR imaging provides more accurate evaluation of the extent of involvement, staging, prognosis, and complications. A strong correlation exists between the contrast-enhancing areas on MR imaging and the viable tissue of the femoral epiphysis, which is an important factor in predicting prognosis.[7] MR imaging features are variable, depending on the different stages of the disease (ie, necrotic, revascularization, and reparative phase).[8]

Early (necrotic) stage of the disease

On T1-weighted images, linear hypointensity along the periphery of the epiphysis, multiple hypointense lines traversing the epiphysis, or loss of the high signal intensity (normal fat signal) may be seen. On T2-weighted or STIR images, hypointense signal is usually seen in the epiphysis, but bone marrow edema can sometimes cause

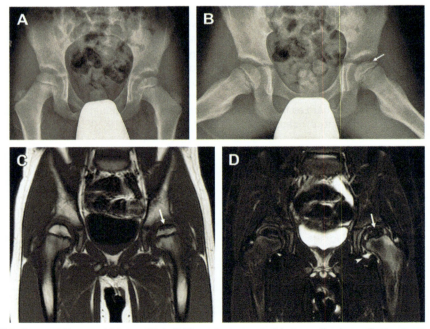

Fig. 1. (A) AP radiograph 7-year-old boy with left hip pain, now unable to walk, shows flattening and sclerosis of the left femoral head. (B) Frog-leg view reveals the same findings in addition to the crescent sign (arrow). (C) Coronal T1-weighted image shows flattening of left femoral epiphysis with hypointense signal (arrow). (D) Coronal T2-weighted fat-saturated image shows the subchondral hypointensity representing the fracture (arrow) surrounded by bone marrow edema medially and laterally. Note the reactive left hip effusion (arrowhead).

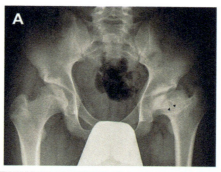

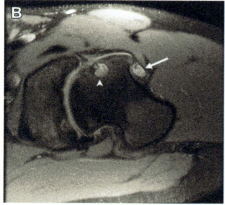
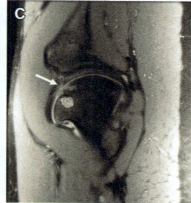

Fig. 2. (*A*) AP radiograph in a15-year-old boy with old LCP disease shows the deformity of the left femoral head (coxa magna and coxa plana) with cystic changes (*arrowheads*). (*B*) Axial proton-density fat-saturated image shows the widened femoral head with the subchondral cyst (*arrowhead*) and reactive effusion (*arrow*). (*C*) Sagittal proton-density fat-saturated image shows ill-defined and irregular labrum (*arrow*).

hyperintense signal (see **Fig. 1**C, D). In some cases, the subchondral fracture shows a curvilinear T1 signal hypointensity and T2 signal hyperintensity (crescent sign).[8] The contrast-enhanced images show nonperfusion of the infarcted areas. Reactive synovitis of the involved hip is a constant finding on MR imaging.[9] It is manifested by hypointense T1 signal and hyperintense T2 signal hip effusion with synovial enhancement.

Revascularization and reparative stages of the disease

Resorption and replacement of the dead bone occur simultaneously in these phases, giving the fragmented appearance. Heterogeneous signal intensity is usually seen on T1- and T2-weighted sequences and heterogeneous enhancement correlates with the reossification process. The new vascularized deposited bone shows high signal (marrow fat) on T1 and enhances after gadolinium administration. MR imaging can be used to assess the various deformities of the epiphysis, physis, and metaphysis that may be seen in these stages, and can help predict the outcome of LCP disease (see **Fig. 2**B, C). More than 50% involvement of the epiphysis or more than 20% of lateral

extrusion of the epiphyseal cartilage is associated with poor prognosis.

The treatment of LCP disease is rest and restricted physical activity until the reparative phase has been established, in which the epiphyseal fragmentation has stabilized and the epiphyseal height is slowly restored.

SCFE

SCFE is a Salter-Harris type 1 shearing fracture of the proximal femoral physis caused by the repetitive stress of weight-bearing. It is the most common hip disorder in adolescents during the period of accelerated growth.[10] The rate of incidence is 10.8 per 100,000 children.[11] SCFE is 2 to 4 times more common in boys than girls.[6] The age of presentation is different between the genders because of difference in puberty; for girls it ranges from 8 to 15 years, with the average incidence at 11 to 12 years; for boys it ranges from 10 to 17 years, with the average incidence at 13 to 14 years.[12] SCFE can be bilateral in 37% of cases, with 18% of them diagnosed simultaneously in both hips at the initial presentation.[13] Most second hip slips occur within 18 months of the first slip.[13]

SCFE is more common in black children and observed more frequently in warm weather.[14] SCFE has several predisposing factors, but obesity is the most significant factor; approximately half of the affected children are heavier than the 95th percentile for their age.[6] Other factors include endocrine disorders (primary hypothyroidism, pituitary dysfunction, growth hormone deficiency, and hypogonadism), metabolic disorders (rickets and malnutrition), renal failure osteodystrophy, radiation therapy, chemotherapy, prior hip dysplasia, and Down syndrome.[12] When SCFE is diagnosed in a child younger than 10 years of age, an underlying metabolic or endocrine disorder should be strongly considered.[15]

Children with SCFE usually present with limping and hip or thigh pain, but one-fourth complain of knee pain.[6] Clinical examination may show limited internal rotation and flexion of the hip.

Depending on the degree of femoral head displacement, the slip is classified as preslip (no displacement), mild (displacement less than one-third the diameter of the metaphysis), moderate (displacement between one-third and two-thirds the diameter of the metaphysis), and severe (displacement more than two-thirds the diameter of the metaphysis).[14]

Radiographic Findings

Standard radiologic evaluation should include supine AP projection and a true lateral view. It is better to avoid the external rotation-abduction (frog-leg) position to avoid the stress on the displaced epiphysis.[6] Before the actual slip occurs (preslip phase), the growth plate of the femoral head becomes wide and indistinct on the AP view (**Fig. 3**A). After the slip occurs, a dense line parallel to the physis appears on the metaphyseal side on the AP view (double-density). In a normal hip, a tangential line drawn along the lateral margin of the femoral neck bisects a small portion of the epiphysis (Klein's line). In SCFE, the portion of the epiphysis lateral to Klein's line may be absent. When the slippage occurs, the epiphysis moves medial and posterior in respect to the metaphysis. Therefore, the lateral view (or the frog-leg view if obtained) usually delineates the slip much better than the AP view (see **Fig. 3**B). In the chronic SCFE cases, periosteal new bone formation can be seen along the femoral neck (**Fig. 4**).

MR Imaging Findings

MR imaging is helpful in preslip cases or when radiographs are equivocal. The MR imaging findings of SCFE include focal or diffuse physeal widening, periphyseal bone marrow edema, joint effusion, and synovitis (see **Fig. 3**C, D).[15] Bone marrow edema is not a constant finding on MR imaging.[15] T1 and water-sensitive sequences should be obtained in all planes to evaluate the slip, its extent, and associated abnormalities, such as osteonecrosis. The axial oblique plane through the long axis of the femoral neck is essential to evaluate subtle slippage (see **Fig. 3**E).[15] MR imaging is also helpful to evaluate the complications of SCFE and its treatment, such as slip progression, early degenerative disease, labral tears, osteonecrosis, chondrolysis, and hardware failure.[14,15]

The goal of SCFE treatment is to stabilize the slip and prevent further progression, which is achieved through in situ pinning without reduction.

DDH

DDH is a term that includes a spectrum of conditions, from hip instability, anatomic dysplasia (changes in shape and dimensions), to dislocation of the hip (usually posterosuperiorly in relation to the acetabulum).[16] It is defined as a deformity of the acetabulum with associated proper or improper location of the femoral head (congruent, subluxed of dislocated).[17] Lax ligamentous support to the hip may also allow excessive motion and facilitate the dysplasia. Morphologic changes may occur in a newborn or during the early hip development, and the term congenital hip dysplasia should be avoided.[18] The acetabular deformity shifts the expected vertical component of the hip joint force away from the acetabular bone surface toward the superolateral capsular-labrum-complex, which acts as a secondary stabilizer, leading to excessive tension and shear stresses.[19] DDH may be associated with changes of soft tissues, including fibrocartilaginous hypertrophy of the labrum (denominated limbus), hypertrophy of the ridge of acetabular cartilage (neolimbus),[20] ligamentum teres thickening, weakening of the cartilage, and hypertrophy of the acetabular fibro-fatty tissue (pulvinar). Although the exact cutoff separating normal from abnormal morphologic findings is not entirely clear, and because there is likely a continuum of this process, early diagnosis of the disease using modern imaging tests is important to minimize future harm to the hip joint[21] and the development of premature osteoarthritis.[16]

The prevalence of DDH is approximately 1.3 per 1000 children, and 1.2 per 1000 newborns require treatment in North America and Western Europe. Genetic and environmental factors, breech positioning, and being first born are associated with an increased prevalence of DDH. An estimated 80% of persons with DDH are girls.[22]

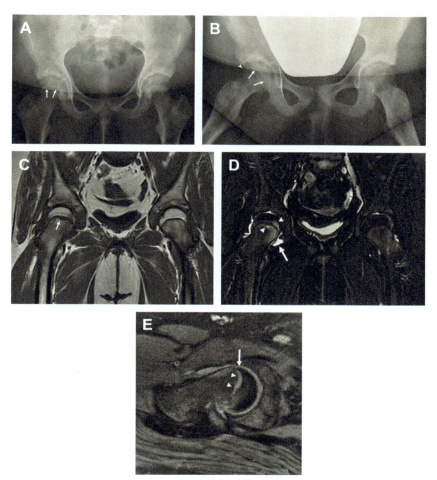

Fig. 3. (*A*) AP radiograph in a12-year-old obese girl with a 3-week history of right hip pain and who is unable to bear weight shows the widened growth plate of the right femoral head (*arrows*). (*B*) Frog-leg view reveals the widened physis (*arrows*) and the mild slip (*arrowhead*). (*C*) Coronal T1-weighted image reveals the widened physis (*arrow*). (*D*) Coronal T2-weighted fat-saturated image shows the periphyseal marrow edema (*arrowheads*) and the reactive hip effusion (*arrow*). (*E*) Axial-oblique proton-density fat-saturated image delineates the widening of the physis (*arrowheads*) and the slip (*arrow*).

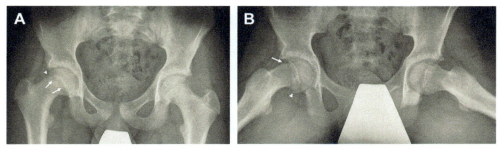

Fig. 4. (*A*) AP radiograph in 12-year-old boy with chronic mild SCFE shows the widened ill-defined physis (*arrows*) and the very subtle slip (*arrowhead*). (*B*) Frog-leg view shows the widened physis and the mild slip (*arrowhead*). Note the periosteal reaction along the lateral margin of the metaphysis (*arrow*).

Screening of DDH in newborns is performed routinely through the physical examination, including the maneuvers of Ortolani (which attempts to reduce a dislocated hip) and Barlow (which attempts to dislocate an unstable hip). The examination may be repeated periodically until the age of 12 months, because the initial examination may fail to diagnose this disorder.[23] Ultrasound and radiographs have not been supported as screening tests. Imaging tests are used for equivocal cases with suspicious physical findings (ultrasound at 6 weeks or pelvic radiography at 4 months). Their use for high-risk cases (girls and boys in breech presentation and girls with a positive family history) is controversial.[23,24]

Ultrasound Findings

Typically ultrasound is the preferred method for evaluating clinically suspected neonatal dysplasia. Advantages of ultrasound include absence of ionizing radiation, static and dynamic evaluation of the hip, low cost, and portability. The main disadvantage is the need for expertise in obtaining and interpreting the images. The study includes the evaluation of

- Acetabular roof angle, labrum angle, and acetabular rim shape
- Congruency of the joint, including a dynamic evaluation
- Acetabular coverage (equivalent of the radiographic migration percentage)
- Soft tissues: pulvinar hypertrophy and limbus interposition for reduction on the dynamic study
- Ossification center of the femoral head: asymmetry in dimensions and vascularization of the head

The constellation of parameters helps stage the development of the hip, and may be used in follow-up studies. Ultrasound also evaluates the congruency of the head in patients with the Pavlik harness and after its removal, and during and after closed reduction. The exact protocol to follow may vary among different institutions and societal recommendations.

Radiographic Findings

Radiographs are most useful after 3 to 6 months of age. A frontal supine projection is performed with neutral position of the hips (standing in older children). The absence of ossification during the first months of life and the ionizing radiation are major limitations of radiographic evaluation. Accessory lines of Hilgenreiner (horizontal line through the top of the triradiate cartilages) and Perkins (perpendicular to Hilgenreiner line crossing the lateral margin of the acetabular roof) are used. Some evaluated parameters are

- Dimensions and position of the ossification centers of the femoral heads (some asymmetry in dimensions is tolerable). The femoral head ossification center may be smaller in the affected side. The ossification center and the superomedial margin of the femoral metaphysis should project over the inner lower quadrant of the intersection of Hilgenreiner and Perkin lines.
- Shenton line: normal when a continuous arch is formed by the lower aspect of the superior pubic ramus and the medial margin of the femoral neck (**Fig. 5**).
- Acetabular index (or inclination angle): angle between the line of Hilgenreiner and the acetabular roof (variable with development; normal below 24° for 1 year of age and below 10° for adults) (see **Fig. 5**).
- Center-edge angle of Wiberg: angle between a vertical line perpendicular to the transverse axis of the acetabulum (as Hilgenreiner line) and a line between the center of the head and the lateral margin of the acetabular roof. This angle should be at least 26° in adults (see **Fig. 5**).
- Von Rosen line: superior extension of the femoral shaft, which should intersect the acetabulum.

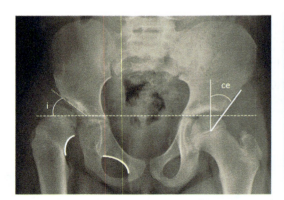

Fig. 5. Pelvic AP radiograph 10-year-old patient with right hip DDH shows (A) disruption of the Shenton line (*solid arches*) on the right, (B) acetabular angle (i) formed between Hilgenreiner line (*dashed line*) and the acetabular roof line (*dotted line*), and the (C) center-edge angle (ce), which is the angle between a line perpendicular to the transverse axis of the pelvis (*thin solid line*) and a line through the center of the femoral head and the margin of the acetabular roof (*thick solid line*). The left side has normal center-edge angle value, but an abnormal center-edge angle is seen on the right.

- Lateral line: normal when there is a continuous arch from the lateral margins of the iliac wing and the femoral neck.
- Migration percentage: percentage of the femoral head lateral to the Perkin line. It should be zero in patients younger than 3 years, and up to 22% for older subjects.
- Medial joint space: distance between the medial margin of the ossification center and acetabular wall. This distance should be less than 1.5 mm.[17]

Radiographs may be used before and after treatment at any age. An arthrogram of the hip may rarely be performed during closed reduction to determinate what is preventing the reduction, such as a limbus (hypertrophied labrum with fibrous and cartilaginous overgrowth)[20] or a thickened ligamentum teres.

CT Findings

CT may be used to supplement radiographs or ultrasound before and after surgical management of the hip. The use of CT is infrequent and special care should be used, especially the implementation of a very-low-dose protocol, to decrease the dose of ionizing radiation. Also, CT has a relative high-cost. However, the use of CT is limited by not only its ionizing radiation dose but also its relatively high cost. Advantages of CT include multiplanar and 3-dimensional reconstructions and the relative speed of the study, mitigating the use of sedation.

CT evaluation includes analysis of hip congruency after reduction and casting of the hip (**Fig. 6**) in the axial plane. In the frog-leg position, a smooth continuity should be present between the anterior aspect of the femoral neck and the pubic bone,[25] with this line being disrupted in dislocated hips.

After closed reduction with immobilization in a spica cast, a hip abduction angle greater than 55° is associated with increased risk of AVN of the head.[24,26] The angle may be calculated between the femoral shaft and the sagittal plane, between the pubic symphysis and coccyx.[27] For severe cases or later diagnosis and treatment in adults, the evaluation of acetabular morphology and version and measurement of femoral head-neck offset may also be measured, before pelvic osteotomy.[25,28] Arthro-CT can demonstrate intra-articular lesions, including labral injuries, and is sensitive to the presence of chondral defects.[29]

MR Imaging Findings

The primary workup for DDH does not usually include MR imaging. However, MR imaging has the advantages of the absence of ionizing radiation and direct visualization of soft tissue structures in multiple planes. Disadvantages include the high cost and frequent need for sedation, although a simplified protocol may potentially preclude that.[25,30] Applications for MR imaging include

- Assessment of proper congruency of the hip.[31] As with CT, the position of the head may be evaluated in multiple planes. The degree of abduction may also be calculated. Because the patient is in a cast, motion artifacts are minimal (**Fig. 7**)
- Diagnosis of AVN of the femoral head, a serious complication that may lead to growth disturbances. AVN of the femoral head may occur in 26% to 47% of cases.[32] After reduction, the femoral head should be in the so-called safe zone, reduced but not hyperabducted, because the latter is associated with AVN. Studies with gadolinium-enhanced MR imaging showed that decreased enhancement of the reduced femoral head, in relation to the contralateral

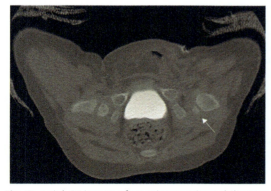

Fig. 6. Axial CT image after spica cast immobilization postreduction in a 1-year-old patient. Persistent left hip incongruence with posterior subluxation is seen (*arrow*).

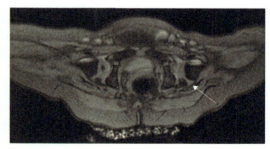

Fig. 7. Axial T2 merge fat-saturated image in a 11-month-old patient after reduction shows the femoral heads to be congruent, but asymmetry in the dimensions is present (*arrow*). (*Courtesy of* Dr. Elka Miller, Ottawa/Canada.)

side, is associated with the development of AVN.[27,31] The presence of an ossification center at the time of the reduction does not seem to protect against AVN, although a tendency is seen toward better outcomes in a recent study.[33]

- Evaluation of soft tissues and their potential impediment to reduction, such as hypertrophy of the pulvinar, ligamentum teres, or transverse ligament; inverted limbus or capsular folds.[31,34] Although previous studies showed better visualization of some of the soft tissues structures with MR imaging arthrography,[34] modern MR imaging scanners, particularly with 3T MR imaging, may preclude the need for intraarticular injection because of improved image quality.[25]

- Labral evaluation in adolescents or adults with late-diagnosed or residual DDH. This finding may be associated with instability or mechanical axis shift from the insufficient acetabular coverage with labral hypertrophy, which is subject to increased stress.

Degenerative labral signal changes with tears and labral shape distortion, with associated hypertrophy or cysts, are typical findings (**Fig. 8**A, B)

- Acetabular and femoral morphology assessment. Both components may present morphologic changes such as acetabular retroversion, coxa profunda, acetabular protrusion, and altered offset of the femoral head and neck. These may be associated with mechanical hip impingement, further increasing the chances of morbidity of the hip joint.

- Hyaline cartilage assessment (see **Fig. 8**C). Patients with DDH are at higher risk for development of osteoarthritis. MR imaging may directly evaluate the hip joint cartilage before the onset of osteoarthritis. A study with mechanically loaded hips showed a decrease in the cartilage T2 signal at outer superficial zones of the acetabulum, representing an area of increased mechanical stress and initial degenerative changes/injury.[35] MR imaging may show areas of chondral injury

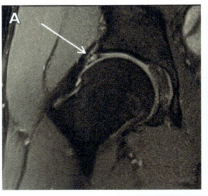
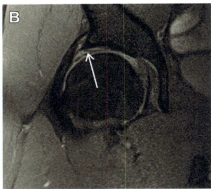
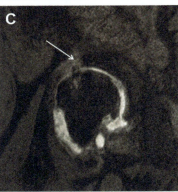

Fig. 8. (A) Coronal proton density fat-suppressed MR imaging shows a labral tear (arrow) in a patient with mild DDH. (B) Coronal proton density fat-suppressed image in the same patient shows early acetabular chondral lesion with thinning and signal changes (arrow) adjacent to the torn labral base. (C) Gradient recalled echo T2 fat-saturated sagittal reformat in a different patient with DDH and severe chondral loss and labral tear (arrow).

before osteoarthritic changes are detected on radiographs. Another study showed a correlation between lower delayed gadolinium-enhanced MR imaging of cartilage index and patients with failed Bernese osteotomy,[36] suggesting that early detection of osteoarthritis may help separate good from poor surgical candidates. However, more studies are needed to demonstrate the real contribution of MR imaging–based cartilage evaluation as a prognostic factor for surgery.[37]

- Contribution to corrective surgery indication. After reduction, residual subluxation may lead to future need for corrective surgery, usually indicated by a constellation of clinical parameters and radiographs. A recent study showed an association between an area of high signal intensity on T2-weighted sequences at the weight-bearing area of the acetabulum and poor acetabular growth, suggesting that this may be a useful parameter in borderline indicated cases for open surgical indication.[38]

TRANSIENT SYNOVITIS

Transient synovitis (toxic synovitis, irritable hip) is a benign transient inflammation of the synovial membrane of the hip. It is one of the most common causes of acute hip pain in children between 3 and 10 years of age.[39,40] It is a self-limited condition and usually resolves within a few days. The cause of transient synovitis is largely unknown. It affects boys more than girls by a ratio of 2:1.[39]

The clinical presentation of transient synovitis may be similar to LCP disease and septic arthritis.[6,39] Therefore, the diagnosis of transient synovitis should be one of exclusion.[39] Affected children present with a recent history of acute hip or knee pain associated with limping. On clinical examination, the hip is usually held in flexion and external rotation with limited range of motion.[39]

The hip radiographs are basically normal in most cases. Occasionally, widening of the medial joint space can be seen, indicating a joint effusion. Ultrasound is excellent to reveal the hip effusion and the synovial thickening but cannot differentiate transient synovitis from septic arthritis (Fig. 9). However, the absence of effusion can exclude septic arthritis of the hip.[41] The MR features of transient synovitis include joint effusion, thickened enhancing synovium, soft tissue signal alterations, and normal bone marrow signal (Fig. 10).[40,42] The main MR finding that differentiates septic arthritis from transient synovitis is the presence of bone marrow edema in the septic hip.[40,42] These areas of bone marrow edema (T1 hypointensity and T2 hyperintensity) enhance after gadolinium injection.[40,42] The absence of joint effusion with enhancing synovium can exclude septic arthritis of the hip with 100% certainty.[43]

The treatment of transient synovitis is symptomatic, involving bedrest and anti-inflammatory medications.

AVN

AVN of the femoral head is an increasingly common cause of musculoskeletal disability. It is the result of bone cell death from interruption of the blood supply.[44] Diagnosis of AVN of the femoral head depends on the combination of clinical symptoms and evaluation of radiographs and/or MR imaging or scintigraphy. The Ficat and the Association Research Circulation Osseous classification are commonly used to assess these imaging modalities.[45]

By convention, the term *avascular (ischemic) necrosis* is generally applied to areas of epiphyseal or subarticular involvement, whereas *bone infarct*

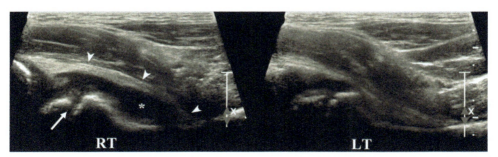

Fig. 9. Young child with transient synovitis of the right hip. Ultrasound image shows effusion in the right hip and normal left hip. The right hip fluid (*asterisk*) is anechoic, displacing the joint capsule (*arrowheads*). Note normal physis of the right hip (*arrow*).

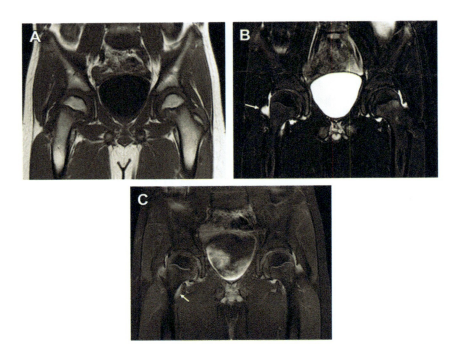

Fig. 10. In a 7-year-old with right hip pain for 6 days not responsive to analgesics, MR imaging was performed to rule out septic arthritis and LCP disease. (*A*) Coronal T1-weighted image shows normal marrow fat signal of the right femoral head. (*B*) Coronal T2-weighted fat-saturated image shows normal signal of the right femoral head and small hip effusion (*arrow*). (*C*) Coronal T1-weighted contrast-enhanced fat-saturated image reveals normal enhancement of the femoral head with subtle increased enhancement of the right hip synovium (*arrow*).

usually is reserved for metaphyseal and diaphyseal involvement. The origin of AVN is multifactorial, although the exact pathophysiology is not fully understood. AVN usually affects bones with a single terminal blood supply, such as the femoral head, carpal bones, talus, and humerus.[45] In practice, AVN is most commonly encountered in the hip.

Pathophysiology

AVN has many causes, including hemoglobinopathies, Cushing syndrome, exogenous steroid use, alcoholism, pancreatitis, HIV, Gaucher disease, and caisson disease, but trauma is the most common cause. AVN of the jaw associated with bisphosphonate use has also been described.[46] AVN may also be idiopathic.

Fifteen thousand new cases of AVN are reported each year in the United States, and AVN accounts for more than 10% of total hip replacement surgeries.[47] The age of onset depends on the underlying cause. Primary AVN most often occurs during the fourth or fifth decade, and is bilateral in 40% to 80% of cases. It has no racial predilection except for cases associated with sickle cell disease and hemoglobin S, which predominantly occur in people of African and Mediterranean descent.

Imaging

Conventional radiographs, CT, nuclear medicine study, and MR imaging can identify AVN. MR imaging is more sensitive than CT, radiography, and even scintigraphy.

Radiographic Findings

Findings on radiographs lag several months behind those of more advanced imaging techniques, and thus radiographs are often unremarkable in the early stages of disease. The earliest findings visible on radiography are sclerosis and changes in bone density. In advanced disease, the subchondral radiolucent line (crescent sign), flattening of the femoral head, and joint space narrowing are seen.[48]

The Ficat staging system is commonly used to classify the radiographic appearance of AVN of the hip.

Radionuclide Findings

In early AVN, decreased uptake on Technetium-99m bone scan occurs in areas of necrosis. Thereafter, an area of increased uptake surrounds the central area of decreased uptake. This "doughnut" sign indicates a reactive zone surrounding the necrotic area.[49] However, bone scans have limitations. In early AVN the findings are less sensitive than MR imaging. The results can be difficult to interpret when the disease is bilateral.

CT Findings

CT is not sensitive in detecting early changes. However, it may be used to assess the extent of more advanced disease.

Osteoporosis is the first visible sign on CT. Later, the central medullary asterisk, which refers to the star-shaped appearance of the normal thickened weight-bearing trabeculae, is distorted, appearing as clumping and fusion of the peripheral asterisk rays. This structure has been termed the *asterisk sign*,[50] and roughly corresponds to the double-line sign seen on MR imaging.

MR Imaging Findings

MR imaging has been accepted as the most sensitive modality in the early detection of AVN. It has a sensitivity of 97% and specificity of 98% for diagnosing AVN of the hip.[51] The high frequency of bilateral osteonecrosis supports the use of large field-of-view sequences of the entire pelvis.

In early AVN, diffuse bone marrow edema occurs, which is seen as decreased signal intensity with poorly defined margins on T1-weighted images. A serpiginous line of low signal intensity is seen on T1-weighted images. A classic appearance of AVN is the double-line sign, which occurs later in the disease process after the onset of osseous repair.[51,52] This sign describes a focal area of high or intermediate signal intensity (white) that is surrounded by a rim of low signal intensity (black) on T1 and T2 images (**Fig. 11**). A peripheral high-signal-intensity line may represent hypervascular granulation tissue, and a low-signal-intensity line correlates with the histologic reactive zone at the outer margin of a necrotic lesion. The double-line sign is seen in up to 80% of cases. Bony collapse and sclerosis are seen as focal areas of low signal on T1-weighted images and of variable signal on T2-weighted images.

The MR imaging findings of AVN of the hip may be classified according to a system proposed by Mitchell and colleagues[51]:

- Class A lesion: signal intensity characteristics analogous to those of fat on T1-weighted images and intermediate signal intensity on T2-weighted images.
- Class B lesion: signal intensity characteristics that are similar to those of blood, with high signal intensity on T1- and T2-weighted images.
- Class C lesion: signal intensity properties that are similar to those of fluid, with low signal intensity on T1-weighted images and high signal intensity on T2-weighted images.
- Class D lesion: signal intensity is similar to that of fibrous tissue, with low signal intensity on T1- and T2-weighted images.

MR imaging also helps quantify the percentage of involvement of the femoral head, extent of articular cartilage involvement, presence and extent femoral head collapse, joint effusion, and secondary osteoarthritic changes in the hip joint.[53,54]

DIFFERENTIAL DIAGNOSES
Transient Osteoporosis of the Hip

Transient osteoporosis of the hip (TOH) is a self-limiting condition that resolves over time. Although it was first described in women in the third trimester of pregnancy, it primarily affects middle-aged men.[55] Evidence of osteoporosis extending from the head to intertrochanteric region is seen on conventional radiographs. Bone scintigraphy shows increased uptake, reflecting the increased bone turnover and inflammatory change, but imaging findings are nonspecific. MR imaging shows diffuse bone marrow edema involving the femoral head and neck region with or without a lesion in the subchondral region, which appears as a hypointense line on both T1 and T2 sequences (**Fig. 12**A, B).[56,57] Subchondral fractures have been identified in patients with transient osteoporosis of the hip, suggesting that subchondral fractures play a role in the pathophysiology of the disorder.[58]

Subchondral Stress Fracture

Subchondral fractures occur as stress fractures in young adults and insufficiency fracture in those

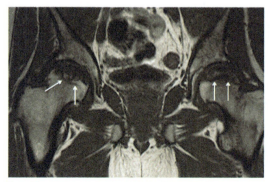

Fig. 11. Bilateral osteonecrosis. Coronal T1-weighted image shows focal areas of bilateral osteonecrosis with a double-line sign (*arrows*). The osteonecrosis involves 100% of the articular surface. No evidence of collapse of the femoral head or secondary osteoarthritis.

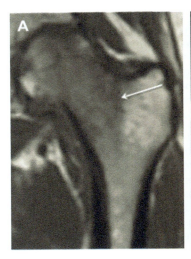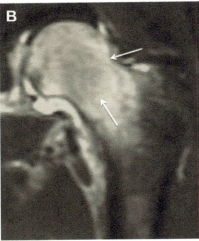

Fig. 12. Transient osteoporosis of the hip in a middle-aged man with increasing hip pain. (*A*) Coronal T1 and (*B*) coronal proton density–weighted fat-saturated images show evidence of extensive marrow edema involving the femoral head and neck (*arrows*). No definite fracture line is seen. A small joint effusion is noted.

who are elderly. On MR imaging, these fractures appear as a linear low-signal area surrounded by high signal consistent with marrow edema on T2-weighted images, with eventual collapse and resorption of the femoral head and development of secondary osteoarthritis.[59]

OSSEOUS INJURIES

Fractures of the hip are common in adults and often lead to significant morbidity and mortality, particularly in the elderly population. Fractures involving the hip can be stress and insufficiency fractures, but most occur after a fall.

Acute posttraumatic femoral head and neck fractures can be capital, subcapital, transcervical, basicervical, intertrochanteric, and subtrochanteric. The obvious fracture can be easily identified on an AP and lateral radiograph. CT scan can better delineate these fractures and has a definitive role in preoperative evaluation.

Occult Fractures

Although the displaced hip fracture can be visualized easily on plain radiography, the nondisplaced fracture may be radiographically occult and require further imaging. Occult fractures in elderly patients as a result of trauma or chronic stress are often seen in the femoral neck, greater trochanter, and acetabulum. In patients with osteoporosis, conventional radiographs may not demonstrate the fracture and CT may be helpful in detecting the fracture. Bone scintigraphy has a lower sensitivity than MR imaging, and may demonstrate increased uptake only days after trauma.[60]

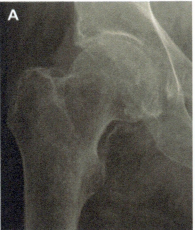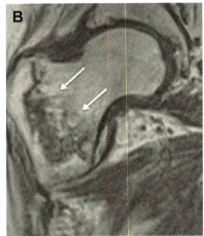

Fig. 13. Occult femoral neck fracture. (*A*) AP radiograph of an elderly patient with a history of fall and unable to weight-bear shows osteoporosis with no definite fracture. (*B*) Coronal T1-weighted image shows a definite nondisplaced femoral neck fracture (*arrow*).

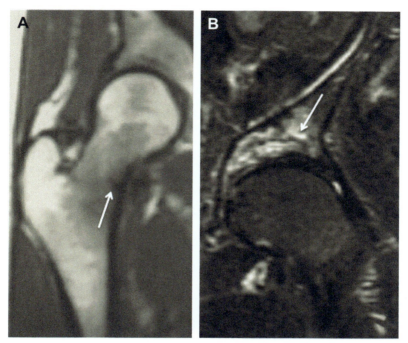

Fig. 14. (*A*) Coronal T1-weighted image showing a stress fracture of the medial femoral neck (*arrow*). (*B*) Coronal short T1 inversion recovery image in a different patient shows evidence of insufficiency fracture (*arrow*) in the supraacetabular region with surrounding edema.

MR imaging has emerged as a sensitive and specific imaging modality with its ability to detect the fracture line and the surrounding edema.[61,62] MR imaging is particularly useful in detecting incomplete femoral neck fractures, which are not evident on conventional radiographs. The detection of these fractures is important, because they may progress to a complete and displaced fracture if the patient continues weight-bearing.[63]

Although some studies have shown that a coronal T1-weighted sequence is sufficient to identify a fracture (**Fig. 13**A, B), the addition of a coronal T2-weighted or a short T1 inversion recovery coronal sequence permits superior visualization of the surrounding bony edema and soft tissue injuries.[59,62–64]

Fatigue-type stress fractures are more frequently seen in young adults who participate in strenuous activity, and are more common in military recruits or athletes. Fatigue fractures are related to the inability of weakened bony trabeculae to withstand physical stresses. Unusually high physical demands on normal bone over the long term can lead to mechanical failure of the bone trabeculae, resulting in a compression-type fracture involving the cancellous bone of the medial inferior femoral neck without disruption of cortical bone.[65,66]

Insufficiency fractures of the femoral neck are the result of normal stresses of everyday activity placed on structurally compromised bone. These fractures are often incomplete, and on MR imaging are seen as low signal intensity areas with surrounding edema. Similar insufficiency fractures can also be seen in the supraacetabular region (**Fig. 14**A, B).[59,66,67]

SUMMARY

The superior resolution and sensitivity in depicting the osseous and soft tissue structures surrounding the hip joint makes MR imaging an ideal modality for assessing the manifestations and sequelae of congenital and traumatic conditions around the hip. MR imaging plays an important role in the evaluation and diagnosis of pediatric hip conditions without the use of ionizing radiation. In adults, it helps provide prompt diagnosis, which allows for early treatment.

REFERENCES

1. Wenger DR, Ward WT, Herring JA. Legg-Calve-Perthes disease. J Bone Joint Surg Am 1991;73(5): 778–88.

2. Guille JT, Lipton GE, Szoke G, et al. Legg-Calve-Perthes disease in girls. A comparison of the results with those seen in boys. J Bone Joint Surg Am 1998; 80(9):1256–63.

3. Barker DJ, Hall AJ. The epidemiology of Perthes' disease. Clin Orthop Relat Res 1986;(209):89–94.

4. Harrison MH, Turner MH, Jacobs P. Skeletal immaturity in Perthes' disease. J Bone Joint Surg Br 1976; 58(1):37–40.

5. Vosmaer A, Pereira RR, Koenderman JS, et al. Coagulation abnormalities in Legg-Calve-Perthes disease. J Bone Joint Surg Am 2010;92(1):121–8.

6. Ozonoff MB. Pediatric orthopedic radiology. 2nd edition. Philadelphia: Saunders; 1992.

7. Mahnken AH, Staatz G, Ihme N, et al. MR signal intensity characteristics in Legg-Calve-Perthes disease. Value of fat-suppressed (STIR) images and contrast-enhanced T1-weighted images. Acta Radiol 2002;43(3):329–35.

8. Dillman JR, Hernandez RJ. MRI of Legg-Calve-Perthes disease. AJR Am J Roentgenol 2009; 193(5):1394–407.

9. Hochbergs P, Eckerwall G, Egund N, et al. Synovitis in Legg-Calve-Perthes disease. Evaluation with MR imaging in 84 hips. Acta Radiol 1998;39(5):532–7.

10. Crawford AH. Slipped capital femoral epiphysis. J Bone Joint Surg Am 1988;70(9):1422–7.

11. Lehmann CL, Arons RR, Loder RT, et al. The epidemiology of slipped capital femoral epiphysis: an update. J Pediatr Orthop 2006;26(3):286–90.

12. Donnelly LF. Diagnostic imaging. Pediatrics. 1st edition. Salt Lake City (UT): Amirsys; 2005.

13. Loder RT, Aronson DD, Greenfield ML. The epidemiology of bilateral slipped capital femoral epiphysis. A study of children in Michigan. J Bone Joint Surg Am 1993;75(8):1141–7.

14. Boles CA, el-Khoury GY. Slipped capital femoral epiphysis. Radiographics 1997;17(4):809–23.

15. Kan JH, Kleinman PK. Pediatric and adolescent musculoskeletal MRI: a cased-based approach. New York: Springer; 2007.

16. Roposch A, Wright JG. Increased diagnostic information and understanding disease: uncertainty in the diagnosis of developmental hip dysplasia. Radiology 2007;242(2):355–9.

17. Gerscovich EO. A radiologist's guide to the imaging in the diagnosis and treatment of developmental dysplasia of the hip. I. General considerations, physical examination as applied to real-time sonography and radiography. Skeletal Radiol 1997;26(7):386–97.

18. Donaldson JS, Feinstein KA. Imaging of developmental dysplasia of the hip. Pediatr Clin North Am 1997;44(3):591–614.

19. Tschauner C, Hofmann S. Labrum lesions in residual dysplasia of the hip joint. Biomechanical considerations on pathogenesis and treatment. Orthopade 1998;27(11):725–32 [in German].

20. Landa J, Benke M, Feldman DS. The limbus and the neolimbus in developmental dysplasia of the hip. Clin Orthop Relat Res 2008;466(4):776–81.

21. Tschauner C, Sheikh MA, Khaldoun K, et al. Labrum lesions and residual dysplasia of the hip joint. Definition and prospectives. Orthopade 1998;27(11):772–8 [in German].

22. Wilkinson JA. A post-natal survey for congenital displacement of the hip. J Bone Joint Surg Br 1972;54(1):40–9.

23. Patel H. Preventive health care, 2001 update: screening and management of developmental dysplasia of the hip in newborns. CMAJ 2001; 164(12):1669–77.

24. Carey T. Current concepts in the treatment of DDH. Available at: http://www.coa-aco.org/library/clinical-topics/current-concepts-in-the-treatment-of-ddh.html. Accessed August 1, 2012.

25. Grissom L, Harcke HT, Thacker M. Imaging in the surgical management of developmental dislocation of the hip. Clin Orthop Relat Res 2008;466(4):791–801.

26. Stanton RP, Capecci R. Computed tomography for early evaluation of developmental dysplasia of the hip. J Pediatr Orthop 1992;12(6):727–30.

27. Tiderius C, et al. Post-closed reduction perfusion magnetic resonance imaging as a predictor of avascular necrosis in developmental hip dysplasia: a preliminary report. J Pediatr Orthop 2009;29(1):14–20.

28. Fayad LM, Johnson P, Fishman EK. Multidetector CT of musculoskeletal disease in the pediatric patient: principles, techniques, and clinical applications. Radiographics 2005;25(3):603–18.

29. Langlais F, et al. Hip pain from impingement and dysplasia in patients aged 20-50 years. Workup and role for reconstruction. Joint Bone Spine 2006; 73(6):614–23.

30. Conroy E, et al. Axial STIR MRI: a faster method for confirming femoral head reduction in DDH. J Child Orthop 2009;3(3):223–7.

31. Jaramillo D, et al. Gadolinium-enhanced MR imaging of pediatric patients after reduction of dysplastic hips: assessment of femoral head position, factors impeding reduction, and femoral head ischemia. AJR Am J Roentgenol 1998;170(6):1633–7.

32. Brougham DI, et al. Avascular necrosis following closed reduction of congenital dislocation of the hip. Review of influencing factors and long-term follow-up. J Bone Joint Surg Br 1990;72(4):557–62.

33. Roposch A, et al. The presence of an ossific nucleus does not protect against osteonecrosis after treatment of developmental dysplasia of the hip. Clin Orthop Relat Res 2011;469(10):2838–45.

34. Kawaguchi T, et al. Reproductive and developmental toxicity study of gadobenate dimeglumine

formulation (E7155) (2)–Combined study of effects on fertility and embryo-fetal toxicity in female rats by intravenous administration. J Toxicol Sci 1999; 24(Suppl 1):71–8 [in Japanese].

35. Nishii T, et al. Loaded cartilage T2 mapping in patients with hip dysplasia. Radiology 2010;256(3): 955–65.

36. Cunningham T, et al. Delayed gadolinium-enhanced magnetic resonance imaging of cartilage to predict early failure of Bernese periacetabular osteotomy for hip dysplasia. J Bone Joint Surg Am 2006; 88(7):1540–8.

37. Kim YJ, et al. Assessment of early osteoarthritis in hip dysplasia with delayed gadolinium-enhanced magnetic resonance imaging of cartilage. J Bone Joint Surg Am 2003;85(10):1987–92.

38. Wakabayashi K, et al. MRI findings in residual hip dysplasia. J Pediatr Orthop 2011;31(4):381–7.

39. Do TT. Transient synovitis as a cause of painful limps in children. Curr Opin Pediatr 2000;12(1):48–51.

40. Yang WJ, Im SA, Lim GY, et al. MR imaging of transient synovitis: differentiation from septic arthritis. Pediatr Radiol 2006;36(11):1154–8.

41. Zawin JK, Hoffer FA, Rand FF, et al. Joint effusion in children with an irritable hip: US diagnosis and aspiration. Radiology 1993;187(2):459–63.

42. Lee SK, Suh KJ, Kim YW, et al. Septic arthritis versus transient synovitis at MR imaging: preliminary assessment with signal intensity alterations in bone marrow. Radiology 1999;211(2):459–65.

43. Hopkins KL, Li KC, Bergman G. Gadolinium-DTPA-enhanced magnetic resonance imaging of musculoskeletal infectious processes. Skeletal Radiol 1995; 24(5):325–30.

44. Vogler JB 3rd, Murphy WA. Bone marrow imaging. Radiology 1988;168:679–93.

45. Ficat RP, Arlet J. Necrosis of the femoral head. In: Hungerford DS, editor. Ischemia and necrosis of bone. Baltimore (MD): Williams & Wilkins; 1980. p. 171–82.

46. Woo SB, Hellstein JW, Kalmar JR. Review: bisphosphonates and osteonecrosis of the jaws. Ann Intern Med 2006;144(10):753–61.

47. Tofferi JK, Gilliland W. Avascular necrosis. Available at: http://emedicine.medscape.com/article/3333364. Accessed August 1, 2012.

48. Imhof H, Breitenseher M, Trattnig S, et al. Imaging of avascular necrosis of bone. Eur Radiol 1997;7(2):180–6.

49. Aiello MR. Avascular necrosis of the femoral head. Available at: http://emedicine.medscape.com/article/386808. Accessed August 1, 2012.

50. Dihlmann W. CT analysis of the upper end of the femur: the asterisk sign and ischemic necrosis of the femoral head. Skeletal Radiol 1982;8:251.

51. Mitchell DG, Rao VM, Dalinka MK, et al. Femoral head avascular necrosis: correlation of MR imaging, radiographic staging, radionuclide imaging, and clinical findings. Radiology 1987;162:709–15.

52. Mitchell DG, Kressel HY, Rao VM, et al. The unique MRI appearance of the reactive interface in avascular necrosis: the double-line sign. Magn Reson Imaging 1987;5(Suppl 1):41.

53. Beltran J, Knight CT, Zuelzer WA, et al. Core decompression for avascular necrosis of the femoral head: correlation between long-term results and preoperative MR staging. Radiology 1990;175:533–6.

54. Koo KH, Kim R. Quantifying the extent of osteonecrosis of the femoral head. A new method using MRI. J Bone Joint Surg Br 1995;77:875–80.

55. Potter H, Moran M, Schneider R, et al. Magnetic resonance imaging in diagnosis of transient osteoporosis of the hip. Clin Orthop 1992;(280):223–9.

56. Grimm J, Higer HP, Benning R, et al. MRI of transient osteoporosis of the hip. Arch Orthop Trauma Surg 1991;110:98–102.

57. Guerra JJ, Steinberg ME. Distinguishing transient osteoporosis from avascular necrosis of the hip. J Bone Joint Surg Am 1995;77(4):616–24.

58. Miyanishi K, Yamamoto T, Nakashima Y, et al. Subchondral changes in transient osteoporosis of the hip. Skeletal Radiol 2001;30:255–61.

59. Beltran J, Opsha O. MR imaging of the hip: osseous lesions. Magn Reson Imaging Clin N Am 2005;13(4): 665–76.

60. Holder LE, Schwarz C, Wernicke PG, et al. Radionuclide bone imaging in the early detection of fractures of the proximal femur (hip): multifactorial analysis. Radiology 1990;174:509–15.

61. Rizzo PF, Gould E, Lyden JP, et al. Diagnosis of occult fractures about the hip: magnetic resonance imaging compared with bone-scanning. J Bone Joint Surg Am 1993;75:395–401.

62. Verbeeten KM, Hermann KL, Hasselqvist M, et al. The advantages of MRI in the detection of occult hip fractures. Eur Radiol 2005;15(1):165–9.

63. Haramati N, Staron RB, Barax C, et al. Magnetic resonance imaging of occult fractures of the proximal femur. Skeletal Radiol 1994;23:19–22.

64. Pandey R, McNally E, Ali A, et al. The role of MRI in the diagnosis of occult hip fractures. Injury 1998;29:61–3.

65. Daffner RH, Pavlov H. Stress fractures: current concepts. AJR Am J Roentgenol 1992;159:245–52.

66. Dorne HL, Lander PH. Spontaneous stress fractures of the femoral neck. AJR Am J Roentgenol 1985; 144:343–7.

67. Devas MB. Stress fractures of the femoral neck. J Bone Joint Surg Br 1965;47:728–38.

MR Imaging of Hip Infection and Inflammation

Luke Maj, MD, MHA[a], Yuliya Gombar III, MS[b],
William B. Morrison, MD[c],*

KEYWORDS

- Hip inflammation • Hip infection • Degenerative arthropathies of the hip • Postoperative hip

KEY POINTS

- Infection and other inflammatory processes involving the hip can look similar on imaging exams.
- Knowledge of MR imaging characteristics of the different conditions can help differentiate them.
- Hip prostheses are prone to various complications; MRI can be a useful adjunct to other modalities.

INTRODUCTION

Inflammation of the hip may be due to infectious and noninfectious causes. The various conditions are difficult to differentiate clinically and by most imaging examinations. A high suspicion for infection is necessary when an unexplained monarticular joint effusion is noted. Hip joint infections can potentiate a medical emergency because of the risk of joint damage as well as local and distant spread. Infections of the hip can occur in any demographic; however, high-risk populations include patients with comorbidities (ie, chronic arthritis, immunosuppression, sickle-cell disease, and diabetes) and postoperative patients. Patient outcomes are positively influenced by early, accurate diagnosis. Magnetic resonance (MR) imaging is highly effective in establishing the presence and underlying cause of inflammatory and degenerative arthropathies.[1] This article discusses the use of MR imaging for the evaluation of various inflammatory conditions of the hip, both infectious and noninfectious.

INFECTION
Modes of Inoculation

Hematogenous

Synovial tissue is highly vascularized and is particularly vulnerable to hematogenous seeding of microbes. Enriched synovial transudative joint fluid and hyaluronic acid from the synovial surface cells establish an ideal medium for pathogens. Blood-borne pathogens advance swiftly through synovial membranes, activating the inflammatory process. Elastases and collagenases released by pathogens and the body's own polymorphonuclear neutrophils break down the protective properties of the articular cartilage matrix.[2]

Contiguous extension

Paralyzed patients are prone to contiguous extension of infection arising from decubitus ulceration. Periarticular bursae, underlying bones, and the hip and sacroiliac joints are vulnerable to infection caused by communication with ulcers that commonly form over the adjacent ischeal tuberosity, sacrum, or greater trochanter. Infection arising in this manner often spread along fascial planes into the adjacent sciatic notch, through the gluteus musculature and along the bones of the pelvis and femur, resulting in extensive infection with abscess formation and necrosis. Infection may also extend along paraspinal muscles and fascia to the facet joints and even into the intervertebral disks.[3]

Direct implantation

This mechanism is usually the result of surgical intervention. Interventions include hip arthroplasty

[a] Division of Musculoskeletal Imaging and Intervention, Thomas Jefferson University Hospital, 111 South 11th Street, Philadelphia, PA, USA; [b] Philadelphia College of Osteopathic Medicine, 717 South Columbus Boulevard, Unit 1215, Philadelphia, PA 19147, USA; [c] Division of Musculoskeletal Imaging and Intervention, Thomas Jefferson University Hospital, 132 South 10th Street, Suite 1079a, Philadelphia, PA 19107, USA
* Corresponding author.
E-mail address: william.morrison@jefferson.edu

Magn Reson Imaging Clin N Am 21 (2013) 127–139
http://dx.doi.org/10.1016/j.mric.2012.09.009
1064-9689/13/$ – see front matter © 2013 Published by Elsevier Inc.

mri.theclinics.com

(ie, arthroscopy, implantation of allograft material, arthrocentesis, and hemi and total hip replacements) and even misplaced attempts at vascular catheter insertion. Septic arthritis caused by hip joint injection is, however, exceedingly rare, with a frequency of 1:25,000.[4] Septic processes anterior to the hip joint (such as pyomyositis or fasciitis) may mimic septic arthritis clinically, which may occur when attempts to aspirate what is actually a sterile joint may result in septic arthritis of the hip due to cross-contamination as pathogens are unintentionally introduced into a sterile joint space.

Postoperative

Introduction of a foreign material (ie, prosthetics) into the body may be a source of infection, either acutely due to contamination of the surgical bed or in delayed fashion as the implant serves as a nidus for hematogenous infection. Evaluation of computed tomographic (CT) and MR images is complicated by beam hardening and magnetic susceptibility artifact. Aspiration is often required to confirm the diagnosis.[5] Other noninfectious processes such as particle disease and aseptic lymphocytic vasculitis-associated lesion (ALVAL) can cause effusion, synovitis, erosion, and mass effect, and can result in prosthesis loosening. These findings can also simulate infection.[6]

Imaging Findings: Infection

Cellulitis

Cellulitis is defined as an acute infectious inflammation of the skin and subcutaneous tissues. MR imaging is useful in ruling out underlying myositis, abscess, sinus tract, fasciitis, septic arthritis, and osteomyelitis. Indicators of cellulitis on MR imaging include infiltration of subcutaneous tissues with edema signal[7] due to the inflammatory response and production of serous exudate.

Fat in the soft tissues is metabolized, leading to an ill-defined region of low T1 signal and high T2 signal. Contrast is useful to differentiate "bland" or noninflammatory edema from true cellulitis with associated hyperemia (**Fig. 1**).

Infectious fasciitis

Infectious fasciitis is a life-threatening, invasive soft-tissue infection that is characterized by widespread, rapidly developing necrosis of the subcutaneous tissue and fascia.[8] The severity of the infection and accelerated deterioration of the infection site warrants rapid surgical intervention including debridement and decompression, as well as aggressive antibiotic therapy. MR imaging is sensitive for the evaluation of this process, seen as fascial edema and enhancement; however, without appropriate clinical context fascial edema is not specific for infection and is seen in many conditions (**Fig. 2**). In addition, sick patients with renal compromise may not be able to tolerate intravenous gadolinium contrast. Therefore, unless clinical suspicion is high or soft-tissue gas is seen on radiographs, fascial edema is normally attributed to innocuous causes. Considering that true infectious fasciitis is a surgical emergency, the long acquisition time of MR imaging may preclude the modality as a sufficient diagnostic tool in this setting. Although MR imaging continues to be useful for evaluating the extent of infection and the existence of underlying abscess or osteomyelitis, CT may be the preferred diagnostic imaging study because of its wide availability, rapid acquisition, and high sensitivity for fascial gas.

Abscess

An abscess is a localized collection of necrotic tissue, fluid, and inflammatory cells that is walled off by a highly vascular and typically irregular inflammatory pseudocapsule. The surrounding

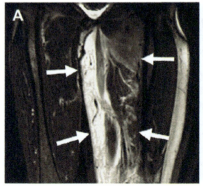
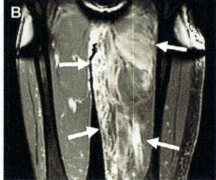

Fig. 1. Cellulitis and myositis. Atypical organism (*Candida albicans*) in a patient with human immunodeficiency virus. Coronal STIR (*A*) and postcontrast T1-weighted fat-saturated (*B*) images show diffuse edema and enhancement (*arrows*) of the subcutaneous muscles compatible with extensive infection.

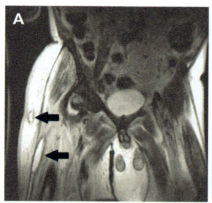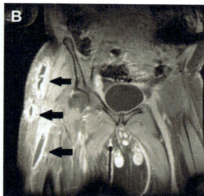

Fig. 2. Polymyositis. Coronal T2-weighted (*A*) and postcontrast T1-weighted fat-saturated (*B*) Images show edema of the anterior compartment muscles with scattered focal fluid collections demonstrating rim enhancement (*arrows*) representing intramuscular vastus lateralis abscesses and fasciitis.

soft tissue is also typically involved and displays a variable degree of edema/cellulitis.

On MR imaging, the central cavity of the abscess appears hypointense to muscle on T1-weighted images because of its liquefactive properties. Most abscesses are hyperintense on T2-weighted or short T1 inversion recovery (STIR) images with a variable degree of surrounding soft tissue edema (see **Fig. 2**). Fluid-sensitive sequences tend to show heterogeneous signal within the abscess. Owing to the hypervascular nature of the inflammatory tissue at the margins of the abscess, thick enhancement of the margins is demonstrated following contrast administration. The central portion remains hypointense, making the abscess cavity stand out on fat-suppressed, postcontrast images. The multiplanar capability

of MR imaging and its soft-tissue contrast make it the ideal modality for planning of surgery or percutaneous drainage.

Heterotopic bone formation[9–11] is important in the differential diagnosis for abscess in the pelvis, especially in paralyzed patients. In the early stages of development, heterotopic ossification demonstrates T2 hyperintensity and rim enhancement after gadolinium administration similar to abscess. Careful distinction is warranted in patients with spinal cord injury, who are concomitantly at increased risk of decubitus ulcers and thus abscess formation, as well as heterotopic bone formation. The use of gradient-echo images, which demonstrate blooming artifact with early rim calcification, as well as correlation with radiographs or CT, is useful (**Fig. 3**).

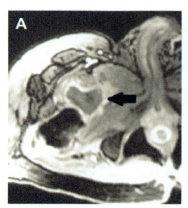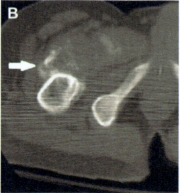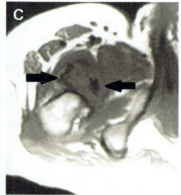

Fig. 3. Heterotopic ossification mimicking abscess on an MR image in a paralyzed patient. (*A*) Axial postcontrast T1-weighted fat-saturated image shows thick rim enhancement (*arrow*) in the region of the iliopsoas bursa, raising concern for abscess formation or septic bursitis. (*B*) Axial CT image verifies linear calcification around the rim (*arrow*), compatible with early heterotopic ossification rather than abscess. (*C*) T1-weighted noncontrast image demonstrates signal loss (*arrows*), representing areas of calcification not well depicted on the postcontrast imaging.

Pyomyositis

Muscle is inherently resistant to infection. Therefore, hematogenous pyomyositis is relatively uncommon. The incidence is increased in the setting of acquired immunodeficiency syndrome[12] or iatrogenic immunosuppression (associated with solid organ transplantation, bone marrow transplantation, or chemotherapy), as well as intravenous drug abuse. The most common site of involvement is the lower extremity, in particular the thigh. Multifocal involvement is seen in slightly less than half the cases. Secondary muscle infection may also occur as a result of contiguous spread from adjacent structures. MR imaging is highly sensitive for detecting pyomyositis. Hyperintensity is seen on T2-weighted or STIR images. Diffuse disease (stage 1) most commonly responds to conservative (antibiotic) therapy. On T1-weighted images, the muscle may appear enlarged but the signal may appear normal.[13] Perifascial fat infiltration may be seen on both T1-weighted and T2-weighted sequences. Postcontrast imaging may show diffuse enhancement in the early stages of disease and therefore help separate this process from other entities such as diabetic myonecrosis. In later stages, however, superimposed necrosis may occur, resulting in abscess formation and subsequently heterogeneous enhancement. With disease progression, more focal fluid collections may be observed (stage 2 disease). Postcontrast images demonstrate rim enhancement, suggestive of small abscesses. Stage 2 disease often warrants a more aggressive approach, with surgical drainage and debridement of necrotic tissue. Contrast-enhanced sequences can often provide the surgeon with a roadmap, helping to delineate fluid collections, sinus tracts, and areas of necrosis (see **Fig. 2**).[14] Stage 3 disease is defined as the extension to adjacent structures, resulting in septic arthritis, osteomyelitis, or septicemia. Pyomyositis of the muscle adjacent to the hip requires an accurate diagnosis, as it may be mistaken for septic arthritis of the hip[15] and lead to complications if aspiration is attempted. Muscle edema on MR imaging is nonspecific and often results in a wide differential diagnosis including but not limited to injury, denervation, rhabdomyolysis, infarction, diabetic myonecrosis, polymyositis, and tumoral infiltration (sarcoma, lymphoma, or metastatic disease). Therefore, the value of clinical correlation is of utmost importance.

Septic bursitis

Hematogenous septic bursitis at the hip is rare; usually it is due to the contiguous spread of infection, especially in paralyzed patients at an increased risk for ulcers or patients with penetrating trauma. With respect to the hip, the greater trochanteric bursa is most frequently involved, secondary to trochanteric ulceration. Septic arthritis of the hip joint may decompress through the hip capsule into the iliopsoas bursa, causing iliopsoas septic bursitis (**Fig. 4**). Bursae are lined by synovium similar to joints, making MR imaging manifestations of bursal infection similar to those seen in septic arthritis. Focal fluid signal corresponding to the bursal location with thick rim enhancement is characteristic. However, this finding is not specific, and mechanical bursitis or inflammatory bursitis related to rheumatoid arthritis can appear identical and should be ruled out by further evaluation. Obese patients often demonstrate small amounts of incidental fluid in

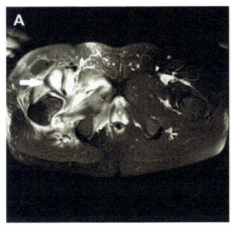
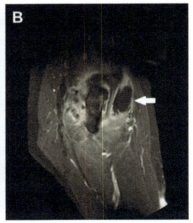

Fig. 4. Septic bursitis. Axial T2-weighted (*A*) and sagittal T1-weighted postcontrast (*B*) fat-saturated images of the right hip show marked distention of the illiopsoas bursa with extensive rim enhancement (*arrow*) and surrounding muscle edema.

the greater trochanteric bursae, generally bilateral and symmetric. Paralyzed patients are prone to the development of heterotopic ossification at the hip bursae, which, as mentioned in the abscess section earlier, may appear similar to infection with fluid signal and rim enhancement in its early stages.[9,16]

Septic arthritis

MR imaging is sensitive for the detection of joint effusion, which is a hallmark feature of any type of arthritis. In septic arthritis, fluid is often complex, particularly in chronic infection.[17,18] However, complex effusion is also found in noninfectious inflammatory arthropathies such as rheumatoid arthritis. On postcontrast imaging thick rim enhancement is characteristic of septic arthritis. In a study examining transient synovitis and septic arthritis, the presence of signal alteration of normal bone marrow on both contrast-enhanced fat-suppressed T1-weighted and T2-weighted sequences was seen in septic arthritis and excluded the diagnosis of transient synovitis.[19] The hyperemia induced in septic arthritis can lead to subchondral edema. Contrast use can help localize extra-articular collections and sinus tracts, helping to delineate extent of infection (**Fig. 5**). Marrow edema and enhancement beyond the subchondral bone into the medullary cavity denotes possible osteomyelitis.[20] MR imaging can assess the status of the articular cartilage, which is quickly eroded in septic arthritis. In later stages, erosions occur at the femoral neck and frank bone destruction may occur. Early detection and treatment of hip joint infection is essential to avoid chondrolysis and rapid development of osteoarthritis. Joint

aspiration and antibiotic coverage is paramount in suspected septic arthritis of the hip.

Osteomyelitis

MR imaging is the ideal imaging modality for detection of marrow infection and extension because of its high tissue contrast resolution and multiplanar capability coupled with high spatial resolution. Sensitivity and specificity of MR imaging for detecting osteomyelitis reaches 90% to 100%.[21,22] Osteomyelitis is demonstrated on T1-weighted images by marrow hypointensity (ie, replacement of marrow fat signal) with edema and enhancement (see **Fig. 5**).

Unlike infection, hematopoietic marrow is symmetrically distributed. It also retains minimal fat signal and enhances minimally, if at all. Clinical findings should be incorporated with the imaging features because cellular infiltration from tumor, as well as trauma and infarction, may produce similar T1 and T2 marrow signal abnormalities. A linear pattern of edema with enhancement along the outer cortex is characteristic of associated periosteal reaction. Periostitis is not as prominent in flat bones such as the iliac bone, so it may be absent in infection around the hip unless the proximal femoral shaft is involved. Bony destruction may be seen in later stages of disease progression, characterized by loss of the low-signal cortical line and mass effect from phlegmon or abscess.

For situations in which osteomyelitis requires surgical debridement, MR imaging is valuable in defining the extent of osseous involvement. Usually the margin of infected bone is well demonstrated on all sequences, although the extent may

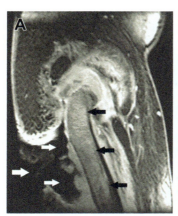
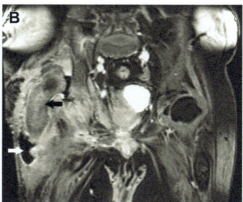

Fig. 5. Septic arthritis and osteomyelitis. Sagittal (*A*) and coronal (*B*) T1-weighted postcontrast fat-saturated images show a chronic extensive ischeal ulcer (*white arrows*) extending to the proximal femoral diaphysis with involvement of the dislocated right hip. There is deformity of the femoral head contour and loss of the articulating cartilage with diffuse synovial and surrounding soft tissue enhancement. Note alteration of marrow fat signal in the femoral head, neck, and proximal diaphysis (*black arrows*) consistent with osteomyelitis.

appear more prominent on STIR or fat-suppressed T2-weighted images compared with T1-weighted images, due to the high sensitivity of these sequences for reactive hyperemia of the surrounding bone. Soft-tissue extent may also be demonstrated, including sinus tracts, septic arthritis, and periarticular abscesses.

Despite the poor spatial resolution the STIR sequence is extremely sensitive to fluid. Thus, the absence of signal abnormality on STIR images or lack of pathologic contrast enhancement on fat-suppressed T1-weighted images effectively excludes the diagnosis of osteomyelitis. MR imaging may discern between a primary soft-tissue infection and secondary osteomyelitis or vice versa by paying attention to a few distinguishing features. In the former, a soft-tissue phlegmonous mass with cortical erosion and subcortical marrow abnormality can be seen. Absence of T2 signal abnormality virtually excludes superimposed osteomyelitis. Occasionally, reactive edema can extend into the medullary bone beyond the subchondral location. There is evidence that the brighter the T2 signal abnormality, the more likely the edema is secondary to osteomyelitis rather than to reactive hyperemia.[23]

However, in this situation, the MR imaging examination must still be considered suspicious for osteomyelitis regardless of the intensity.

MR imaging is also useful for diagnosing active infection in areas complicated by trauma or prior surgery. Despite artifact, adjacent fluid collections, periostitis, and marrow replacement can be delineated. Contrast enhancement can be useful in this setting; precontrast and postcontrast imaging can be performed to detect subtle areas of hyperemia around areas of susceptibility. Contrast can also distinguish nonenhancing areas of infarction from rapidly enhancing hyperemia due to infection.[24] In the setting of sickle-cell disease, the 2 are difficult to distinguish, because reactive hyperemic zones often marginate areas of infarction. These hyperemic zones enhance and may even have periosteal reaction if the infarct is acute.

Chronic osteomyelitis, commonly seen in paralyzed patients, can present with atypical patterns on MR imaging because of the wide spectrum of chronicity, activity, and the body's response. It is often characterized radiographically by a mixed pattern of lysis, sclerosis, and cortical thickening, typically at the ischeal tuberosity, sacrum, and greater trochanter. Sclerosis may be a low signal on both T1-weighted and T2-weighted images, with granulation tissue representing active infection, demonstrating hyperintensity on T2-weighted images and enhancement on contrast-enhanced images. Sequestrum formation, which is seen as intraosseous foci of hypointensity on all sequences surrounded by enhancing inflammatory tissue, is important to recognize. These foci represent avascular fragments of necrotic bone that may be a source for continuous infection and often require debridement. Cortical thickening representing long-standing periostitis may also demonstrate low signal intensity; active periostitis, as earlier, is seen on MR imaging as linear edema and enhancement along the outer cortical margin. Sinus tracts are often present in patients with active chronic osteomyelitis, visualized as irregular, linear T2-hyperintense streaks through the soft tissues with surrounding fat replacement and tram-track enhancement. These tracts arise from ulcers and dissect through the soft tissues. Tracts often communicate with abscess cavities. Infections often extend far from the source; because of the complicated patterns of spread through the soft tissues, MR imaging is an essential part of the preoperative algorithm.

Infection of the Postoperative Hip

Infection is an uncommon complication after hip arthroplasty, seen after less than 1% of procedures.[25] Patients may present shortly after surgery (assuming implantation) or in delayed fashion, presumably related to hematogenous spread, with the implant acting as a nidus. Patients present with pain and difficulty bearing weight. There may be a low-grade fever, but in early stages this is not common. Laboratory values such as sedimentation rate, leukocyte count, and other markers are nonspecific. Aspiration with fluid analysis is essential, but MR imaging is a useful adjunct to the workup.

Assessing a patient for suspected infection postoperatively can present as a challenge, particularly in cases of total hip arthroplasty. Imaging is problematic because of metallic susceptibility artifact. To reduce the effect of metallic artifact in such cases, various changes are applied to the imagining protocol[26]:

- Maximizing bandwidth
- Using STIR instead of fat-saturated T2-weighted sequences
- Using fast-spin echo instead of spin echo (SE) sequences[27]
- Avoiding gradient-echo sequences
- Lowering time to echo (TE) on STIR and fat-saturated SE sequences, that is, change to 30 to 40 ms
- Using a large field of view and increasing the matrix
- Performing precontrast and postcontrast T1-weighted non–fat-saturated sequences

Despite artifact, MR imaging remains useful for the evaluation of the periprosthetic soft tissues (particularly for detection of abscesses and sinus tracts) and the adjacent marrow, as well as for defining the spread of infection (**Fig. 6**).[28] By implementing metal artifact reduction techniques mentioned earlier, adequate images can be acquired with most prosthesis types. Equipment vendors are developing new metal artifact reduction sequences that will likely make this less of an issue in the future.

A positive culture result from a hip aspirate remains necessary to make a definitive diagnosis of infection. However, a negative aspiration result does not exclude the presence of infection,[29–31] and false-positives (usually secondary to skin contamination) must also be considered. The use of imaging for guidance in collecting a sample continues to play a pivotal role in making a correct diagnosis. Arthrography, along with aspiration, is the standard method for evaluation of a suspected hip prosthesis infection, but MR imaging can play a role in evaluating the location and size of fluid collections around the prosthesis, as well as help differentiating infection originating in the joint, versus one arising in the soft tissues that may be missed on fluoroscopic-guided aspiration alone.

Imaging Findings: Inflammation

Rheumatoid arthritis

Among the numerous types of arthropathies, rheumatoid arthritis is the most common noninfectious inflammatory arthritis. As with most other forms of autoimmune disease, rheumatoid arthritis affects women more often than men. Pathoetiologically, rheumatoid arthritis is a type III hypersensitivity reaction that typically has onset of symptoms in the 20s to 40s. Eighty percent of patients suffering from rheumatoid arthritis have a positive rheumatoid factor and strong association with HLA-DR4, putting them at an increased risk for other autoimmune disorders.[2] Although most patients have a positive rheumatoid factor, a small subset is factor-negative but fulfill other criteria characteristic of rheumatoid arthritis; these patients may subsequently turn rheumatoid factor-positive. Symptoms at presentation classically include joint stiffness, especially in the morning, with pain lasting greater than 30 minutes and improving with use. Pain and swelling is most commonly polyarticular and symmetric, indicating the systemic nature of the disease.[32] Often the symptoms are insidious, with slow progression over months until treatment is sought.[33] During this period, intermittent arthralgias may occur in one or more joints (monoarticular or pauciarticular), and severity of involvement may be asymmetric. Systemic manifestations are nonspecific and include fatigue and weight loss. Some patients have rapid progression of disease, causing severe debilitation, but in many patients the disease becomes quiescent for long periods, with occasional flare-ups.

The basic pathologic finding of rheumatoid arthritis is inflammation and proliferation of the synovium (called pannus), which leads to the various radiological appearances. Rheumatoid arthritis can affect any synovial structure, including bursae and tendon sheaths. Rheumatoid nodules, which are fibrinoid necroses surrounded by palisading histiocytes,[2] occur in approximately 15% of all rheumatoid patients but are not commonly seen at the pelvis and hip. Although hip involvement is uncommon (compared with hands, feet, and the upper spine), when the hip joints are affected findings tend to be bilateral and symmetric. This symmetric bilateral distribution along with a masslike synovial pannus is characteristic of rheumatoid arthritis and is helpful in diagnostic confirmation. With that in mind, MR image evaluation for synovitis at the hip should include sequences of the whole pelvis so that

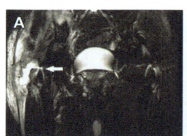 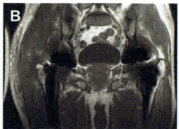 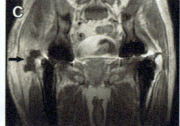

Fig. 6. Infected hip arthroplasty in a patient with fever and inability to bear weight. Coronal STIR (*A*), T1-weighted precontrast without fat saturation (*B*), and T1-weighted postcontrast without fat saturation (*C*) images in a patient with bilateral total hip arthroplasties show complex rim-enhancing fluid collection (*black arrow*) superficial and superior to the right greater trochanter communicating with the prosthetic hip joint via a thin tract on STIR imaging (*white arrow*). Findings are compatible with prosthetic hip infection.

both hips may be compared. This technique also aids in the evaluation of periarticular disease such as bursitis, as well as the sacroiliac joints, which may also become involved.

In patients with known rheumatoid arthritis, MR imaging is useful for the evaluation of effusion, erosions, and synovial pannus formation, as well as of the underlying cartilage.[34] Chronologic changes can be used as objective evidence of disease progression or improvement with response to treatment.

The synovial proliferation that occurs in rheumatoid arthritis is seen on MR imaging as a masslike prominence of tissue within the joint capsule, low signal on T1-weighted images, and hyperintense on T2-weighted or STIR sequences (although less intense than fluid). The pannus may be homogeneous or heterogeneous and may demonstrate hemorrhage, with low signal areas representing hemosiderin. On postcontrast images, the fibrovascular nature of the pannus results in vivid enhancement, similar to that seen with other synovial inflammatory or hyperemic processes such as infection. This finding itself is nonspecific, whereas the masslike morphology and symmetry of the process is more useful as a discriminatory feature.

The inflammatory nature of the synovial process in rheumatoid arthritis causes the underlying bone to become hyperemic, which may result in subchondral marrow edema and enhancement, resembling septic arthritis. The pannus causes a mass effect on the margins of the articular surfaces, at the junction with the capsule (the bare area), which can cause erosion at the femoral neck. Focal areas of bone marrow edema are characteristic in the early stages before discrete erosion occurs. Pannus may also extend from the joint along the facial planes. Effusion is almost universal, but the extent of the effusion varies. At times, the extent of the pannus into the joint is so prominent that it leaves little to no fluid in the space to be aspirated. In the setting of effusion, minor amounts of synovial proliferation are seen

on MR imaging as "dirty fluid" or a complex signal on T2-weighted or STIR images (**Fig. 7**).

Subchondral cysts are common at involved joints, and as mentioned earlier, pannus may erode into the central aspect of the acetabulum, simulating a cyst on radiographs and CT and making it difficult to distinguish between the two. Intraosseous pannus can be differentiated from cystic change on MR imaging: the pannus has a signal lower than the fluid on T2-weighted images and enhances brightly; cysts should have fluid signal and demonstrate marginal enhancement.

Another finding seen in rheumatoid arthritis is uniform cartilage loss; joint narrowing is classically concentric (diffuse), with axial migration of the femoral head (acquired coxa profunda). With more advanced disease, the iliopectineal line bows inward and the central acetabulum thins, an appearance called "protrusio acetabulae."[35]

The chondrolytic effect of rheumatoid arthritis leads to the early development of advanced secondary osteoarthritis in the hip joints. The end-stage hip may be so degenerated that it is difficult to determine the source of the initial insult without clinical information or evaluation of other joints. Large osteophytes form at the femoral head–neck junction, especially laterally. Cysts become prominent, and subchondral edema and enhancement are readily observed on MR images.

Involvement of the greater trochanteric bursa or iliopsoas bursa often occurs and is seen as a complex fluid signal in the distended bursa, with intense enhancement on postcontrast imaging.

Pigmented villonodular synovitis

Pigmented villonodular synovitis (PVNS) is a benign, uncommon monoarticular process of hypertrophic and hemorrhagic synovial proliferation. The condition usually affects individuals in late adolescence or early adulthood. The knee is the most common joint involved, with the hip being the second. Hypertrophic proliferation of the synovium is villous, nodular, or villonodular, which

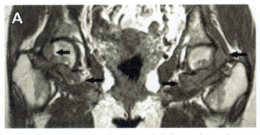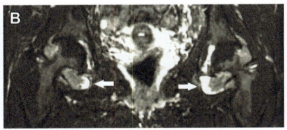

Fig. 7. Rheumatoid arthritis with bilateral involvement of the hips. (*A*) Coronal T1-weighted image demonstrates a masslike synovial proliferation symmetrically involving the hip joints bilaterally (*arrows*) with erosion at the femoral necks. (*B*) Coronal T2-weighted fat-saturated image of the hips shows complex fluid in the joint (*arrows*) representing synovial pannus.

largely depends on the amount of hemosiderin present. An MR image appearance of intra-articular hemosiderin deposition and single joint involvement is highly suggestive.

MR imaging demonstrates characteristic features of a heterogeneous, diffuse, synovial based, masslike or nodular thickening. A villous appearance is seen less frequently. Joint effusion is variable. On T1-weighted images, the signal intensity of the thickened synovium is intermediate to low. On T2-weighted images, the signal is generally low because of the hemosiderin content; however, the amount of hemosiderin varies (**Fig. 8**). "Blooming" or accentuation of low signal resulting from hemosiderin is best seen on gradient-echo images. Extrinsic erosion of bone may also be seen on both sides of the joint, with prominent cysts. PVNS may be confused with synovial hemangioma and hemophiliac arthropathy on MR imaging. Intra-articular PVNS can be distinguished from these conditions because it is monoarticular and not associated with serpentine vascular channels (hemangioma) or a clinical history of hemophilia.[36,37]

Diagnosis of PVNS is not complete until the location and the exeunt are defined for guidance of treatment and surgical intervention. MR imaging is the modality of choice for diagnosis and evaluation of disease extension for complete surgical resection. Rare malignant transformation of PVNS has been reported, resulting in poor outcomes due to the typically high-grade nature.[38]

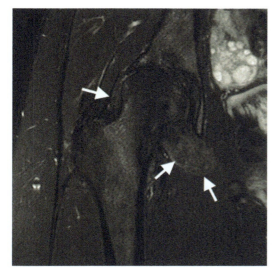

Fig. 8. Pigmented villonodular synovitis. Coronal T2-weighted fat saturated image shows extensive synovial proliferation (*white arrows*) with low signal due to hemosiderin deposition.

Synovial osteochondromatosis

Synovial osteochondromatosis (SOC), like PVNS, is an uncommon monoarticular arthritis, characterized by chondroid metaplasia of the synovial lining forming nodules that often calcify.[39] These cartilage nodules may detach from the synovium and be free floating in the joint fluid or may remain attached to the synovial capsule. SOC is not limited to the joint and can form in tendon sheaths or bursae.[40–42] The pathognomonic characteristic of SOC on any modality is the presence of numerous intra-articular bodies of similar size in a joint that lacks proportionate osteoarthritis. Although the MR imaging appearance has a high degree of variability depending on extent and degree of calcification, identifying multiple chondral or osteochondral bodies is often enough to solidify the suspected diagnosis (**Fig. 9**).[36,37,43–45]

The appearance of primary synovial chondromatosis was well documented by Kramer and coworkers[46] and categorized by their 3 distinct presentations, as listed in the following order of commonality.

1. Lobulated, homogeneous, intra-articular signal with intermediate intensity, which can give the impression of muscle on T1-weighted images. On T2-weighted images there is high signal intensity that may have focal areas of low signal intensity with all pulse sequences that correspond to regions of calcification.
2. Same as (1) with the absence of low-signal-intensity focal areas.
3. Same as (2) with or without the presence of low-signal-intensity focal areas but includes high-signal-intensity foci isointense to fat with a peripheral rim of low signal intensity, representing mature ossification.

At the hip bone, erosion occurs in 73%, typically at the femoral neck.[45] When intravenous contrast is introduced, heterogeneous enhancement is seen, with hyperintense synovium and nonenhancing regions representing hyaline cartilage nodules.[47]

Transformation of primary synovial chondromatosis to chondrosarcoma is rare but reported; rapid progression, bone destruction, increasing mass effect, or deteriorating clinical course warrants a workup for malignant transformation.[48]

Conditions Affecting Hip Prostheses

Wear-induced synovitis (particle disease)

MR imaging is a useful adjunct to radiographs, aspiration, and CT in the evaluation of the patient with a painful hip replacement. One condition affecting hip arthroplasty in the later stages is

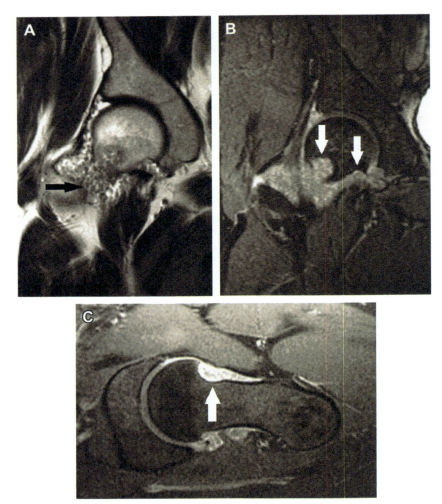

Fig. 9. Synovial osteochondromatosis. Coronal T2-weighted (*A*), coronal (*B*), and oblique axial (*C*) T1-weighted fat-saturated postcontrast images of the hip show innumerable dark bodies (*black arrow*) adherent to the synovium with synovial proliferation and marginal femoral head/neck erosions (*white arrows*).

wear of components. Shedding of the liner/spacer or other components related to use may result in synovitis as synovial macrophages attempt to digest the material; mass effect and effusions or periarticular fluid collections can result. Osteoclastic activity causes bone resorption around the prosthesis and can lead to component loosening with breakage and/or migration. The appearance of bone erosion and destruction can simulate infection (**Fig. 10**).[49]

Histologic examination from specimens taken at revision surgery correlates with wear-induced synovial response seen on MR imaging. Synovial proliferation with intermediate signal foci on proton density-weighted sequences suggests polymeric debris, which may represent polyethylene and/or polymethyl methacrylate on histology. The presence of mixed intermediate- and low-signal debris on MR imaging correlates with the presence of mixed polymeric and metallic debris at histology.[50]

MR imaging can be used to demonstrate the expansion of the pseudocapsule and decompression to adjacent bursae; the iliopsoas bursa is a common site of decompression and may present as a palpable mass or manifest as symptoms of femoral nerve compression. Synovitis may also communicate with the trochanteric bursa via dehiscence of the surgical site. Thus, fluid seen in either bursa posthip arthroplasty should be further investigated for communication and source of the joint.[26]

Differential diagnosis

Joint effusion and synovial proliferation have a wide differential. When considering the differential diagnosis for hip inflammatory disease, the

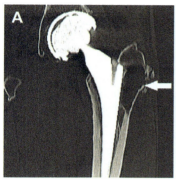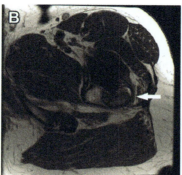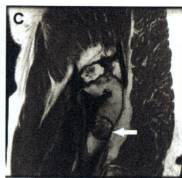

Fig. 10. Wear-induced synovitis (particle disease). (*A*) Coronal CT in bone window demonstrates a well-defined lytic lesion (*arrow*) adjacent to the left prosthesis involving the greater trochanter. Axial T1-weighted (*B*) and sagittal proton density-weighted (*C*) images show low internal signal lesion (*arrow*) defined by low signal intensity line consistent with biopsy/surgically proved particle disease.

distribution and extent of synovial pannus are valuable. Active rheumatoid arthritis involving the hips typically has masslike synovial proliferation, with bilateral involvement indicating a systemic disease. Ankylosing spondylitis can also have a symmetric distribution in the hips, but the sacroiliac joints should also be evaluated. The presence of sacroiliac dysfunction with hip involvement suggests the rheumatoid factor negative ankylosing spondylitis, whereas rheumatoid arthritis rarely involves the sacroiliac joints. Gout, reactive arthritis (previously known as Reiter disease), and psoriatic arthritis can all be in the differential diagnosis for inflammatory arthritis but are uncommon at the hip. Hemophiliacs, in the early stages of articular disease, can also demonstrate synovial proliferation that is generally bilateral in weight-bearing joints such as the hips. A thorough history and appropriate laboratory workup can help confirm the diagnosis. Monoarticular entities such as infection, SOC, and PVNS can generally be differentiated using a combination of clinical information and the specific MR imaging appearance (eg, calcification and hemosiderin).

Similarly, aggressive or advanced degenerative arthritis can also show synovial proliferation. The end stage of osteoarthritis often presents on MR imaging with joint effusion and synovial enhancement that can mimic an inflammatory arthropathy. However, identification of large osteophytes disproportionate to the extent of effusion or synovitis should raise suspicion of degeneration as the primary condition. That being said, arthritic joints can become superinfected, and severe osteoarthritis is often seen in late stages of rheumatoid arthritis as a result of destruction of cartilage, so the clinical context must always be considered when generating a deferential diagnosis.

In paralyzed patients, heterotopic ossification in the early stages can simulate abscess, with focal fluid signal and rim enhancement (see **Fig. 3**). The correct diagnosis can be reached by inspecting the margins of low signal representing zonal calcification, as well as typical location, around the hips, especially in the region of the iliopsoas or greater trochanteric bursa. Confirmation of rim calcification, typical of heterotopic bone can be made by comparison with CT scan or radiographs. In mature heterotopic ossification, the focus demonstrates corticomedullary differentiation, with internal fatty marrow signal. At this stage of ossification, the difference between infection and heterotopic ossification is straightforward, with little room for misinterpretation.

SUMMARY

With its superior anatomic resolution and high sensitivity in depicting pathologic processes of the joint, bone marrow, and surrounding soft-tissue structures, MR imaging is the ideal modality for demonstrating the manifestations and sequelae of the infectious and other inflammatory conditions involving the hip. Although the MR imaging features of these conditions may overlap, imaging findings combined with the clinical history yields a high degree of specificity, ultimately enhancing the confidence of the radiologist.

REFERENCES

1. Anon. NIH consensus conference: total hip replacement. NIH Consensus Development Panel on Total Hip Replacement. JAMA 1995;273(24):1950–6.
2. Robbins SL, Cotran R, Kumar V, et al. Diseases of immunity. In: Robbins SL, Kumar V, editors. Robbins

and Cotran pathologic basis of disease. 8th edition. Philadelphia: Elsevier; 2008. p. 205, 810–811.

3. Moran KM, Finkbeiner AA. Iliopsoas abscess following catheterization of the femoral artery: diagnostic and treatment strategies. Am J Orthop 1997; 26:446–8.

4. Freiberger RH. Introducing arthrography. In: Freiberger RH, Kaye JJ, editors. Arthrography. Norwalk (CT): Appleton-Century Croft; 1979. p. 1.

5. Savarino L, Baldini N, Tarabusi C, et al. Diagnosis of infection after total hip replacement. J Biomed Mater Res B Appl Biomater 2004;70:139–45.

6. Takagi M, Santavirta S, Ida H, et al. High-turnover periprosthetic bone remodeling and immature bone formation around loose cemented total hip joints. J Bone Miner Res 2001;16:79–88.

7. Beltran J. MR imaging of soft-tissue infection. Magn Reson Imaging Clin N Am 1995;3:743–51.

8. Kotrappa KS, Bansal RS, Amin NM. Necrotizing fasciitis. Am Fam Physician 1997;55(2):448.

9. Ledermann HP, Schweitzer ME, Morrison WB. Pelvic heterotopic ossification: MR imaging characteristics. Radiology 2002;222:189–95.

10. Parikh J, Hyare H, Saifuddin A. The imaging features of post-traumatic myositis ossificans, with emphasis on MRI. Clin Radiol 2002;57:1058–66.

11. Kransdorf MJ, Meis JM, Jelinek JS. Myositis ossificans: MR appearance with radiologic-pathologic correlation. AJR Am J Roentgenol 1991;157:1243–8.

12. Rodgers WB, Yodlowski ML, Mintzer CM. Pyomyositis in patients who have the human immunodeficiency virus. Case report and review of the literature. J Bone Joint Surg Am 1993;75:588–92.

13. Struk DW, Munk PL, Lee MJ, et al. Imaging of soft tissue infections. Radiol Clin North Am 2001;39:277–303.

14. Rahmouni A, Chosidow O, Mathieu D, et al. MR imaging in acute infectious cellulitis. Radiology 1994;192:493–6.

15. King RJ, Laugharne D, Kerslake RW, et al. Primary obturator pyomyositis: a diagnostic challenge. J Bone Joint Surg Br 2003;85:895–8.

16. Haritides J, Christodoulou P, Tsakonas A. Tuberculous trochanteric bursitis. Chir Organi Mov 2004; 89:177–80.

17. Brower AC. Septic arthritis. Radiol Clin North Am 1996;34:293–309.

18. Resnick D, Niwayama G. Osteomyelitis, septic arthritis and soft tissue infection. In: Resnick D, Niwayama G, editors. Diagnosis of bone and joint disorders, vol. 3, 4th edition. Philadelphia: WB Saunders; 2002. p. 2419–35.

19. Lee SK, Suh KJ, Kim YW, et al. Septic arthritis versus transient synovitis at MR imaging: preliminary assessment with signal intensity alterations in bone marrow. Radiology 1999;211:459–65.

20. Greenspan A, Tehranzadeh J. Imaging of infectious arthritis. Radiol Clin North Am 2001;39:267–76.

21. Morrison WB, Schweitzer ME, Bock GW, et al. Diagnosis of osteomyelitis: utility of fat-suppressed contrast-enhanced MR imaging. Radiology 1993; 189:251–7.

22. Kaiser S, Jorulf H, Hirsch G. Clinical value of imaging techniques in childhood osteomyelitis. Acta Radiol 1998;39:523–31.

23. Craig JG, Amin MR, Wu K, et al. Osteomyelitis of diabetic foot: MR imaging pathologic correlation. Radiology 1997;203:849–55.

24. Gylys-Morin VM. MR imaging of pediatric musculoskeletal inflammatory and infectious disorders. Magn Reson Imaging Clin N Am 1998;6:537–59.

25. Antti-Poika I, Josefsson G, Konttinen Y, et al. Hip arthroplasty infection. Current concepts. Acta Orthop Scand 1990;61:163–9.

26. Potter HG, Foo LF. Magnetic resonance imaging of joint arthroplasty. Orthop Clin North Am 2006;37: 361–73, vi–vii.

27. White LM, Kim JK, Mehta M, et al. Complications of total hip arthroplasty: MR imaging-initial experience. Radiology 2000;215:254–62.

28. Potter HG, Foo LF, Nestor BJ. What is the role of magnetic resonance imaging in the evaluation of total hip arthroplasty? HSS J 2005;1:89–93.

29. Kraemer WJ, Saplys R, Waddell JP. Bone scan, gallium scan and hip aspiration in the diagnosis of infected total hip joint arthroplasty. J Arthroplasty 1993;8:611–6.

30. Tehranzedeh J, Gubernick I, Blaha D. Prospective study of sequential technetium 99m phosphate and gallium imaging. Clin Nucl Med 1988;13:229–36.

31. Maus TP, Berquist TH, Bender CE, et al. Arthrographic study of painful total hip arthroplasty: refined criteria. Radiology 1987;162:721–7.

32. Kaarela K. Prognostic factors and diagnostic criteria in early rheumatoid arthritis. Scand J Rheumatol Suppl 1985;57:1–54.

33. Molenaar ET, Voskuyl AE, Dinant HJ, et al. Progression of radiologic damage in patients with rheumatoid arthritis in clinical remission. Arthritis Rheum 2004;50:36–42.

34. Peterfy CG. New developments in imaging in rheumatoid arthritis. Curr Opin Rheumatol 2003;15:288–95.

35. Damron TA, Heiner JP. Rapidly progressive protrusio acetabuli in patients with rheumatoid arthritis. Clin Orthop Relat Res 1993;289:186–94.

36. Kransdorf MJ, Murphey MD. Synovial tumors. In: Imaging of soft tissue tumors. 2nd edition. Philadelphia: Lippincott Williams & Wilkins; 2006. p. 381–436.

37. Dorfman HD, Czerniak B. Synovial lesions. In: Bone tumors. St Louis (MO): Mosby; 1998. p. 1041–86.

38. Murphey MD, Rhee JH, Lewis RB, et al. Pigmented villonodular synovitis: radiologic-pathologic correlation. Radiographics 2008;28:1493–518.

39. Mark M, Jorge V, Julie F, et al. From the archives of the AFIP: imaging of synovial chondromatosis with

radiologic-pathologic correlation. Radiographics 2007;27(5):1465–88.

40. Patel MR, Desai SS. Tenosynovial osteochondromatosis of the extensor tendon of a digit: case report and review of the literature. J Hand Surg Am 1985;10:716–9.

41. Bui-Mansfield LT, Rohini D, Bagg M. Tenosynovial chondromatosis of the ring finger. AJR Am J Roentgenol 2005;184:1223–4.

42. Covall DJ, Fowble CD. Synovial chondromatosis of the biceps tendon sheath. Orthop Rev 1994;23:902–5.

43. Crotty JM, Monu JU, Pope TL Jr. Synovial osteo-chondromatosis. Radiol Clin North Am 1996;34:327–42.

44. Resnick D. Tumors and tumor-like lesions of soft tissues. In: Diagnosis of bone and joint disorders. 4th edition. Philadelphia: Saunders; 2002. p. 4204–73.

45. Shanley DJ, Evans EM, Buckner AB, et al. Synovial osteochondromatosis demonstrated on bone scan: correlation with CT and MRI. Clin Nucl Med 1992; 17:338–9.

46. Kramer J, Recht M, Deely DM, et al. MR appearance of idiopathic synovial osteochondromatosis. J Comput Assist Tomogr 1993;17:772–6.

47. Kim SH, Hong SJ, Park JS, et al. Idiopathic synovial osteochondromatosis of the hip: radiographic and MR appearances in 15 patients. Korean J Radiol 2002;3:254–9.

48. Davis RI, Hamilton A, Biggart JD. Primary synovial chondromatosis: a clinicopathologic review and assessment of malignant potential. Hum Pathol 1998;29:683–8.

49. Malchau H, Potter HG. How are wear-related problems diagnosed and what forms of surveillance are necessary? J Am Acad Orthop Surg 2008; 16(Suppl 1):S14–9.

50. Hayter CL, Potter HG, Padgett DE, et al. MRI assessment of wear-induced synovitis. In: Proceedings of the 19th Annual Meeting ISMRM. Montreal (Canada); 2011.

Magnetic Resonance Imaging of Hip Tumors

Laura W. Bancroft, MD*, Christopher Pettis, MD,
Christopher Wasyliw, MD

KEYWORDS

- MR imaging • Tumor • Hip • Femur • Pelvis • Metastases • Solitary bone cyst • Sarcoma

KEY POINTS

- After initial evaluation with radiography, magnetic resonance (MR) imaging is the most common modality used to establish the diagnosis and characterize osseous and soft tissue tumors of the hip.
- Tumors involving the proximal femur are often benign, and MR imaging can be specific in diagnosing solitary bone cyst, osteochondroma, and chondroblastoma.
- Osseous metastases and myeloma are the most common causes of malignancy in patients older than 40 years, with metastases being 25 to 30 times more common than primary malignancy of bone.
- Benign and malignant soft tissue tumors about the hip are often nonspecific in their MR imaging appearances, but knowledge of the patient's age may direct a more limited differential diagnosis.
- Fibrosarcoma and rhabdomyosarcoma are common in young children, and liposarcoma and undifferentiated pleomorphic sarcoma are more common in middle-aged and elderly populations.

INTRODUCTION

Magnetic resonance (MR) imaging of hip tumors is often obtained for imaging finding discovered on radiographs or for further evaluation of a soft tissue mass found on clinical examination. MR imaging is the most common modality used to establish the diagnosis and characterize osseous and soft tissue tumors of the hip. Tumors involving the proximal femur are often benign, and MR imaging can be fairly specific in diagnosing lesions such as solitary bone cyst, osteochondroma, and chondroblastoma. Osseous metastases and myeloma are the most common causes of malignancy in patients older than 40 years of age, and should be suspected when multiple lesions are present. Benign and malignant soft tissue tumors about the hip vary according to age, and their MR imaging features are often times nonspecific. This report will provide an MR imaging pictorial for some of the more common tumors of the hip.

IMAGING PROTOCOL

MR imaging has emerged as the preferred modality for evaluating both osseous and soft tissue masses of the hip by providing information for both diagnosis and staging. Lesions should be imaged in at least 2 orthogonal planes, using fast spin echo T1-weighted and fluid-sensitive MR pulse sequences in at least 1 of these planes. Fat suppression on T2-weighted images is useful to increase lesion-to-background signal intensity differences for high signal intensity lesions that are located within the marrow or fatty soft-tissue. Fat suppression imaging is also useful in

Dr Bancroft receives book royalties from Lippincott and is a speaker for the Institute for International Continuing Medical Education. Drs Pettis and Wasyliw do not have any financial disclosures.
University of Central Florida School of Medicine, Florida Hospital, Florida State University School of Medicine, 601 East Rollins, Orlando, FL 32803, USA
* Corresponding author.
E-mail address: Laura.Bancroft.md@flhosp.org

mri.theclinics.com

decreasing or eliminating the MR signal from fat, allowing increased conspicuity of lesions containing paramagnetic substances (eg, methemoglobin) on T1-weighted images, and in identifying contrast enhancement. Gradient-echo imaging in a single plane may be a useful adjunct in demonstrating hemosiderin in lesions that have hemorrhaged.

In general, a small field of view is preferred; however, imaging of the entire pelvis in at least 1 plane is advised for appropriate staging. It is useful to place a marker over the area of clinical concern to ensure that it is appropriately imaged, especially in cases of suspected subcutaneous lipoma or lipomatosis, in which case the lesion may not be appreciated as distinct from the adjacent adipose tissue. Contrast enhancement is often not required; however, we find it useful in the detection of underlying tumors in the presence of hemorrhage.

BENIGN OSSEOUS TUMORS

Most tumors involving the proximal femur are benign. The most common primary tumors and pseudotumors of the hip include fibrous dysplasia, solitary bone cyst, osteoid osteoma, chondroblastoma, giant cell tumor, osteochondroma, aneurysmal bone cyst, and Langerhans cell histiocytosis.[1]

Solitary Bone Cyst

Solitary (or unicameral) bone cyst is most commonly found in the proximal humerus but is located in the proximal femur in up to 21% of cases.[1] Solitary bone cysts are nonaggressive, unilocular lesions that have a predilection for the metaphyses of long bones. Lesions can have associated cortical thinning; mild expansile remodeling; well-defined or sclerotic margins on radiography, computed tomography (CT), or MR imaging; and absent internal matrix on radiography (**Fig. 1**).[2] In

the proximal femur, it may be difficult to differentiate from the cystic variant of fibrous dysplasia on both imaging and pathologic evaluation.[1]

Osteochondroma/Multiple Hereditary Exostosis

Osteochondroma is the most common bone tumor and is categorized as a developmental lesion as opposed to a true neoplasm.[3] Osteochondroma accounts for 20% to 50% of all benign bone tumors and 10% to 15% of all bone tumors.[3,4] Osteochondromas are composed of cortical and medullary bone with an overlying hyaline cartilage cap, have medullary and cortical continuity with the parent bone, and may be sessile or penducu-lated. The femur is the most commonly affected bone (30% of cases), with the distal femur affected 3 times more often than the proximal femur.[3]

MR imaging confirms the cortical and medullary continuity with the parent bone, and the medullary component will closely approximate the signal of the adjacent marrow on all sequences (**Fig. 2**). The hypointense cortical margin can be variable in thickness. The cartilaginous cap is variable in signal depending on its water content, mineralization, and age of the patient; young patients with active growth may demonstrate marked heterogeneity of the cartilaginous cap on all sequences.[3] Because malignant transformation can occur in 1% of solitary osteochondromas and in 3% to 5% of patients with hereditary multiple exostoses, MR imaging can be helpful in assessing malignant features. Continued lesion growth and a hyaline cartilage cap greater than 2 cm in thickness after skeletal maturity is suggestive of malignant transformation.[3,5] MR imaging has 100% sensitivity and 98% specificity for differentiating osteochondromas and chondrosarcoma when cartilage cap thickness of 2 cm was used as a threshold.[5] MR imaging is also helpful in assessing complications

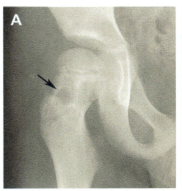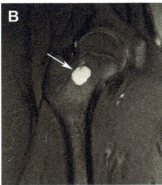

Fig. 1. Solitary bone cyst in a 6-year-old boy presents with enlarging femoral neck lucency on radiographs. (A) Anteroposterior radiograph of the right hip shows a lucency (*arrow*) in the femoral neck with thin sclerotic margins. (B) Fast spin echo T2-weighted fat-suppressed coronal image shows a hyperintense cystic lesion (*arrow*) without nodular components or adjacent marrow edema. Lesion proved to be solitary bone cyst and was treated with curettage and bone grafting.

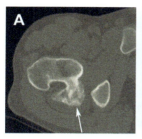
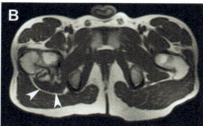

Fig. 2. Osteochondroma in a 23-year-old man with a 3-year history of right hip mass, discomfort, and snapping. (*A*) Axial CT demonstrates a pendunculated osteochondroma (*arrow*) extending posterior to the right femoral neck, with marrow continuity and no complicating features. (*B*) Axial T1-weighted image shows the isolated osteochondroma with a uniform cartilage cap (*arrowheads*) measuring less than 1.5 cm. The osteochondroma was excised via a posterior approach.

such as fractured stalk of a pendunculated osteochondroma, neurovascular compromise by mechanical compression, and overlying bursitis.

Hereditary multiple exostoses (HMEs) (also known as diaphyseal aclasis or familial ostechondromatosis) is an autosomal dominant disorder in which multiple osteochodromas are present. Osseous deformities involving the proximal femur are relatively common, with a 25% prevalence rate of coxa valga deformity.[3] Axial T1-weighted imaging will show the characteristic MR imaging features of osteochondromas (as discussed previously) but with multiplicity and often deformity of the involved and adjacent bones (**Fig. 3**).

Chondroblastoma

Chondroblastoma accounts for less than 2% of benign primary bone tumors and usually involves the epiphyseal or apophyseal regions in skeletally immature patients.[6] Chondroblastoma occurs twice as often in male patients, and most lesions occur between the ages of 5 and 25 years.[6] The most common clinical presentation is protracted pain, and some patients may have some loss of joint function. The most common anatomic location of this tumor is in the proximal femur, followed by the distal femur, proximal tibia, proximal humerus, hands, and feet (**Fig. 4**A).[7] Chondroblastoma presents on radiographs as a lucent lesion in

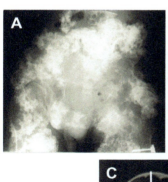
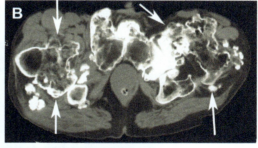
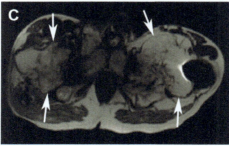

Fig. 3. Multiple osteochondromas in a 45-year-old man with multiple hereditary exostoses, worsening right hip pain and enlarging masses. (*A*) Anteroposterior pelvic radiograph shows multiple calcified masses involving the pelvis and imaged portions of the proximal femurs. (*B*) CT better delineates the multiple calcified masses emanating from the femoral necks (*arrows*) and remainder of the pelvis. (*C*) Axial T1-weighted image shows the predominantly hyperintense fatty marrow signal intensity throughout the femoral neck osteochondromas (*arrows*).

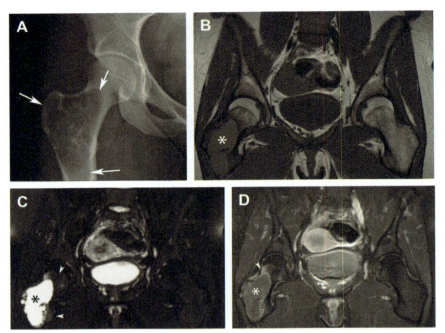

Fig. 4. Chondroblastoma of right proximal femur in a 19-year-old woman presenting with a 2-year history of right hip pain that was worse at night and not elicited by walking. (*A*) Anteroposterior radiograph of the right hip demonstrates a lytic lesion with narrow zone of transition and chondroid calcifications (*arrows*). (*B–D*) Coronal MR images demonstrate a corresponding lesion (*asterisk*), which is hyperintense to skeletal muscle on T1-weighted imaging (*B*), markedly hyperintense on fast spin echo T2-weighted fat-suppressed imaging (*C*), and peripherally enhancing (*D*). Note the involvement of the greater trochanter and surrounding edema-like signal changes and enhancement in the proximal femoral marrow (*arrowheads*). The chondroblastoma was treated with curettage, phenolization, bone grafting, and prophylactic fixation.

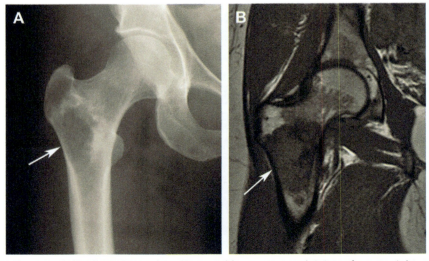

Fig. 5. Metastatic non–small cell carcinoma in a 43-year-old woman complaining of severe right groin pain and weakness. (*A*) Anteroposterior radiograph of the right hip shows a predominantly lytic lesion (*arrow*) in the right intertrochanteric and subtrochanteric femur, with partially sclerotic margin. (*B*) Coronal T1-weighted image through the right hip shows the extent of the marrow-replacing mass (*arrow*), which proved to be metastatic non–small cell carcinoma on needle biopsy. Patient underwent prophylactic cephalomedullary nail fixation.

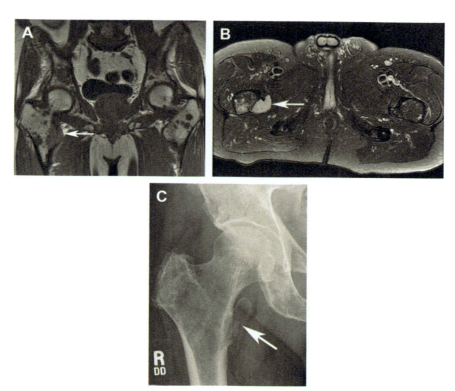

Fig. 6. Myeloma with pathologic fracture of the lesser trochanter of the right femur in a 67-year-old man. (*A, B*) Coronal T1-weighted (*A*) and axial fast spin echo T2-weighted fat-suppressed (*B*) images show multiple marrow-replacing lesions throughout the skeleton in this patient with recurrent myeloma, with dominant lesion destroying the lesser trochanter of the right femur (*arrow*) at the iliopsoas attachment. (*C*) Anteroposterior radiograph of the right hip shows the lytic destructive lesion (*arrow*) with superior displacement of the lesser trochanteric fragment.

the epiphysis or apophyseal equivalent and may have subtle chondroid matrix, adjacent periosteal reaction and expansile remodeling if secondary aneurysmal bone cyst is present (which can occur in 15% of cases) (see **Fig. 4**A).[6] MR imaging accurately demonstrates the extent of the actual tumor and the classic, adjacent marrow edema-like signal changes (see **Fig. 4**B–D). Rarely, the lesion may extend extraosseously into the hip joint, resulting in reactive synovitis.[8] The differential diagnosis of chondroblastoma includes giant cell tumor. Patients are often treated with curettage and bone grafting, although there is a report in the literature about further supplementation with vascularized fibular graft.[9,10]

MALIGNANT OSSEOUS TUMORS

Metastases and myeloma are the most common causes of malignancy in the proximal femur in patient older than 40 years of age, because the proximal femurs contain hematopoietic marrow. However, the most common primary malignant osseous tumors are chondrosarcoma (24%), Ewing

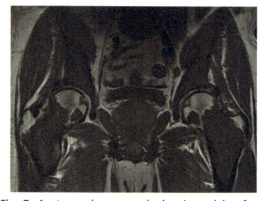

Fig. 7. Acute myelogeneous leukemia evolving from myelodysplastic syndrome and chronic myelomonocytic leukemia in a 61-year-old man. T1-weighted coronal image shows symmetric, near-complete marrow replacement of the pelvis and proximal femurs. Note the marrow is slightly hypointense to skeletal muscle and involves portions of the femoral heads.

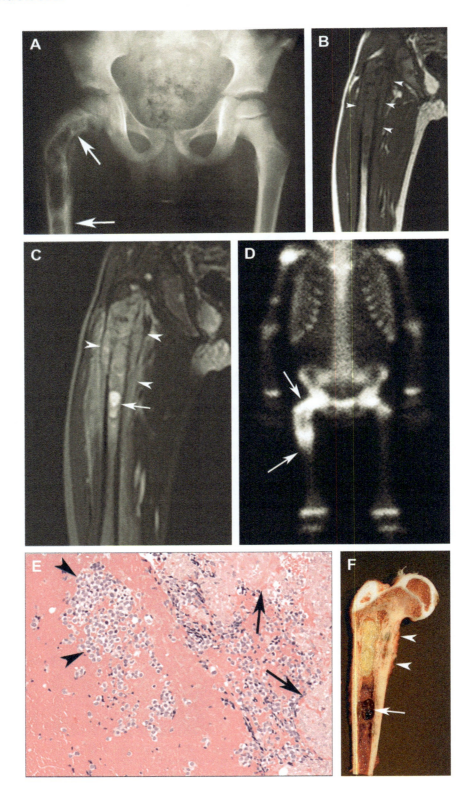

sarcoma (16%), osteosarcoma (9%), and fibrosarcoma/malignant fibrous histiocytoma (5%).[1]

Metastasis

Osseous metastasis is the most common bone malignancy, occurring 25 to 30 times more frequently than primary malignant tumors of bone.[11] In children younger than 2 years, neuroblastoma should be highly considered. It will appear as multifocal lytic lesions on radiographs and marrow-replacing lesions on MR imaging, and it may simulate the appearance of osteomyelitis.[1] Whole-body MR imaging can substitute for skeletal scintigraphy in detecting skeletal metastases in children and is helpful in evaluating initial tumor staging and early treatment response, but it has only a complementary role with conventional oncologic imaging methods for the detection of extraskeletal metastases.[12] In the adult population, the MR imaging characteristics of multiple marrow-replacing lesions are often nonspecific, and correlation with the primary source of malignancy should be sought (Fig. 5).

Myeloma

Plasma cell myeloma (more commonly known as myeloma) is the most common primary bone malignancy. It is a malignant clonal neoplasm of plasma cells of B-lymphocyte origin, resulting in the overproduction of monoclonal immunoglobulins.[13] Myeloma is characterized by osteolytic lesions, bone pain, hypercalcemia, monoclonal gammopathy, and disorders caused by amyloid deposition.[14] Plasma cell myeloma most commonly presents in the 6th and 7th decades, and men and women are affected equally.[14] The diagnosis is made in a clinical setting of symptomatic and progressive disease using a combination of bone marrow biopsy, serum IgG and IgA levels, urine immunoglobulin levels, and lytic bone lesions.[14]

Imaging can detect the extent of intramedullary disease, any extramedullary myelomatous foci, complications, and treatment response. Bones containing red marrow are most frequently involved, such as the vertebrae, ribs, skull, pelvis, femur, clavicle, and scapula. Imaging findings of multiple myeloma include osteopenia, lytic lesions, and pathologic fracture. The lytic lesions are typically "punched out" but can exhibit expansile remodeling of the adjacent bone. In the sclerotic form of myeloma, there is usually a mixed pattern of lytic and sclerotic lesions; the number of sclerotic foci is usually limited but can be extensive.[15] Osteosclerotic myeloma can also be associated with POEMS (polyneuropathy, organomegaly, endocrinopathy, monoclonal gammopathy, skin changes) syndrome.[16] On MR imaging, myeloma can have several patterns – focal lesions (localized), complete replacement of the marrow (diffuse), or innumerable small marrow-replacing lesions (variegated) (Fig. 6).[17] Plasmacytoma is a solitary myelomatous lesion that is typically isointense to skeletal muscle on T1-weighted imaging and hyperintense to muscle on T2-weighted imaging. Isolated reports of a "mini-brain" MR appearance of plasmacytoma in the spine and proximal femur describe the enhancing, radial distribution of tumor separated by thickened bony trabeculae.[17]

Tumor burden detected on imaging is generally predictive of patient survival. MR imaging is excellent in evaluating the extent of disease at diagnosis, during and after treatment (see Fig. 6). The Durie/Salmon PLUS staging system is currently used to stage patients with multiple myeloma and is based on radiographs, MR imaging, and positron-emission tomography (PET)/CT.[15,18] Stage IA is a normal skeletal survey or a single lesion. Stage IB is less than 5 focal lesions or mild diffuse spine disease. Stage II is 5 to 20 focal lesions or moderate diffuse spine disease (vertebral body signal intensity greater than disc on T1-weighted imaging). Stage III is more than 20 focal lesions or severe diffuse spine disease (vertebral body signal intensity isointense or hypointense to the adjacent disc on T1-weighted imaging). Whole body diffusion-weighted imaging with apparent diffusion coefficient analysis has

Fig. 8. Ewing sarcoma of right proximal femur in a 5-year-old, limping boy complaining of intermittent right thigh pain. (A) Anteroposterior radiograph delineates the extensive lytic lesion involving the right proximal femoral neck and diaphysis (arrows). (B, C) Coronal T1-weighed (B) and fast spin echo T2-weighted fat-suppressed (C) images show a long segment marrow replacing lesion involving the proximal half of the femur, with inferior cystic component (arrow), proximal cortical destruction, and periosteal reaction (arrowheads). (D) Skeletal scintigraphy reveals marked radiotracer uptake of the lesion (arrows) with central photopenia, which is consistent with tumor necrosis. (E) Microscopic section shows sheets of uniform tumor cells (arrowheads) with small round nuclei and scant clear cytoplasm and focal area of necrotic tumor cells (arrows) (hematoxylin and eosin, original magnification ×400). Preoperative chemotherapy was administered, the proximal femur was resected, and Repiphysis expandable implant (Wright Medical Technology, Arlington, TN) was placed. (F) Bivalved resected specimen shows tumor involvement throughout the proximal femoral diaphysis and neck, with prominent periosteal reaction (arrowheads) and focal tumoral necrosis (arrow) corresponding to MR and histologic findings.

proved useful in the short-term treatment response in patients with myeloma.[19]

Leukemia

Acute myeloid leukemia (AML) is a clonal expansion of myeloid blasts in the bone marrow, blood, or other tissue and accounts for 70% of all cases of acute leukemia.[20] Most cases occur in adults (median age of 60 years) and there is an equal prevalence among men and women.[20] Leukemia and multiple other hematopoietic tumors can demonstrate nonspecific marrow infiltration, with hypointense T1 signal and hyperintense T2 signal (Fig. 7).[21] Use of in-phase and out-of-phase imaging can be helpful, because signal intensity loss of more than 20% on out-of-phase imaging is highly worrisome for malignant marrow infiltration.[22] Investigators studying patients with AML have correlated results of iron oxide–enhanced imaging studies with bone marrow angiogenesis.[23] Change in gradient echo relaxation time maps has shown prominent areas of highly vascularized bone marrow in patients with AML, whereas control subjects had only moderately vascularized bone marrow with homogeneous vessel distribution.[24]

Chronic myelogeneous leukemia (CML) is the most common myeloproliferative disease (15%–20% of all cases of leukemia), has a slight male predominance, and has a median age of diagnosis in the 5th and 6th decades.[24] Patients with CML (as well as any of the leukemias) can demonstrate diffuse osteopenia on radiographs and marrow infiltration evident on MR imaging. Chronic lymphocytic leukemia (CLL) is a neoplasm of monomorphic B-lymphocytes in the peripheral blood, bone marrow, and lymph nodes.[25] The median age of patients with CLL is 65 years old, and men are afflicted twice as often as women.[25] Extensive lytic lesions simulating multiple myeloma on radiography have been reported in cases of CLL.[26] As with any of the leukemias, MR imaging appearance of chronic lymphocytic leukemia can reveal homogeneous or heterogeneous marrow infiltrative patterns.

Ewing Sarcoma

Ewing sarcoma is the second most common bone malignancy in children and adolescents, accounting for approximately 3% of all pediatric cancers.[27] Ewing sarcoma may arise in bone or soft tissue and is more common in boys and in white and Hispanic children.[28] The most common sites of osseous involvement include the pelvis (26%), femur (20%), tibia/fibula (18%), chest wall (16%), upper extremity (9%), and spine (6%).[29]

Nine percent of cases involve the proximal femur.[1] When involving the long bones, Ewing sarcoma preferentially involves the diaphyses. Ewing sarcoma is typically lytic and can have circumferential periosteal reaction on radiographs (Fig. 8A). On MR imaging, Ewing sarcoma is hypointense or isointense to skeletal muscle and best assessed for lesion extent on T1-weighted imaging and variable in signal on T2-weighted images with periosteal reaction (see Fig. 8B, C)[30] Because it is a rapidly growing neoplasm, Ewing sarcoma may have large areas of tumor necrosis, reflected as cystic change (see Fig. 8D–F).[31] MR imaging can detect intraosseous skip lesions, but sometimes these may be difficult to differentiate from physiologic hematopoietic marrow, especially in children. Dalrup-Link and colleagues compared the diagnostic accuracy of whole-body MR imaging, bone scintigraphy, and FDG-PET in the detection of bone metastases in children.[32] They found that PET with ^{18}F-fluorodeoxyglucose positron emission tomography (^{18}F FDG-PET) was superior to both whole-body MR imaging and bone scintigraphy, with sensitivity of 90% for FDG-PET in comparison with sensitivities of 82% and 71% for whole-body MR imaging and bone scintigraphy, respectively.[32] Dynamic MR imaging, diffusion-weighted MR imaging, and whole-body fast inversion recovery MR imaging may also prove useful in staging patients, and monitoring the extent of tumoral necrosis.[33,34]

Chondrosarcoma

Chondrosarcoma is a malignant cartilaginous tumor that accounts for 3.6% of all primary bone malignancies in the United States; it may arise from bone or soft tissue.[28] Chondrosarcoma is most common in middle-aged patients and has a predilection for the proximal femur and pelvis, with 11% of cases occurring in the proximal femur.[1] Although rare (2% of all chondrosarcoma), clear cell chondrosarcoma typically occurs in the proximal epiphysis of the femur.[1] A fraction (0.5%–5%) of cases may arise in a preexisting lesion, such as osteonchodroma or enchondroma.[28] It is difficult to reliably differentiate enchodroma and grade 1 chondrosarcoma with radiographs and histology. Pain related to the lesion, deep endosteal scalloping (more than two-thirds the cortical thickness), cortical destruction and soft tissue mass, periosteal reaction, and marked uptake of radionuclide are all worrisome features of chondroid lesions that are suggestive of chondrosarcoma.[35,36] Increased risk of malignant degeneration occurs in patients with multiple osteochondromas or enchondromas, axial location, and lesions larger than 5 cm.[28,37] Noncontrast T1-weighted images are helpful in distinguishing the true extent of the tumor from the peritumoral edema that may be present (**Fig. 9**). Dynamic MR imaging of the primary tumor may reflect tumor perfusion, microcirculation, and tumor interstitium and may correlate with potential effectiveness of drug delivery.[28] Up to 11% of chondrosarcomas will undergo dedifferentiation, which is highly malignant with a poor prognosis.[38] These tumors demonstrate dimorphic features, often with dominant lytic lesion adjacent to a mineralized tumor and large, unmineralized soft tissue mass associated with intraosseous chondroid-containing tumor on CT or MR imaging (**Fig. 10**).[38]

BENIGN SOFT TISSUE TUMORS

Benign soft tissue tumors at the hips and adjacent pelvis vary according to patient age. More common tumors include fibrous hamartoma of infancy and lipoblastoma in young children, lipoma and a variety of fibrous tumors in middle-aged patients, and lipoma, myxomas, and neurofibroma in the elderly.[39]

Desmoid

Deep fibromatosis, also known as desmoid tumor, is a benign neoplasm that has aggressive biologic behavior and arises from connective tissue in muscle, fascia, or aponeuroses (**Fig. 11**A).[40] An increased incidence of desmoid tumors has been found in patients with familial adenomatous polyposis and Gardner syndrome, but most extremity lesions are idiopathic.[41] Desmoids can be ovoid (52%) or infiltrative (35%) or have an irregular or lobulated contour (76%) on MR imaging and a "fascial tail" evident in 80% of cases.[42,43] MR imaging signal characteristics will depend on the composition of the desmoid, in which early-stage lesions are often more cellular and evolved lesions have more collagen deposition. Lesions are generally isointense or mildly hyperintense to skeletal muscle on T1-weighted images (see **Fig. 11**B). Hypocellular lesions with dense collagenous

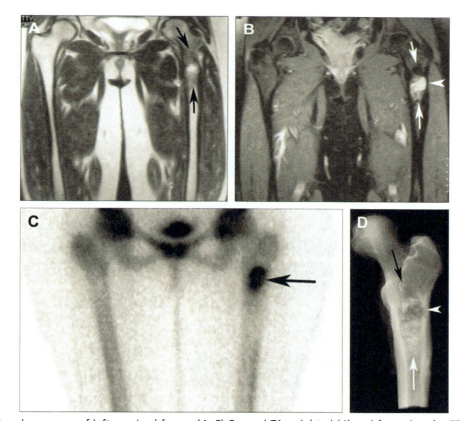

Fig. 9. Chondrosarcoma of left proximal femur. (*A*, *B*) Coronal T1-weighted (*A*) and fast spin echo T2-weighted fat-suppressed (*B*) images show a heterogeneous mass (*arrows*) in the subtrochanteric femur with deep endosteal scalloping of the lateral cortex (*arrowhead*). (*C*) Skeletal scintigraphy demonstrates marked radiotracer uptake within the lesion (*arrow*). (*D*) Resected specimen radiograph demonstrates the proximal femoral mass (*arrows*) with chondroid calcifications and areas of deep endosteal scalloping (*arrowhead*).

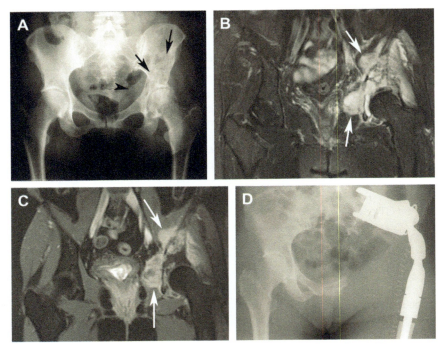

Fig. 10. Dedifferentiated chondrosarcoma of left acetabulum and iliac body in a 47-year-old woman with a 6-month history of left hip pain and inability to bear weight. (*A*) Anteroposterior radiograph displays a lytic lesion with chondroid matrix destroying the left acetabulum and most of the iliac body (*arrows*), with extraosseous soft tissue extension (*arrowhead*) displacing the obturator fat plane. (*B, C*) Coronal fast spin echo T2-weighted fat-suppressed (*B*) and enhanced T1-weighted fat-suppressed (*C*) images show the corresponding destructive soft tissue mass (*arrows*) with marked enhancement of most of the lesion. (*D*) Postoperative anteroposterior radiograph obtained after left hemipelvectomy, proximal femoral resection, and placement of saddle prosthesis onto the sacrum.

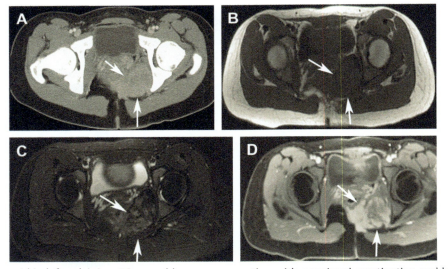

Fig. 11. Desmoid in left pelvis in a 26-year-old woman presenting with occasional constipation and left buttock pain after prolonged sitting. (*A*) Axial enhanced CT scan demonstrates an enhancing, infiltrating soft tissue mass (*arrows*) in the left lateral pelvis abutting the acetabulum and invading the rectum and vagina. (*B–D*) Corresponding axial MR images demonstrate signal characteristics that are primarily isointense to muscle on T1-weighted imaging (*B*), relative hypointense with more discrete areas of signal loss on T2-weighted fat-suppressed imaging (*C*), with avid enhancement (*D*). Needle biopsy confirmed a desmoid and patient underwent excision of the mass through a combined approach, although clear margins were not achievable.

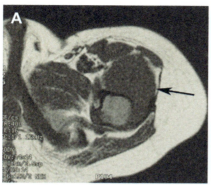
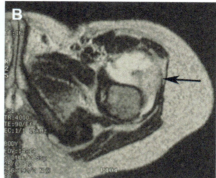

Fig. 12. Rhabdomyosarcoma of left proximal quadriceps muscle in a 5-year old boy. (*A, B*) Axial images of the left proximal thigh shows a mass in the quadriceps muscle that is isointense to skeletal muscle on T1-weighted images (*A*) and heterogeneously hyperintense on T2-weighted images (*B*). Mass was biopsied and proved to be rhabdomyosarcoma.

components will have lower T2-weighted signal than lesions with more extracellular myxoid matrix (see **Fig. 11**C).[43] Desmoid tumors will avidly enhance, except for the more hypointense, fibrotic portions (**Fig. 11**D). MR imaging is useful in defining the size and compartmental extension of these infiltrative tumors.[43] Thirty-one percent of lesions will cross major fascial boundaries on MR imaging, 77% of patients will have residual or recurrent tumor after surgical resection, and 66% of patients are followed with MR imaging as a result of recurrent disease.[42,44]

MALIGNANT SOFT TISSUE TUMORS

Malignant soft tissue tumors of the hips and adjacent pelvis also vary according to patient age. More common sarcomas include fibrosarcoma and rhabdomyosarcoma in young children and liposarcoma and undifferentiated pleomorphic sarcoma in the middle-aged population and elderly.[45]

Rhabdomyosarcoma

Rhabdomyosarcoma is the most common soft tissue sarcoma in children younger than 15 years old, is the third most common extracranial solid childhood tumor after neuroblastoma and Wilms tumor, and accounts for approximately 7% of malignancies in childhood.[46] Rhabdomyosarcoma arises from immature mesenchymal cells with skeletal cell lineage; however, this tumor may arise anywhere in the body, often in sites lacking striated muscle.[46] Twenty percent of tumors will arise in the extremities and masses can be extensive because they tend to spread along the facial planes.[46] There are 5 subtypes of rhabdomyosarcoma: undifferentiated, alveolar, embryonal, botryoid, and spindle cell. However, no MR imaging characteristics have been described to reliably differentiate these subtypes.[47] Rhabdomyosarcoma tends to be a nonspecific soft tissue mass on MR imaging, with intermediate signal intensity on T1-weighted imaging (**Fig. 12**A) and

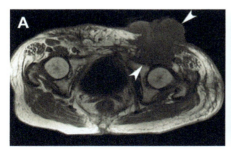
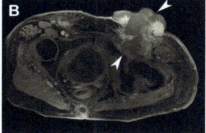

Fig. 13. Radiation-induced sarcoma in an 82-year-old woman presenting with left inguinal mass and radiation therapy 18 and 7 years earlier for endometrial and squamous cell carcinoma of the vagina. Axial T1-weighted (*A*) and enhanced T1-weighted fat-suppressed (*B*) images show a large, fungating left inguinal mass (*arrowheads*) abutting the left anterior femoral head and anterior column of the acetabulum. Histology demonstrated high-grade sarcoma, consistent with radiation-induced sarcoma, and external hemipelvectomy was performed.

intermediate-to-high signal on T2-weighted images (see **Fig. 12**B).[48] Tumors strongly enhance and rarely have cystic components.[48]

Radiation-Induced Sarcoma

Radiation-induced sarcoma is a complication of radiation therapy that occurs more often in soft tissue than in bone, and patients typically present with an enlarging mass.[49] Undifferentiated pleomorphic sarcoma is the most common postradiation sarcoma of the soft tissues (67%), followed by extraskeletal osteosarcoma (13%) and fibrosarcoma (11%). Great variability is reported in the latent period of radiation-induced sarcoma, with occurrence generally ranging between 4 and 30 years after radiation, with a mean of 8 to 12 years.[50] The reported radiation dose also varies, but in general, the mean reported dose is approximately 50 Gy, which is in keeping with current therapeutic practices.[50] As with other soft-tissue sarcomas, small lesions may seem innocuous on initial MR imaging and the MR imaging features of larger lesions are often nonspecific soft tissue masses (**Fig. 13**A, B).

SUMMARY

There are multiple benign and malignant osseous and soft tissue tumors of the hip, some of which have characteristic imaging findings on MR imaging. Tumors involving the proximal femur are most often benign, and MR imaging can be fairly specific in diagnosing solitary bone cyst, osteochondroma, and chondroblastoma. Osseous metastases and myeloma are the most common causes of malignancy in patients older than 40 years, with metastases being 25 to 30 times more common than primary malignancy of bone. Benign and malignant soft tissue tumors about the hip are often nonspecific in their MR imaging appearances, but knowledge of the patient's age may direct a more limited differential diagnosis. Fibrosarcoma and rhabdomyosarcoma are common in young children, and liposarcoma and undifferentiated pleomorphic sarcoma are more common in the middle-aged and elderly populations. Finally, MR imaging is commonly used to stage tumors and follow patients postoperatively in the setting of malignancy.

REFERENCES

1. Bloem JL, Reidsma II. Bone and soft tissue tumors of hip and pelvis. Eur J Radiol 2011. [Epub ahead of print].
2. Wada R, Lambert RG. Deposition of intraosseous fat in a degenerating simple bone cyst. Skeletal Radiol 2005;34(7):415–8.
3. Murphey MD, Choi JJ, Kransdorf MJ, et al. Imaging of osteochondroma: variants and complications with radiologic-pathologic correlation. Radiographics 2000;20(5):1407–34.
4. Douis H, Saifuddin A. The imaging of cartilaginous bone tumours. I. Benign lesions. Skeletal Radiol 2012;41(10):1195–212.
5. Bernard SA, Murphey MD, Flemming DJ, et al. Improved differentiation of benign osteochondromas from secondary chondrosarcomas with standardized measurement of cartilage cap at CT and MR imaging. Radiology 2010;255(3):857–65.
6. Motamedi K, Seeger LL. Benign bone tumors. Radiol Clin North Am 2011;49(6):1115–34.
7. Robbin M, Murphey MD. Benign chondroid neoplasms of the bone. Semin Musculoskelet Radiol 2000;4:45–8.
8. Kaneko H, Kitoh H, Wasa J, et al. Chondroblastoma of the femoral neck as a cause of hip synovitis. J Pediatr Orthop B 2012;21(2):179–82.
9. Paloski MD, Griesser MJ, Jacobson ME, et al. Chondroblastoma: a rare cause of femoral neck fracture in a teenager. Am J Orthop (Belle Mead NJ) 2011;40(9):E177–81.
10. Riedel B, Franklin C, Seal A, et al. Free vascularized fibula graft to treat chondroblastoma of the hip. Orthopedics 2012;35(2):e259–61.
11. Kim SH, Smith SE, Mulligan ME. Hematopoietic tumors and metastases involving bone. Radiol Clin North Am 2011;49(6):1163–83.
12. Goo HW, Choi SH, Ghim T, et al. Whole-body MRI of paediatric malignant tumours: comparison with conventional oncological imaging methods. Pediatr Radiol 2005;35(8):766–73.
13. Angtuaco EJ, Fassas AB, Walker R, et al. Multiple myeloma: clinical review and diagnostic imaging. Radiology 2004;231:11–23.
14. Grogan TM, Van Camp B, Kyle RA, et al. Plasma cell neoplasms. In: Jaffe ES, Harris NL, Stein H, et al, editors. Pathology and genetics: tumours of haematopoietic and lymphoid tissues. Lyons (France): IARC Press; 2001. p. 142–56.
15. Mulligan ME, Badros AZ. PET/CT and MR imaging in myeloma. Skeletal Radiol 2007;36:5–16.
16. Chong ST, Beasley HS, Daffner RH. POEMS syndrome: radiographic appearance with MRI correlation. Skeletal Radiol 2006;35:690–5.
17. Subhas N, Bauer TW, Joyce MJ, et al. The "mini brain" appearance of plasmacytoma in the appendicular skeleton. Skeletal Radiol 2008;37(8):771–4.
18. Durie B. The role of anatomic and functional staging in myeloma: description of Durie/Salmon PLUS staging system. Eur J Cancer 2006;42:1539–43.
19. Horger M, Weisel K, Horger W, et al. Whole-body diffusion-weighted MRI with apparent diffusion coefficient mapping for early response monitoring in

multiple myeloma: preliminary results. AJR Am J Roentgenol 2011;196(6):W790–5.

20. Brunning RD, Matutes E, Harris NL, et al. Acute myeloid leukemia: introduction. In: Jaffe ES, Harris NL, Stein H, et al, editors. Pathology and genetics: tumours of haematopoietic and lymphoid tissues. Lyons (France): IARC Press; 2001. p. 77–80.

21. Hwang S, Panicek DM. Magnetic resonance imaging of bone marrow in oncology. Part 2. Skeletal Radiol 2007;36:1017–27.

22. Zajick DC Jr, Morrison WB, Schweitzer ME, et al. Benign and malignant processes: normal values and differentiation with chemical shift MR imaging in vertebral marrow. Radiology 2005;237:590–6.

23. Matuszewski L, Persigehi T, Wall A, et al. Assessment of bone marrow angiogenesis in patients with acute myeloid leukemia by using contrast-enhanced MR imaging with clinically approved iron oxides: initial experience. Radiology 2006;242:217–24.

24. Vardiman JW, Pierre R, Thiele J, et al. Chronic mye-logeneous leukemia. In: Jaffe ES, Harris NL, Stein H, et al, editors. Pathology and genetics: tumours of haematopoietic and lymphoid tissues. Lyons (France): IARC Press; 2001. p. 20–6.

25. Muller-Hermelink HK, Catovsky D, Montserrat E, et al. Chronic lymphocytic leukaemia/small lympho-cytic lymphoma. In: Jaffe ES, Harris NL, Stein H, et al, editors. Pathology and genetics: tumours of haematopoietic and lymphoid tissues. Lyons (France): IARC Press; 2001. p. 127–30.

26. Greenfield HM, Hunt R, Lee LK, et al. B-cell chronic lymphocytic leukaemia with extensive lytic lesions. Eur J Haematol 2006;76:356–7.

27. Bestic JM, Peterson JJ. Bancroft LW Pediatric FDG PET/CT: physiologic uptake, normal variants, and benign conditions. Radiographics 2009;29(5): 1487–500.

28. Kaste SC. Imaging pediatric bone sarcomas. Radiol Clin North Am 2011;49(4):749–65, vi–vii. [Epub 2011 Jun 16].

29. Ludwig JA. Ewing sarcoma: historical perspectives, current state-of-the-art, and opportunities for tar-geted therapy in the future. Curr Opin Oncol 2008; 20(4):412–8.

30. Rajiah P, Ilaslan H, Sundaram M. Imaging of sarcomas of pelvic bones. Semin Ultrasound CT MR 2011;32(5):433–41.

31. Hammoud S, Frassica FJ, McCarthy EF. Ewing's sarcoma presenting as a solitary cyst. Skeletal Radiol 2006;35(7):533–5.

32. Daldrup-Link HE, Franzius C, Link TM, et al. Whole-body MR imaging for detection of bone metastases in children and young adults: comparison with skel-etal scintigraphy and FDG PET. AJR Am J Roentgen-ol 2001;177(1):229–36.

33. Mazumdar A, Siegel MJ, Narra V, et al. Whole-body fast inversion recovery MR imaging of small cell

neoplasms in pediatric patients: a pilot study. AJR Am J Roentgenol 2002;179(5):1261–6.

34. Brisse H, Ollivier L, Edeline V, et al. Imaging of malignant tumours of the long bones in children: monitoring response to neoadjuvant chemotherapy and preoperative assessment. Pediatr Radiol 2004; 34:595–605.

35. Murphey MD, Flemming DJ, Boyea SR, et al. Enchon-droma versus chondrosarcoma in the appendicular skeleton: differentiating features. Radiographics 1998;18(5):1213–37.

36. Murphey MD, Walker EA, Wilson AJ, et al. From the archives of the AFIP: imaging of primary chondro-sarcoma: radiologic-pathologic correlation. Radio-graphics 2003;23(5):1245–78.

37. Heffernan EJ, Alkubaidan FO, Munk PL. Radi-ology for the surgeon: musculoskeletal case 42. Chondrosarcoma arising from an osteochondro-ma in a patient with hereditary multiple exostoses (osteochondromatosis). Can J Surg 2008;51(5): 397–8.

38. Littrell LA, Wenger DE, Wold LE, et al. Radio-graphic, CT, and MR imaging features of dedifferen-tiated chondrosarcomas: a retrospective review of 174 de novo cases. Radiographics 2004;24(5): 1397–409.

39. Kransdorf MJ. Benign soft-tissue tumors in a large referral population: distribution of specific diag-noses by age, sex, and location. AJR Am J Roent-genol 1995;164(2):395–402.

40. Weiss SW, Goldblum JR, Enzinger FM. Enzinger and Weiss's soft tissue tumors. 4th edition. St Louis (MO): Mosby; 2001.

41. Oweis Y, Lucas DR, Brandon CJ, et al. Extra-abdom-inal desmoid tumor with osseous involvement. Skel-etal Radiol 2012;41(4):483–7.

42. Lee JC, Thomas JM, Phillips S, et al. Aggressive fibromatosis: MRI features with pathologic correla-tion. AJR Am J Roentgenol 2006;186(1):247–54.

43. Dinauer PA, Brixey CJ, Moncur JT, et al. Pathologic and MR imaging features of benign fibrous soft-tissue tumors in adults. Radiographics 2007;27(1): 173–87.

44. McCarville MB, Hoffer FA, Adelman CS, et al. MRI and biologic behavior of desmoid tumors in children. AJR Am J Roentgenol 2007;189(3):633–40.

45. Kransdorf MJ. Malignant soft-tissue tumors in a large referral population: distribution of diagnoses by age, sex, and location. AJR Am J Roentgenol 1995; 164(1):129–34.

46. Park K, van Rijn R, McHugh K. The role of radiology in paediatric soft tissue sarcomas. Cancer Imaging 2008;8:102–15.

47. Franco A, Lewis KN, Lee JR. Pediatric rhabdomyo-sarcoma at presentation: can cross-sectional imaging findings predict pathologic tumor subtype? Eur J Radiol 2011;80(3):e446–50.

48. Van Rijn RR, Wilde JC, Bras J, et al. Imaging findings in noncraniofacial childhood rhabdomyosarcoma. Pediatr Radiol 2008;38(6):617–34.
49. Lagrange JL, Ramaioli A, Chateau MC, et al. Sarcoma after radiation therapy: retrospective multiinstitutional study of 80 histologically confirmed cases. Radiation Therapist and Pathologist Groups of the Fédération Nationale des Centres de Lutte Contre le Cancer. Radiology 2000;216(1):197–205.
50. Garner HW, Kransdorf MJ, Bancroft LW, et al. Benign and malignant soft-tissue tumors: posttreatment MR imaging. Radiographics 2009;29(1):119–34.

MR Imaging of Metal-on-Metal Hip Prostheses

Carson B. Campe, MD, William E. Palmer, MD*

KEYWORDS

- MR imaging • Metal artifact reduction • Hip arthroplasty • Metal-on-metal • Pseudotumor

KEY POINTS

- Metal-on-metal (MoM) implants are commonly used in total hip arthroplasty, with estimates of more than 1 million placed in the past 20 years.
- Compared with metal-on-polyethylene (MoPoly) implants, MoM implants are associated with elevated serum levels of metal ions, adverse periarticular soft tissue reactions, and increased long-term failure rates.
- In patients with suspected reaction to metal, MR imaging is most valuable when susceptibility artifact is minimized by careful selection and design of pulse sequences. Proton density (PD)-weighted images and T1-weighted images together enable soft tissue discrimination and the characterization of pseudotumors.
- In patients with reaction to metal, MR imaging findings most frequently include (1) juxta-articular collections that communicate with the joint space and (2) thickened periarticular soft tissues with irregular, infiltrative margins and low signal intensity.
- MR imaging complements clinical evaluation and laboratory testing in identification and monitoring of patients with reaction to metal and may help guide management including revision arthroplasty.

INTRODUCTION

Since their introduction in the 1960s as a system for total hip arthroplasty, MoPoly implants have demonstrated excellent long-term results, with some designs yielding approximately 80% implant survival at 25 years, averaged over all patient populations.[1] In this system, the metal ball (cobalt-chrome) of the femoral component articulates with the plastic (polyethylene) liner of the acetabular component. Although there are many reasons for hardware failure, such as infection, loosening, and dislocation, longevity of the MoPoly implant is limited primarily by polyethylene wear, periprosthetic osteolysis caused by the release of plastic debris into the joint, and aseptic loosening.[2,3] In older patients, the expected lifespan of MoPoly

is usually satisfactory. In younger patients, however, implant durability is decreased, likely because of higher activity levels, and implant longevity begins to drop well below that reported in the older population.[1] Given longer life expectancy in the younger population, prosthetic implant durability and osteolysis represent both important preoperative considerations in the choice of implant and potential postoperative complications requiring revision arthroplasty.[1,4]

To combat wear of the plastic liner, other bearing combinations besides MoPoly have been tested, including ceramic ball in ceramic socket and metal ball in metal socket. By eliminating the plastic liner and using hard-on-hard bearing surfaces, the expectation is that implant durability can be extended.

Funding sources: Dr Palmer—Departmental; Dr Campe—None. Conflict of Interest: None.
Division of Musculoskeletal Imaging, Department of Radiology, Massachusetts General Hospital, 55 Fruit Street, Boston, MA 02114, USA
* Corresponding author.
E-mail address: wpalmer@partners.org

Magn Reson Imaging Clin N Am 21 (2013) 155–168
http://dx.doi.org/10.1016/j.mric.2012.09.005
1064-9689/13/$ – see front matter © 2013 Elsevier Inc. All rights reserved.

Compared with MoPoly, MoM arthroplasty has demonstrated lower in vitro wear rates.[5] Two major MoM designs have been developed. In one of these, the implant maintains a conventional design, including a complete femoral component. In the other, the acetabular component is the same but the femoral head is resurfaced rather than removed entirely. In this resurfacing arthroplasty, the stem or peg of the femoral component is short and extends only into the femoral neck, thereby preserving bone. Potential benefits of resurfacing include increased postoperative activity, range of motion, joint stability, and the possibility of more successful revision surgery due to the preservation of the femoral neck.[6] Due to the theoretic superiority and initial promising results with both resurfacing[7,8] and total hip arthroplasty,[9] the use of MoM implants rose steadily. The National Joint Registry (NJR) for England and Wales recorded in 2008–2009 that MoM resurfacing procedures represented 30% of primary hip arthroplasties in patients less than 55 years of age.[10] In the United States, review of the Nationwide Inpatient Sample database from 2005–2006 revealed that 35% of all total hip replacements used MoM bearings, including 69% of replacements in patients under 65 years of age.[11] One group estimated that more than 1 million MoM implants have been placed over the past 2 decades.[12]

Despite early success, more recent data have revealed higher than expected rates of failure after MoM arthroplasty.[13] In 2010–2011, the NJR of England and Wales showed a mean 7-year revision rate of 13.6% for MoM total hip replacement and 11.3% for MoM resurfacing hip replacement compared with 3.4% for MoPoly total hip replacement.[14] The National Joint Replacement Registry in Australia recorded a 7.3% revision rate at 7 years after MoM arthroplasty compared with a 4.8% revision rate after MoPoly arthroplasty.[15] Another report suggested that revision rates and even re-revision rates were higher after MoM resurfacing.[16] Based on data from the NJR of England and Wales, Smith and colleagues[17] concluded that all patients with MoM implants should be carefully monitored for failure. In this same study, the investigators recommended that ceramic-on-ceramic bearings could be continued, but MoM articulations should not be implanted in the future. Current recommendations from the US Food and Drug Administration and the UK Medicines and Healthcare Products Regulatory Agency include restricted use of MoM prostheses and careful monitoring of all patients who have received MoM hip arthroplasty.

In light of these unexpected outcomes, several investigators have attempted to elucidate the reasons for the increased failure rate. The evidence to date indicates that multiple factors are involved, including the design and composition of the bearing surfaces, the alignment of the components achieved by the surgeon at the time of implantation, and the degree of patient-specific sensitivity to metal.[18] Although each factor contributes variably to the development of pathology in an individual patient, the combined effect on local tissues contributes substantially to the increased failure rate. Local reaction to metal involves predominantly periprosthetic soft tissues and, as experience has grown, has been described by different terms in the literature.[19] Most commonly, the soft tissue reaction to metal has been called *pseudotumor*, a borrowed term originally used to describe solid masses resulting from polyethylene wear debris in patients with MoPoly arthroplasty and osteolysis.[20] This review continues to use the generic term, pseudotumor, to encompass the spectrum of local soft tissue abnormalities that reflect reaction to metal. In the setting of MoM arthroplasty, pseudotumor is more likely to refer to complex cystic collections and periprosthetic soft tissue thickening rather than actual solid masses. Osteolysis, similar to that seen with MoPoly components, rarely occurs after MoM arthroplasty.[21,22]

ADVERSE REACTION TO METAL

In patients with MoM implants, the literature currently supports 2 main mechanisms to explain adverse reaction to metal:

1. Excessive wear of bearing surfaces causing metallic debris and periprosthetic soft tissue deposition (dose-dependent reaction depending on the degree of metal wear)
2. Hypersensitivity to metal (reaction to metal does not require substantial wear of bearing surfaces)

Excessive wear of bearing surfaces depends on several factors, such as component composition,[16,23] corrosion,[24,25] and abnormal loading across the implant surfaces.[26–28] At revision surgery in patients with pseudotumors, retrieved implants frequently demonstrate excessive metal wear along the weight-bearing edge of the acetabular component, indicating uneven load distribution that may result from component malposition (such as increased acetabular abduction/inclination or poor acetabular anteversion) and/or decreased head diameter.[12,17,27] Excessive wear is associated with elevated cobalt and chromium levels in serum, red blood cells, urine, and joint fluid.[26,29,30] Animal studies have demonstrated synovial ulceration, necrosis, macrophage infiltration, and lymphocyte response following a single injection of intra-articular cobalt and chromium with effects lasting up to two years.[31] Although MoM failure rates seem to reflect dose-dependent reaction to metal ions, elevated serum levels of cobalt and chromium are not adequate for the diagnosis of implant failure, demonstrating a sensitivity of 63% and specificity of 86% in predicting which patients will present with implant failure and requirement for revision surgery.[32]

Based on the histopathologic appearance of periarticular soft tissue samples retrieved from MoM patients, pathologists have described an aseptic lymphocyte-dominated vasculitis-associated lesion (ALVAL), which seems to represent an immune-mediated type IV delayed hypersensitivity reaction, at least locally.[22,33] This phenomenon suggests that a subpopulation of patients has hypersensitivity to metal and, therefore, is more susceptible to the failure of MoM arthroplasties. In support of this immune-mediated etiology, some patients with failed implants demonstrate appropriate positioning and alignment of components, nonpathologic levels of cobalt and chromium, and minimal wear of retrieved components when evaluated postoperatively.[12,25,34]

Other factors correlating with MoM implant failure include (1) gender: female patients demonstrate a higher risk of implant failure[26,35]; (2) size of the femoral ball: smaller femoral head sizes correlate with increased failure rates because of concentrated load and compromised wear properties compared with larger head sizes[12,35]; and (3) age: patients less than 40 years of age have increased rates of revision likely due to higher levels of activity.[36]

In patients presenting with adverse reaction to metal, clinical symptoms are often nonspecific. Most frequently, lateral hip pain or groin discomfort is present.[25,37] Compressive neurovascular symptoms may result from a palpable mass.[38,39] Because MoM implants may develop infection and loosening similar to MoPoly implants, the work-up should take into account the possibility of other complications besides reaction to metal. Although some inflammatory markers may be elevated in patients with adverse reactions to metal,[40,41] normal or low erythrocyte sedimentation rate and C-reactive protein levels help exclude infection. Imaging plays an important early role in symptomatic patients with MoM implants and suspected reaction to metal.[19,25,35] As experience grows, MR imaging is more frequently requested as a baseline study even in asymptomatic patients with MoM arthroplasties. **Fig. 1** shows an algorithm proposed for the work-up, surveillance, and management of patients with MoM implants (see **Fig. 1**).[18]

The imaging armamentarium can include several modalities, depending on local resources, preferences, and expertise. Radiographs demonstrate the alignment of components, osteolysis, fracture,

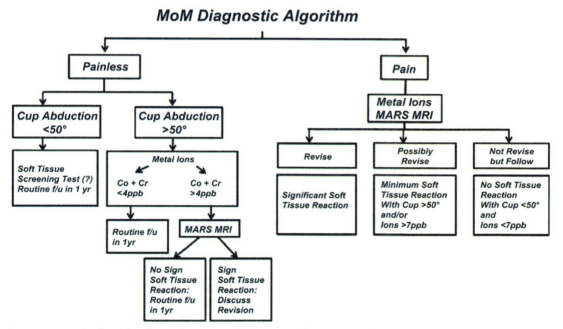

Fig. 1. Diagnostic algorithm for evaluation and treatment of patients with MoM hip arthroplasty. MARS, metal artifact reduction sequence; Co, cobalt; Cr, chromium; ppb, parts per billion. (*Reprinted from* Kwon YM, Jacobs JJ, Macdonald SJ, et al. Evidence-based understanding of management perils for metal-on-metal hip arthroplasty patients. J Arthroplasty 2012;27(Suppl 8):20–5; with permission from Elsevier.)

and loosening. Subsidence and other positional changes can be followed accurately over time. Component orientation, including acetabular inclination, acetabular version, and femoral stem or peg position, can be better quantitated using CT or radiographic views that are carefully standardized. Although radiographs often show the complications of particle disease in MoPoly implants, they are typically unrevealing in MoM implants despite substantial adverse tissue reaction.[25] Whereas particle disease is characterized by osteolysis, reaction to metal is characterized by pseudotumor and other soft tissue abnormalities that are undetectable by radiographic techniques. Ultrasound can demonstrate superficial fluid collections and soft tissues masses in reaction to metal,[42] but the true extent of involvement can be impossible to gauge because of pathologic tissue distortion and spread of tissue reaction into deep, poorly visualized compartments of the thigh and pelvis. Recent data suggest that ultrasound underestimates the prevalence of adverse tissue reaction.[43] CT is more commonly requested in the assessment of periprosthetic osteolysis in MoPoly arthroplasty than for the assessment of periarticular pseudotumor in MoM arthroplasty.

MR imaging has an established role in the evaluation of patients with suspected reaction to metal despite severe susceptibility artifact created by the ferromagnetic properties of metallic implants.[44–46] MR imaging effectiveness depends on the limitation of this artifact. Diagnostic images are more challenging to produce in MoM implants compared with MoPoly prostheses due to the increased metal mass and corresponding susceptibility (**Fig. 2**).

IMAGING TECHNIQUE

At the authors' institution, the MoM MR imaging protocol includes 5 sequences. First, short tau

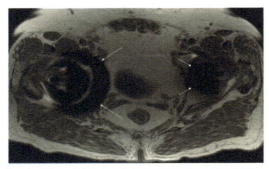

Fig. 2. T1-weighted axial image of pelvis demonstrating greater artifact from MoM resurfacing arthroplasty component in right hip (*long arrows*) compared with artifact from MoPoly total hip component in left hip (*short arrows*).

inversion recovery (STIR) coronal and T1-weighted axial sequences are obtained through the entire pelvis. Subsequently, PD-weighted images are prescribed with a smaller field-of-view in 3 planes through the affected hip. To limit the susceptibility artifact from metal, routine MR sequences and parameters must be modified. Specific parameters are discussed later (**Table 1**).

Susceptibility Artifact

Magnetic susceptibility (or magnetizability) refers to the extent to which a material becomes magnetized when placed in an external magnetic field. Materials placed in a high-strength magnetic field (B_0) react to the effects of B_0 based on their molecular and atomic structure. Ferromagnetic materials, such as those used in orthopedic implants, have the capacity for concentrating and distorting local magnetic forces. Local field inhomogeneities created by a ferromagnetic material result in

1. Dephasing of adjacent proton spins and signal decay through $T2^*$ effect
2. Regional decrease or increase in local precessional frequencies causing erroneous spatial mapping of spins in the readout gradient, ultimately leading to signal dropout in one location and signal pileup in another location
3. Shifts in local phase and frequency gradients and signals, resulting in geometric distortion along both the phase and frequency encoding axes.

Susceptibility Artifact Reduction

Standard commercial hardware and software allow pulse sequence manipulations that reduce susceptibility artifact.[47,48] Several considerations should be made in the design of a MoM protocol:

1. Susceptibility artifact is proportional to B_0. Therefore, low-field systems may have an inherent advantage in the imaging of patients with bulk metal prostheses. Due to the predominance of 1.5-T magnets, a majority of MoM scans are performed using these systems. The parameters listed in this article apply to 1.5-T systems. Ultra–high-field magnets, such as 3-T units, should be avoided.
2. Spin-echo sequences are less affected by susceptibility artifact because the 180° refocusing pulse mitigates spin dephasing. Gradient-echo sequences have limited or no role in MoM imaging.
3. To characterize the T1-weighted signal from structures, the repetition time (TR) should remain in the range appropriate for T1-weighted images (500–600 ms at 1.5 T).

Table 1
Metal artifact reduction imaging protocol. Magnet = 1.5 Tesla. Coil = torso phased-array or appropriate combination of local coils

Sequence	Plane	TR	TE	FOV	Matrix	Slice (mm)	Skip (mm)	NEX	Echo Train	TI	Bandwidth
T1W TSE	Pelvis axial	500–600	22	240 × 340	512 × 216	5	20%	3–4	6	—	350–400
STIR TSE	Pelvis coronal	4100–4500	24	340 × 340	256 × 205	5	20%	2	9	150	200–300
PD TSE	Hip axial	4200–4500	34	200 × 200	512 × 307	4	25%	3	20	—	350–400
PD TSE	Hip coronal	3200–5400	34	200 × 200	512 × 359	4	25%	1	20	—	350–400
PD TSE	Hip sagittal	3200–3400	34	200 × 200	512 × 359	4	25%	3	20	—	350–400

Abbreviations: FOV, field of view; NEX, number of excitations; TE, echo time; TI, inversion time; TSE, turbo spin echo on Siemens/Philips systems or fast spin echo (FSE) on GE/Hitachi/Toshiba systems; T1W, T1-weighted.

4. In fast (turbo) spin-echo sequences, echo train length should be increased, although the trade-off is increased blurring artifact.

5. By minimizing echo time (TE) and echo spacing, there is less time for spin dephasing and the associated loss in signal. The TE in T1-weighted sequences should be lower than 25 ms. PD-weighted sequences (TE <35 ms) are used instead of T2-weighted sequences due to decreased susceptibility artifact and superior anatomic detail.

6. By increasing receiver bandwidth (BW), TE and echo spacing can be decreased. At 1.5-T, BW between 350 and 400 Hz/pixel balances the advantages of decreased susceptibility artifact with the disadvantages of decreased signal-to-noise ratio (SNR).[49]

7. Steeper amplitude of the frequency-encoding gradient diminishes the relative impact of field inhomogeneities.

8. STIR sequences can be used as a fluid-sensitive, fat-suppression technique. Water excitation sequences may also have a role in MoM imaging. Frequency-selective (spectral) fat suppression is suboptimal because local field inhomogeneities prevent homogeneous fat saturation and often lead to the suppression of signal from tissues containing water rather than tissues containing fat.

9. Decreasing voxel size limits diffusion-related signal loss and, by improving the spatial resolution, also improves delineation of the artifact. The trade-off is lower SNR. Parameter modifications include higher matrix (optimally >256 × 256), thinner slices, and smaller field-of-view.

Several investigators have proposed metal artifact reduction (MAR) imaging protocols.[44,45,50,51] In MoM hip implants, the MR parameters listed in **Table 1** are appropriate in any generic 1.5-T system to reduce susceptibility artifact and generate a diagnostic clinical study within a reasonable time frame (see **Table 1**):

FUTURE DEVELOPMENTS AND SEQUENCES UNDER INVESTIGATION

Several newer MR pulse sequences are under development by different vendors and are specifically designed to limit susceptibility artifact. They hold promise in the MR imaging of individuals with bulk metal implants, including joint prostheses. Currently, none of these sequences has been approved for clinical use in the United States. They are yet to be made commercially available.

View angle tilting (VAT) consists of the application of a compensatory slice selection gradient during readout with the effect of projecting spins affected by susceptibility back into the appropriate pixels and decreasing in-plane geometric distortions near the metallic component.[52] The VAT reduction in distortion occurs at the expense of image blurring, although this maybe resolved with modification of the RF pulse.[53]

The MARS sequence is a modification of the VAT technique using a spin-echo sequence with increased strength of the slice selection gradient, increased receiver BW, and increased read frequency encoding gradient combined with VAT. The result is elimination of in-plane distortion but through-plane distortion is not corrected and the increased frequency-encoding gradient results in decreased SNR up to 50% for a 30-cm field of view.[54] Due to the limitations of through-plane distortion, image blurring, and decreased SNR, VAT and MARS sequence are not widely used in clinical investigations.

Slice encoding for metal artifact correction (SEMAC) addresses through-plane distortion by using a 3-D acquisition to encode the profile of all imaged slices and align them to their actual voxel locations during readout.[55] When used in combination with spin-echo technique and a VAT compensation gradient (SEMAC-VAT), robust susceptibility artifact correction can be achieved.[56] Newer permutations of the VAT technique have also emerged, utilizing a 3-D VAT acquisition, Multiple Slab acquisition with VAT (MSVAT), coupled with a 3D TSE sequence with variable flip angle entitled Sampling Perfection with Application-optimized Contrasts using different flip angle Evolution (SPACE). The combined MSVAT-SPACE sequence has yielded similar susceptibility artifact reduction to the SEMAC-VAT technique when compared in preliminary phantom testing.[57]

Multiacquisition with variable-resonance image combination (MAVRIC) also uses a 3-D readout, similar to SEMAC, to eliminate through-plane distortion but uses excitation of limited spectral BWs to address in-plane distortion.[58] The result is robust susceptibility artifact reduction, similar in degree to the SEMAC-VAT technique.[56]

In reaction to metal, a common feature is periarticular soft tissue necrosis. In the brain, physiologic MR imaging using diffusion and perfusion techniques has the potential for characterizing tissues and differentiating regions that are viable, ischemic, or necrotic. Unfortunately, diffusion and perfusion techniques are limited in the environment of bulk metal. MR imaging has yet to demonstrate periarticular abnormalities that correlate closely with the gross necrosis identified during revision surgery and proved histologically on evaluation of tissue specimens. Although MR images can be obtained after intravenous administration of contrast material, fat suppression typically fails in the presence of metallic hardware. Postcontrast T1 fat-suppression has been achieved with reduced artifact using sequences that are designed to take advantage of the opposed phase imaging of water and fat, so-called iterative decomposition of water and fat with echo asymmetry and least-squares estimation (IDEAL).[59]

HISTORICAL BACKGROUND AND TERMINOLOGY

Since first implanted in the 1930s, MoM prostheses have been plagued by unacceptable complications. Those first-generation designs were quickly rejected due to rapid loosening and wear.[60] In the 1970s, revamped MoM designs were also jettisoned because of early failure related to pain, loosening, and periprosthetic soft tissue necrosis.[61] Until recently, the MoPoly design, introduced by Sir John Charnley in the 1960s, dominated clinical practices. Based on advances in manufacturing and metallurgy, the newest generation of MoM implants initially promised improved results. Unfortunately, periprosthetic soft tissue reaction and increased implant failure has resurfaced. In pathology reports, histologic findings reveal necrosis and a lymphocyte-dominated immune response.[33] Although the pathoetiology of this adverse reaction remains unclear, the clinical implications and surgical findings are better recognized.

The term, pseudotumor, has been used to encompass the heterogeneous spectrum of soft tissue lesions, including focal inflammatory reactions, necrotic regions, fluid collections of varying compositions and wall-thicknesses, and solid mass-like nodules. Even as experience has grown and knowledge spread, this term has continued to be used despite controversy regarding the clinical significance of these soft tissue lesions and their associations with symptoms. Some pseudotumors may represent valid surrogate markers of adverse reactions to metal, but the data are inconclusive. They may provide important prognostic information, but supporting longitudinal studies are lacking. They may indicate the need for revision surgery, but the evidence remains anecdotal.

MR IMAGING FINDINGS AFTER MOM ARTHROPLASTY

In patients with MoM implants, early orthopedic publications underestimated the presence of pseudotumor due to the lack of MR imaging in the assessment of both symptomatic and asymptomatic patients. An investigation from 2009 attempted to establish the epidemiology of pseudotumors, reporting a prevalence as low as 0.15% in 670 resurfacing MoM implants.[62] Estimations have steadily risen as more studies have been performed, now approaching 30% in symptomatic MoM resurfacing patients undergoing revision.[63] Whereas one ultrasound study in asymptomatic patients demonstrated 5% prevalence of pseudotumors after resurfacing arthroplasty,[64] another ultrasound study in asymptomatic patients demonstrated 30% prevalence in resurfacing implants and 40% in total arthroplasty implants.[42] When MR imaging was used, 59% of all MoM patients had pseudotumors without a significant difference in prevalences comparing painful (57%) and well-functioning (61%) components.[43] Although the large numbers of p seudotumors in asymptomatic patients raise the possibility that they reflect the mere presence of an implant rather than specifically the presence of a MOM implant, the number of pseudotumors in symptomatic MoPoly hip replacements are far fewer, ranging from 4.6%[65] and 5.8%[66] to 13%.[42]

For the purposes of diagnostic reporting in clinical practice, as well as research designed to

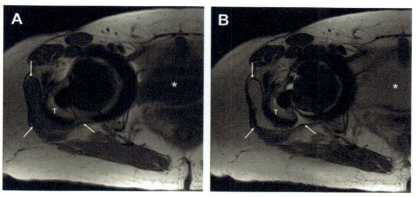

Fig. 3. T1-weighted (*A*) and PD-weighted (*B*) axial images of right hip demonstrating peritrochanteric collection (*arrows*) with signal characteristics similar to urine in the bladder (*asterisk*). Note variable thickness low to intermediate signal wall and posterior communication to the joint. T, trochanter.

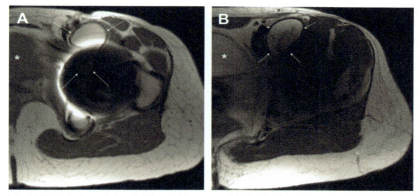

Fig. 4. T1-weighted (*A*) and PD-weighted (*B*) axial images of left hip demonstrating thin-walled iliopsoas collection (*arrows*) with very high T1 signal, greater than both muscle and urine, and PD signal similar to water; compare with bladder (*asterisk*).

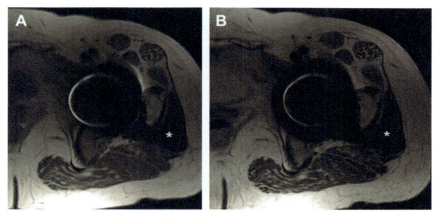

Fig. 5. T1-weighted (*A*) and PD-weighted (*B*) axial images of left hip demonstrating peritrochanteric collection with low T1 and PD signal.

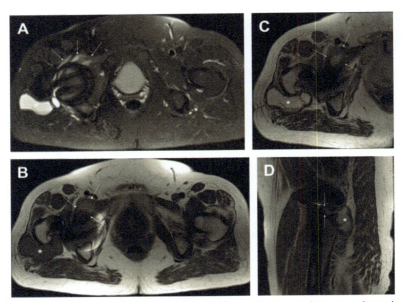

Fig. 6. STIR (*A*) and T1-weighted (*B*) axial images of pelvis demonstrating right posterolateral peri-trochanteric collection (*asterisk*) with posterior communication to the joint and iliopsoas collection (*arrows*) better appreciated on T1/PD-weighted images. Severe atrophy of obturator internus is also seen. (*C*) PD-weighted axial image of right hip demonstrating thin-walled right posterolateral peri-trochanteric collection (*asterisk*) with fluid-fluid level and debris. Thick-walled iliopsoas collection (*arrows*) is also seen. (*D*) PD-weighted sagittal image of right hip demonstrating posterolateral peritrochanteric fluid collection (*asterisk*) with communication to joint space along neck of femoral component (*arrows*).

stratify the significance of specific lesions, several investigators have attempted to develop a system for classifying pseudotumors, grouping them into subcategories based on size, signal characteristics, articular communication, and periarticular versus juxta-articular location.[43,44] Like most classifications systems, the knowledge of exact subcategories is not as important in day-to-day image interpretation as the identification of abnormalities that are relevant to diagnosis and management. In patients with MoM implants, image interpretation can be challenging due to susceptibility artifact, even when the MR protocol is fully optimized. In retrospect, even obvious abnormalities are often overlooked by seasoned musculoskeletal radiologists who lack experience with reaction to metal. It helps to use a systematic approach based on an understanding of

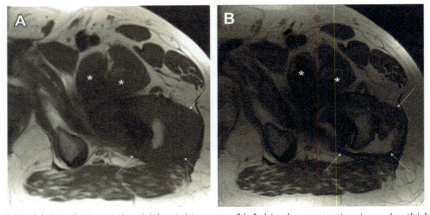

Fig. 7. T1-weighted (*A*) and PD-weighted (*B*) axial images of left hip demonstrating irregular thick-walled peritrochanteric and posterior collection (*arrows*) with low T1 and high PD signal. Anterior, partially intramuscular, bi-lobed iliopsoas collection (*asterisk*) demonstrates low T1 and low PD signal with thick capsule.

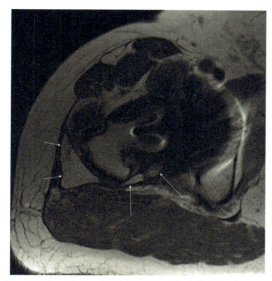

Fig. 8. PD-weighted axial image of right hip demonstrating lateral peri-trochanteric fluid collection (*short arrows*) communicating with joint space posteriorly along neck of femoral component (*long arrows*). Note debris within collection.

pseudotumors and to remember that reaction to metal remains, at the time of this publication, a diagnosis with medicolegal implications. It can be assumed that all patients and their legal representatives are reading the imaging reports.

Fluid collection is the most common subtype of pseudotumor. In symptomatic hips, juxta-articular fluid collections have prevalences approaching 100%.[44,45,67] During image interpretation, the first step is identification of the collection. Even a small collection is important because it can be specific for reaction to metal depending on its location and communication with the prosthesis. Large collections are obvious, but smaller ones are easily missed on PD-weighted images because the signal

intensity can be identical to normal fat. To identify smaller collections with increased sensitivity and confidence, compare PD-weighted images side by side with T1-weighted images, which improves tissue discrimination. Fluid and fat are easily differentiated on T1-weighted images. T1-weighted images also help characterize the fluid signal intensity. In the majority of cases, the collection has a transudative appearance and demonstrates signal intensity similar to the signal from urine in the bladder (**Fig. 3**). In other cases, the signal intensity is greater than the signal from muscle, indicating a complex, exudative collection that may be more specific for reaction to metal (**Fig. 4**). Collections may demonstrate low signal on all sequences suggesting the possibility of metallosis (**Fig. 5**). Occasionally, collections demonstrate internal debris, fluid-debris levels, or fluid-fluid levels, best detected using a combination of PD- and T1-weighted images (**Fig. 6**). On PD-weighted images, wall thickness can be characterized as thin or thick, smooth, or irregular and normal or low in signal intensity. All permutations may be present in reaction to metal (**Fig. 7**).

The location of a collection is critical information for orthopedists who are evaluating a MoM implant and planning to revise a prosthesis that is complicated by reaction to metal. The collection can be lateral, anterior, or posterior to the hip. The exact location may depend on the surgical approach at the time of implant placement, because reactive fluid often dissects preferentially along the surgical tract.[45] If, for example, a posterolateral approach was used, fluid typically leaks through a capsular defect posterior to the greater trochanter, passing laterally and collecting over the greater trochanter, where it may extend cranially or caudally as it enlarges, or spread across the iliotibial band into subcutaneous fat (**Fig. 8**). Posteriorly, the pseudotumor may involve gluteal muscles (**Fig. 9**). Anterior collections may result from the leak of fluid

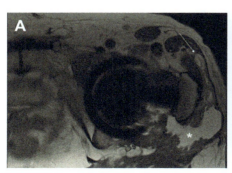
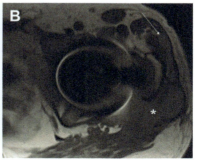

Fig. 9. PD-weighted (*A*) and T1-weighted (*B*) axial images of left hip demonstrating predominantly posterior irregular thick-walled collection (*asterisk*) with posterior communication to the joint space. Collection extends into overlying gluteal musculature. Small peri-trochanteric component extends into lateral soft tissues (*arrow*).

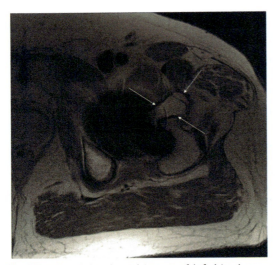

Fig. 10. PD-weighted axial image of left hip demonstrating anterior fluid collection (*arrows*) lateral to the iliopsoas muscle, possibly within the bursa.

implant. This communication may be obvious due to gross capsular stripping and disruption or nearly impossible to identify when the connecting tract is decompressed and collapsed. Because the posterolateral surgical approach is commonly used in hip replacement, and because the trochanteric space is the most common site of fluid collection, it is most important to examine carefully the region posterior to the trochanter (contiguous with bone) for the presence of a subtle, communicating channel. Pseudotumors should also be distinguished from abscesses and neoplasms.

Solid masses develop much less commonly than fluid collections, ranging in prevalence from 6% to 8% in painful MoM implants.[45,67] Solid pseutotumors, when present, may occur in conjunction with a fluid collection and demonstrate decreased signal intensity on all pulse sequences. These findings further improve diagnostic specificity in establishing reaction to metal.

Periprosthetic soft tissue thickening represents another form of pseudotumor and can be detected in the majority of symptomatic MoM implants when the MR imaging protocol is optimized for MAR (**Fig. 11**). This abnormal capsular tissue is contiguous with the prosthesis along the neck of the femoral component and often demonstrates poor margination, suggesting infiltration.[12] The thickest regions are usually posterior and inferior, extending 1 cm to 4 cm from the implant. Low signal intensity may result from either metal deposition or tissue necrosis.

Muscle atrophy reflects a combination of disuse and postoperative change. Depending on the surgical approach, regions of severe fatty atrophy are superimposed on generalized muscle atrophy.

into the iliopsoas muscle or bursa, where they take the path of least resistance and dissect cranially into the pelvis (**Fig. 10**). In all MR imaging studies, follow the course of the femoral and sciatic nerves because pseudotumors can cause neurologic symptoms or other palsies due to local compression and irritation.[68]

Juxta-articular pseudotumors must be distinguished from bursal collections, although imaging overlap occasionally makes the differentiation difficult. Trochanteric and iliopsoas bursal collections can be self-contained. In pseudotumor, because fluid originates from the joint space, the collection always communicates with the

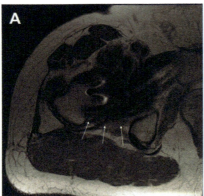
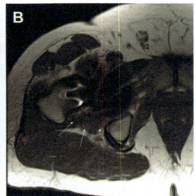

Fig. 11. PD-weighted (*A*) and T1-weighted (*B*) axial images of right hip demonstrating low signal intensity periarticular soft tissue thickening most prominent posterior to the neck of the prosthesis; better appreciated on PD-weighted sequence.

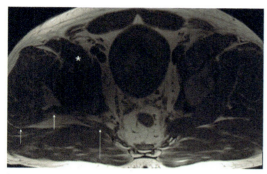

Fig. 12. T1-weighted axial image of pelvis demonstrating severe atrophy ipsilateral to a MoM implant with relatively normal contralateral native hip muscle bulk. Prominent atrophy and fatty replacement involves gluteus medius and minimus (*short arrows*), piriformis (*long arrow*) and iliopsoas (*asterisk*).

In the posterolateral approach, for example, piriformis, gemelli, obturator internis, and obturator externis muscles all show severe fatty atrophy (**Fig. 12**).[45] In lateral approaches that involve tendon attachments to the greater trochanter, gluteus minimus and medius devlop focal atrophic changes. Although a grading system has been proposed,[69] muscle atrophy is not specific for MoM implants or reaction to metal. It is worthwhile reporting atrophic changes because surgeons may take them into account when planning revision arthroplasty.

Periprosthetic bone is especially challenging to evaluate due to susceptibility artifact. After resurfacing arthroplasty, patients may present with femoral neck fractures related to the short prosthetic stems.[35,70] Osteolysis can occur but likely occurs less frequently in MoM implants compared with MoPoly implants (**Fig. 13**). In

a postmortem analysis, MoM femoral components revealed small regions of osteolysis that were radiographically occult.[21]

SUMMARY

MoM hip arthroplasty was expected to provide benefits over the well-established MoPoly systems, promising durability and stability from the all-metal design and large size of the femoral ball. After widespread placement of MoM implants, international outcomes have been disappointing, revealing unacceptable failure rates. Compared with MoPoly implants, MoM implants are associated with elevated serum levels of metal ions, adverse periarticular soft tissue reactions, and increased long-term failure rates. MR imaging complements clinical evaluation and laboratory testing in the monitoring of patients with reaction to metal and may help guide management, including revision arthroplasty. In patients with reaction to metal, MR imaging findings most frequently include (1) juxta-articular collections that communicate with the joint space and (2) thickened periarticular soft tissues with irregular, infiltrative margins and low signal intensity. In patients with suspected reaction to metal, MR imaging is most valuable when susceptibility artifact is minimized by the careful selection and design of pulse sequences. PD- and T1-weighted images together enable soft tissue discrimination and the characterization of pseudotumors. As experience grows, investigations will further reduce susceptibility artifact, enable the quantification of necrotic tissue, and establish criteria that can be used to predict outcomes in MoM implants.

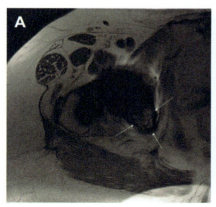
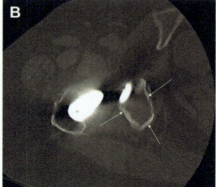

Fig. 13. (*A*) PD-weighted axial image of right hip demonstrating mottled appearance of ischium (*arrows*) consistent with osteolysis also seen on CT. (*B*) CT image of right hip demonstrating lytic process in ischium (*arrows*) consistent with osteolysis.

REFERENCES

1. Berry DJ, Harmsen WS, Cabanela ME, et al. Twenty-five-year survivorship of two thousand consecutive primary Charnley total hip replacements: factors affecting survivorship of acetabular and femoral components. J Bone Joint Surg Am 2002;84(2):171–7.
2. Purdue PE, Koulouvaris P, Potter HG, et al. The cellular and molecular biology of periprosthetic osteolysis. Clin Orthop Relat Res 2007;454:251–61.
3. Harris WH. Wear and periprosthetic osteolysis: the problem. Clin Orthop Relat Res 2001;393:66–70.
4. Sochart DH, Porter ML. The long-term results of Charnley low-friction arthroplasty in young patients who have congenital dislocation, degenerative osteoarthrosis, or rheumatoid arthritis. J Bone Joint Surg Am 1997;79(11):1599–617.
5. Fisher J, Jin Z, Tipper J, et al. Tribology of alternative bearings. Clin Orthop Relat Res 2006;453:25–34.
6. Grigoris P, Roberts P, Panousis K, et al. The evolution of hip resurfacing arthroplasty. Orthop Clin North Am 2005;36(2):125–34, vii.
7. Treacy RB, McBryde CW, Pynsent PB. Birmingham hip resurfacing arthroplasty. A minimum follow-up of five years. J Bone Joint Surg Br 2005;87(2):167–70.
8. Steffen RT, Pandit HP, Palan J, et al. The five-year results of the Birmingham Hip Resurfacing arthroplasty: an independent series. J Bone Joint Surg Br 2008;90(4):436–41.
9. Long WT, Dorr LD, Gendelman V. An American experience with metal-on-metal total hip arthroplasties: a 7-year follow-up study. J Arthroplasty 2004;19(8 Suppl 3):29–34.
10. National Joint Registry England and Wales 6th Annual Report. Available at: http://www.njrcentre.org.uk/NjrCentre/Portals/0/Sixth%20annual%20NJR%20report.pdf. Accessed July 25, 2012.
11. Bozic KJ, Kurtz S, Lau E, et al. The epidemiology of bearing surface usage in total hip arthroplasty in the United States. J Bone Joint Surg Am 2009;91(7):1614–20.
12. Hart AJ, Matthies A, Henckel J, et al. Understanding why metal-on-metal hip arthroplasties fail: a comparison between patients with well-functioning and revised birmingham hip resurfacing arthroplasties. AAOS exhibit selection. J Bone Joint Surg Am 2012;94(4):e22.
13. van der Weegen W, Hoekstra HJ, Sijbesma T, et al. Survival of metal-on-metal hip resurfacing arthroplasty: a systematic review of the literature. J Bone Joint Surg Br 2011;93(3):298–306.
14. National Joint Registry England and Wales 8th Annual Report. Available at: http://www.njrcentre.org.uk/NjrCentre/Portals/0/Documents/NJR%208th%20Annual%20Report%202011.pdf. Accessed July 25, 2012.
15. Australian Orthopaedic Association National Joint Registry 2011. Available at:http://www.dmac.adelaide.edu.au/aoanjrr/documents/AnnualReports2011/AnnualReport_2011_WebVersion.pdf. Accessed July 25, 2012.
16. de Steiger RN, Miller LN, Prosser GH, et al. Poor outcome of revised resurfacing hip arthroplasty. Acta Orthop 2010;81(1):72–6.
17. Smith AJ, Dieppe P, Vernon K, et al. Failure rates of stemmed metal-on-metal hip replacements: analysis of data from the National Joint Registry of England and Wales. Lancet 2012;379(9822):1199–204.
18. Kwon YM, Jacobs JJ, Macdonald SJ, et al. Evidence-based understanding of management perils for metal-on-metal hip arthroplasty patients. J Arthroplasty 2012;27(Suppl 8):20–5.
19. Daniel J, Holland J, Quigley L, et al. Pseudotumors associated with total hip arthroplasty. J Bone Joint Surg Am 2012;94(1):86–93.
20. Griffiths HJ, Burke J, Bonfiglio TA. Granulomatous pseudotumors in total joint replacement. Skeletal Radiol 1987;16(2):146–52.
21. Huber M, Reinisch G, Zenz P, et al. Postmortem study of femoral osteolysis associated with metal-on-metal articulation in total hip replacement: an analysis of nine cases. J Bone Joint Surg Am 2010;92(8):1720–31.
22. Park YS, Moon YW, Lim SJ, et al. Early osteolysis following second-generation metal-on-metal hip replacement. J Bone Joint Surg Am 2005;87(7):1515–21.
23. Mabilleau G, Kwon YM, Pandit H, et al. Metal-on-metal hip resurfacing arthroplasty: a review of periprosthetic biological reactions. Acta Orthop 2008;79(6):734–47.
24. Keegan GM, Learmonth ID, Case CP. Orthopaedic metals and their potential toxicity in the arthroplasty patient: a review of current knowledge and future strategies. J Bone Joint Surg Br 2007;89(5):567–73.
25. Donell ST, Darrah C, Nolan JF, et al. Early failure of the Ultima metal-on-metal total hip replacement in the presence of normal plain radiographs. J Bone Joint Surg Br 2010;92(11):1501–8.
26. Langton DJ, Jameson SS, Joyce TJ, et al. Early failure of metal-on-metal bearings in hip resurfacing and large-diameter total hip replacement: a consequence of excess wear. J Bone Joint Surg Br 2010;92(1):38–46.
27. Kwon YM, Glyn-Jones S, Simpson DJ, et al. Analysis of wear of retrieved metal-on-metal hip resurfacing implants revised due to pseudotumours. J Bone Joint Surg Br 2010;92(3):356–61.
28. De Haan R, Campbell PA, Su EP, et al. Revision of metal-on-metal resurfacing arthroplasty of the hip: the influence of malpositioning of the components. J Bone Joint Surg Br 2008;90(9):1158–63.

29. Kim PR, Beaulé PE, Dunbar M, et al. Cobalt and chromium levels in blood and urine following hip resurfacing arthroplasty with the Conserve Plus implant. J Bone Joint Surg Am 2011;93(Suppl 2):107–17.

30. Rasquinha VJ, Ranawat CS, Weiskopf J, et al. Serum metal levels and bearing surfaces in total hip arthroplasty. J Arthroplasty 2006;21(6 Suppl 2):47–52.

31. Howie DW, Vernon-Roberts B. Long-term effects of intraarticular cobalt-chrome alloy wear particles in rats. J Arthroplasty 1988;3(4):327–36.

32. Hart AJ, Sabah SA, Bandi AS, et al. Sensitivity and specificity of blood cobalt and chromium metal ions for predicting failure of metal-on-metal hip replacement. J Bone Joint Surg Br 2011;93(10):1308–13.

33. Willert HG, Buchhorn GH, Fayyazi A, et al. Metal-on-metal bearings and hypersensitivity in patients with artificial hip joints. A clinical and histomorphological study. J Bone Joint Surg Am 2005;87(1):28–36.

34. Matthies A, Underwood R, Cann P, et al. Retrieval analysis of 240 metal-on-metal hip components, comparing modular total hip replacement with hip resurfacing. J Bone Joint Surg Br 2011;93(3):307–14.

35. Ollivere B, Darrah C, Barker T, et al. Early clinical failure of the Birmingham metal-on-metal hip resurfacing is associated with metallosis and soft-tissue necrosis. J Bone Joint Surg Br 2009;91(8):1025–30.

36. Glyn-Jones S, Pandit H, Kwon YM, et al. Risk factors for inflammatory pseudotumour formation following hip resurfacing. J Bone Joint Surg Br 2009;91(12):1566–74.

37. Pandit H, Glyn-Jones S, McLardy-Smith P, et al. Pseudotumours associated with metal-on-metal hip resurfacings. J Bone Joint Surg Br 2008;90(7):847–51.

38. Counsell A, Heasley R, Arumilli B, et al. A groin mass caused by metal particle debris after hip resurfacing. Acta Orthop Belg 2008;74(6):870–4.

39. Harvie P, Giele H, Fang C, et al. The treatment of femoral neuropathy due to pseudotumour caused by metal-on-metal resurfacing arthroplasty. Hip Int 2008;18(4):313–20.

40. Mahmud T, Satchithananda K, Lewis A, et al. Sterile pseudotumour can explain a high c-reactive protein American Academy of Orthopaedic Surgeons Annual Meeting. Poster No. P086 at the American Academy of Orthopaedic Surgeons Annual Meeting. February 7–11, 2012. San Francisco, CA.

41. Mikhael MM, Hanssen AD, Sierra RJ. Failure of metal-on-metal total hip arthroplasty mimicking hip infection. A report of two cases. J Bone Joint Surg Am 2009;91(2):443–6.

42. Williams DH, Greidanus NV, Masri BA, et al. Prevalence of pseudotumor in asymptomatic patients after metal-on-metal hip arthroplasty. J Bone Joint Surg Am 2011;93(23):2164–71.

43. Hart AJ, Satchithananda K, Liddle AD, et al. Pseudotumors in association with well-functioning metal-on-metal hip prostheses: a case-control study using three-dimensional computed tomography and magnetic resonance imaging. J Bone Joint Surg Am 2012;94(4):317–25.

44. Toms AP, Marshall TJ, Cahir J, et al. MRI of early symptomatic metal-on-metal total hip arthroplasty: a retrospective review of radiological findings in 20 hips. Clin Radiol 2008;63(1):49–58.

45. Sabah SA, Mitchell AW, Henckel J, et al. Magnetic resonance imaging findings in painful metal-on-metal hips: a prospective study. J Arthroplasty 2011;26(1):71–6.

46. Walde TA, Weiland DE, Leung SB, et al. Comparison of CT, MRI, and radiographs in assessing pelvic osteolysis: a cadaveric study. Clin Orthop Relat Res 2005;437:138–44.

47. Peh WC, Chan JH. Artifacts in musculoskeletal magnetic resonance imaging: identification and correction. Skeletal Radiol 2001;30(4):179–91.

48. Lee MJ, Kim S, Lee SA, et al. Overcoming artifacts from metallic orthopedic implants at high-field-strength MR imaging and multi-detector CT. Radiographics 2007;27(3):791–803.

49. Toms AP, Smith-Bateman C, Malcolm PN, et al. Optimization of metal artefact reduction (MAR) sequences for MRI of total hip prostheses. Clin Radiol 2010;65(6):447–52.

50. Hayter CL, Potter HG, Su EP. Imaging of metal-on-metal hip resurfacing. Orthop Clin North Am 2011;42(2):195–205, viii.

51. Mistry A, Cahir J, Donell ST, et al. MRI of asymptomatic patients with metal-on-metal and polyethylene-on-metal total hip arthroplasties. Clin Radiol 2011;66(6):540–5.

52. Cho ZH, Kim DJ, Kim YK. Total inhomogeneity correction including chemical shifts and susceptibility by view angle tilting. Med Phys 1988;15(1):7–11.

53. Butts K, Pauly JM. Reduction of blurring in view angle tilting MRI. Proc Intl Soc Mag Reson Med 2002;10.

54. Olsen RV, Munk PL, Lee MJ, et al. Metal artifact reduction sequence: early clinical applications. Radiographics 2000;20(3):699–712.

55. Lu W, Pauly KB, Gold GE, et al. SEMAC: slice encoding for metal artifact correction in MRI. Magn Reson Med 2009;62(1):66–76.

56. Chen CA, Chen W, Goodman SB, et al. New MR imaging methods for metallic implants in the knee: artifact correction and clinical impact. J Magn Reson Imaging 2011;33(5):1121–7.

57. Ai T, Padua A, Goerner F, et al. SEMAC-VAT and MSVAT-SPACE sequence strategies for metal artifact reduction in 1.5T magnetic resonance imaging. Invest Radiol 2012;47(5):267–76.

58. Koch KM, Lorbiecki JE, Hinks RS, et al. A multispectral three-dimensional acquisition technique for imaging near metal implants. Magn Reson Med 2009;61(2):381–90.

59. Gerdes CM, Kijowski R, Reeder SB. IDEAL imaging of the musculoskeletal system: robust water fat separation for uniform fat suppression, marrow evaluation, and cartilage imaging. AJR Am J Roentgenol 2007;189(5):W284–91.

60. Ostlere S. How to image metal-on-metal prostheses and their complications. AJR Am J Roentgenol 2011; 197(3):558–67.

61. Jones DA, Lucas HK, O'Driscoll M, et al. Cobalt toxicity after McKee hip arthroplasty. J Bone Joint Surg Br 1975;57(3):289–96.

62. Malviya A, Holland JP. Pseudotumours associated with metal-on-metal hip resurfacing: 10-year Newcastle experience. Acta Orthop Belg 2009;75(4):477–83.

63. Grammatopolous G, Pandit H, Kwon YM, et al. Hip resurfacings revised for inflammatory pseudotumour have a poor outcome. J Bone Joint Surg Br 2009; 91(8):1019–24.

64. Kwon YM, Ostlere SJ, McLardy-Smith P. "Asymptomatic" pseudotumors after metal-on-metal hip resurfacing arthroplasty: prevalence and metal ion study. J Arthroplasty 2011;26(4):511–8.

65. Tallroth K, Eskola A, Santavirta S, et al. Aggressive granulomatous lesions after hip arthroplasty. J Bone Joint Surg Br 1989;71(4):571–5.

66. Howie DW, Cain CM, Cornish BL. Pseudo-abscess of the psoas bursa in failed double-cup arthroplasty of the hip. J Bone Joint Surg Br 1991;73(1):29–32.

67. Hart AJ, Sabah S, Henckel J, et al. The painful metal-on-metal hip resurfacing. J Bone Joint Surg Br 2009;91(6):738–44.

68. Clayton RA, Beggs I, Salter DM, et al. Inflammatory pseudotumor associated with femoral nerve palsy following metal-on-metal resurfacing of the hip. A case report. J Bone Joint Surg Am 2008;90(9): 1988–93.

69. Bal BS, Lowe JA. Muscle damage in minimally invasive total hip arthroplasty: MRI evidence that it is not significant. Instr Course Lect 2008;57: 223–9.

70. Shimmin AJ, Back D. Femoral neck fractures following Birmingham hip resurfacing: a national review of 50 cases. J Bone Joint Surg Br 2005;87(4): 463–4.